Current Topics in Pathology

Ergebnisse der Pathologie

51

Edited by

H.-W. Altmann, Würzburg · K. Benirschke, Hanover · K. M. Brinkhous, Chapel Hill
A. Bohle, Tübingen · P. Cohrs, Hannover · H. Cottier, Bern · M. Eder, München · P. Gedigk,
Bonn · W. Giese, Münster · Chr. Hedinger, Zürich · S. Iijima, Hiroshima · W. H. Kirsten,
Chicago · I. Klatzo, Bethesda · K. Lennert, Kiel · H. Meessen, Düsseldorf · W. Sandritter,
Freiburg · G. Seifert, Hamburg · H. C. Stoerk, New York · H. U. Zollinger, Basel

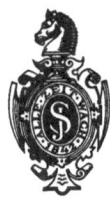

Springer-Verlag Berlin · Heidelberg · New York 1970

ISBN-13: 978-3-642-99965-9   e-ISBN-13: 978-3-642-99963-5
DOI: 10.1007/978-3-642-99963-5

Current Topics in Pathology

With Volume 51, "Current Topics in Pathology" takes a new direction in an effort to keep up with the rapid evolution of science, and pathology in particular. Current Topics has evolved from the "Ergebnisse der Allgemeinen Pathologie und pathologischen Anatomie des Menschen und der Tiere" which began publication in 1896. Its original editors, LUBARSCH and OSTERTAG, conceived of this series as complementary to the classical and more static Handbook of Pathology, the "HENKE-LUBARSCH".

Such complementation, if at all necessary, is no longer conceived to be the essential function of this publication. With the changing nature of international scientific endeavors, with the broadening of the concept of what constitutes pathology, and with English as the predominant language of communication, Current Topics will now endeavor to serve as a more international publication than in the past. A group of European and North American Editors will bring to pathologists and other biologists comprehensive reviews of current aspects of this discipline, primarily in English. By rapid publication, and through solicitation of truly up-to-date work, the editors hope that it will be possible to keep readers abreast of exciting developments in investigative pathology. As the contents of the first issue show, the concept of pathology is not conceived narrowly. Pathology has ceased to be a discipline merely concerned with anatomic alterations in man, rather, it encompasses all of abnormal biology. And in this manner the editors hope to broaden the reading experience of pathologists, to bring into contact seemingly dissociated disciplines and also, in a manner of speaking, to bridge the Atlantic.

The Editors   The Publishers

Contents

Department of Pathology, Dartmouth Medical School, Hanover,
New Hampshire 03755, U.S.A.

Spontaneous Chimerism in Mammals
A Critical Review*

Kurt Benirschke

With 10 Figures

Table of Contents

* Financial support by Grant GM 10210 of the National Institutes of Health
is gratefully acknowledged.

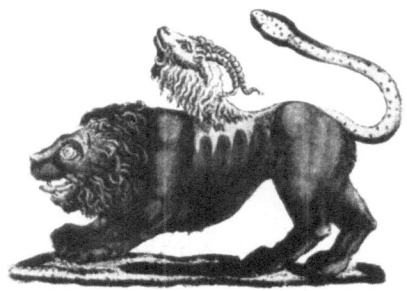

This illustration of a "Chimära" comes from an old German text on "Fabelhafte Thiere" and depicts the composite nature of this animal as a mixture of lion/goat/serpent under "Vermischte Gegenstände".

I. Introduction and History

The rapid developments of human cytogenetics in the last decade and, more recently, that of other mammals, has demonstrated that chromosomal abnormalities are frequent biological occurrences. Not only have numerical errors of human and animal zygotes been defined, many other irregularities of the genome, such as deletions, translocations and inversions have been recognized. The genetic study of some such individuals has shown clearly that some are the result of faulty gametogenesis, *i.e.*, the maldistribution of chromosomes during first and second maturation divisions of meiosis.

As methods improved and larger samples were scrutinized in greater detail it was found that admixtures of different cell lines occurred in certain abnormal individuals, findings which could not be readily traced to irregular gametogenesis. In particular, among patients with developmental disturbances of sex organs such "mosaicism" is often seen. This applies equally to domestic animals with sexual anomalies. In addition, the detailed study of twins and spontaneous abortuses has shown further most complex interrelationships. These findings have aided materially in the understanding of the pathogenesis of the complex phenomena known as mosaicism and chimerism.

It is the purpose of this paper to review all of the pertinent data on mammalian *chimerism*, to define its contribution to abnormal development and to set it apart from *mosaicism*. The review endeavors to show that chimerism is but one step in a biological continuum which can be envisaged to encompass hybridization at one end of its spectrum to genic mosaicism at the other.

II. Terminology

The term chimerism derives from the Greek chimera (χίμαιρα) "she goat or monster" (Oxford Universal Dictionary 1955), a firebreathing monster, with lion's head, a goat's body and a serpent's tail. This composition of different animals has not been taken too literally as the frontispiece shows and the Greek mythology has created many other wonders of admixture (the Centaur, Sphinx, Sirena, Gryllus, etc.), many of which were the creation of Typhon, who himself was thought to be so frightful that Zeus set him afire and buried him alive, burning under Mount Aetna. The offspring under consideration here, the chimera, was devastating Lycia at a time when Bellerophon was sent out, to be killed for his misbehavior. Having tamed previously the winged horse Pegasus though, Bellerophon overcame the chimera as well and it is undoubtedly because of this charming fable that the term is still with us, in its "ordinary modern use (1587) being a mere wild fancy, an unfounded conception".

The term "chimerism" is used widely in biology for a variety of phenomena. As was already pointed out by COTTERMAN (1958) it is difficult to separate chimerism clearly from mosaicism. This is particularly the case when an attempt is made to distinguish these two distinct biological events in papers of different disciplines and written without giving adequate definitions. Today, many articles still appear in which the terms are used interchangeably. Because of the entirely different developmental sequelae, however, it is suggested that the two terms be separated whenever possible. If such a genetical definition of the two events is impossible, then it is suggested that the less committal term *"admixture"* be employed.

The *definition of chimerism* here employed then follows that used previously and succinctly delineated by CHU *et al.* (1964) and by RUSSELL and WOODIEL (1966). The former authors suggest the following usage:

"A *mosaic* is an individual with cell populations of more than one genotype (*e.g.*, karyotype) derived from a single zygotic genotype through mutational or zygotic events (*e.g.*, somatic mutation, somatic crossing over, mitotic loss, mitotic nondisjunction, etc.). A *chimera* is an individual with cell populations of more than one genotype arising through mixture of different zygotic genotypes (*e.g.*, transplantation, chorionic vascular anastomosis, double fertilization and subsequent participation of both fertilized meiotic products into one developing embryo, etc.)".

RUSSELL and WOODIEL (1966) stated that "true chimerism may be defined as the condition in which two separately derived *genomes* coexist in the same individual". This, they suggested "may be contrasted with mosaicism in which the individual derives from a single zygote nucleus but shows two or more *genotypes* either as a result of genetic changes during somatic cell divisions, or a result of heterozygosis of the DNA in one of the gametes". They

1*

chose to indicate the presence of different cell lines of both, mosaics and chimeras, by triple dividing lines (e.g. XX///XY, or XO///XY).

In a recent publication, Corey and Miller (1966) have proposed what I consider an unfortunate alternative. They describe all such cellular admixtures as "mosaics" and then proceed to subdivide their "chimeras" into: 1a) post-zygotics (the typical mosaics by the present nomenclature); 1b) different zygotes (the chimeras) and here only those produced by chorionic vascular anastomoses, by transplacental exchange, by postnatal transplantation or radiation, while 2b) constitute the "perizygotic chimeras", the true fusion products of zygotes. It must be admitted that categorization of individual cases may be difficult or impossible at times. I feel, however, that a useful distinction between mosaics and chimeras can usually be made according to the suggestion by the first authors and, therefore, I prefer to adhere to these terms (Benirschke, 1967).

The term chimera has been used widely by botanists to describe the fascinating results of grafting different species, but Corey and Miller (1966) are not correct when they suggest that Winkler (1907) was the first to employ the term in a biological context. Thus, among cartilaginous fishes of the subclass Holocephali exists the order of *Chimaerae* variously called ratfish (Romer, 1967), seacats, Kingfisch (Brehm, 1892) whose name, not because of cellular admixture but because of their peculiar structure, was introduced by Linnaeus.

So far as mammalian chimerism is concerned, tribute must be paid to R. D. Owen (1945, 1946) who demonstrated the phenomenon of blood chimerism in cattle twins for the first time. He referred to it as erythrocyte mosaicism. Only subsequently has it been named blood (group) chimerism under which name it is now known. This laid the fundamental intellectual basis for the concept of "acquired tolerance". Owen noted the following: a) a twin bull failed to transmit some of his blood antigens to twenty progeny (while these antigens were possessed by his twin); b) in a case of superfecundation leading to heterosexual twins, these possessed identical blood groups whose antigens could not all have come from the respective sires but could be explained from cell admixture before birth, and c) by developing an immunological method he could discern two distinct populations of red blood cells in cattle twins. What was innovative in Owen's contribution was his recognition of the permanency of the state of blood admixture, that is, it persisted throughout the adult life of cattle twins. The embryonic origin and the importance to the development of freemartins by this blood exchange were first suggested by Tandler and Keller (1911) in their study of freemartins. Owen thus deduced that a heifer whose blood type was "the same" as her twin brother's would probably be a freemartin.

Keller and Tandler (1916) and, simultaneously Lillie (1917) demonstrated in impressive studies of the placentas of cattle twins that chorionic vascular fusion correlated with freemartinism in the females of heterosexual twins. These deductions have subsequently been confirmed on numerous occasions, and they were then expanded to include other multiple gestations and other ruminants. As will be seen, it formed also the basis for the early results in tissue transplantation. Moreover, the phenomenon has been observed in double-yolked bird eggs, in experimental parabiosis of rodents and it remains a challenging experiment of nature. To date the exact pathogenesis of the sterilizing influence in bovine twins is not fully understood, but in recent years renewed interest has been accorded this phenomenon because of the discovery of blood chimerism in man and marmoset monkeys who do not suffer the freemartin effect of ruminants. Furthermore, a variety of mammalian hermaphrodites, including some human, were shown to be chimeric composites of XX and XY cell lines whose formal morphogenesis needs explanation. Finally, with the recent advent of experimental fusion of blastocysts, first described by TARKOWSKI (1961), methods are now available which may soon yield more insight into these problems than was ever possible through analysis of nature's accidents.

It is seen then that chimerism is of varied extent. In some cases it affects exclusively circulating cells and is produced through the aegis of chorionic vascular anastomoses in twins (notably ruminants and marmoset monkeys); in some cases of chimerism all somatic tissues are involved. For the purpose of this review it will be easiest to discuss the subject along the line of species, rather than with respect to the various tissues involved. It is recognized, however, that broad overlaps exist in these topics which will be considered at the end.

III. Artiodactyla

A. Cattle

1. Freemartinism, Marrow Chimerism, Tolerance

The fact that the female co-twin of a bull calf is likely to be barren has apparently been an ancient observation, as numerous specific terms for this condition exist in many languages, witness the Roman: taura. The origin of the familiar English term "freemartin" is not exactly known, although it has been the subject of numerous publications, best known and most comprehensive of which is that by FORBES (1946). Interesting statements concerning the precise etymology of this name are also to be found in letters to the British Medical Journal (1887). The German "Zwicke" and the French "vache-bœuf" are other well-known connotations, but to this author one of the most descriptive and interesting is the French "vache mule" (BERTRAND, 1965) which combines the cow with the notorious sterility of the mule. Interesting reviews of the topic are also to be found in the papers by BALLANTYNE (1910) and particularly by PRICE (1967).

The mechanism of female twin sterility was totally unexplained until TANDLER and KELLER's (1911) first note describing placental blood vessel communications among these twins. They observed the notable fact that in the one set of twins they examined and whose female partner was normally developed such anastomoses were absent. Doubtless, this observation led them to inquire more systematically into the nature of afterbirths of cattle twins. In their major thesis (Keller and Tandler, 1916) they came forth with a formal explanation of the phenomenon. First, these authors proved the dizygotic nature of such twins by ascertaining the presence of two corpora lutea. They were then able to demonstrate that of 120 binovular twins 109 had only common chorionic sacs but also, that they possessed well developed vascular anastomoses connecting the fetal circulations. These were conveniently demonstrated by injection with methylene blue. In 84 heterosexual twins with one partner being a freemartin there were well developed anastomoses. In 5 cases none were present, and in only one additional case was there a malformation of the female genitalia without demonstrably patent cross-circulation. The finding was compatible with the assumption that a previously existing anastomosis had obliterated in embryonic life. These results encouraged the authors to postulate that male endocrine substances were exchanged before birth and that these were most likely to blame for the female sexual maldevelopment. The extreme variations of these ovarian and uterine abnormalities are only cursorily described and, since they will be the subject of a more comprehensive review by Professor A. Gropp, they will not be considered further. Suffice it to say that phallus-like structures and testis-like gonads were observed in some freemartins of this series. In a subsequent communication Keller (1920) expanded his collection to 103 freemartins and seven normally formed twins. Also, he described an analogous case in a goat in this study.

At nearly the same time Lillie (1916) issued his first publication along similar lines of thought, describing wide arterial anastomoses between the fetal circulations of bovine twins and the unusual and unexplained sex ratios (14 ♂♂; 21 ♂♀; 6 ♀♀) among cattle twins found at slaughter. This initial description was followed by his extensive and well-illustrated account of the freemartin problem (Lillie, 1917) and the analytical study of the gonadal changes by his student Chapin (1917). These are entirely in agreement with the findings of the Austrian investigators.

Since these pioneering studies, numerous investigations have supported these findings. The frequency of twinning in cattle varies between one and four percent, depending on the race. Further, only about ten percent of like-sex twins in cattle are monozygous (Johansson and Rendel, 1968), so that freemartinism is a common event. The frequency of multiple ovulation is, of course, greatly increased when FSH (largely pregnant mare serum gonadotropin) is administered to cows in the common effort to increase the number of offspring (see Hafez et al., 1964). In such multiple births, complicated chimerism and also freemartinism have been seen. Thus, Owen (1946) reported in quadruplets three blood groups admixed in all four and in a set of quintuplets his group reported so complex an admixture that the erythrocyte genotype could not be established for any individual animal (Owen et al., 1946). In this litter four males were associated with one female which was severely masculinized, having a penile structure and the red cell group analysis suggested that anastomoses must have existed among all quintuplets. The degree of the genital malformation in this freemartin is comparable to that described by BUYSE (1936) in which one female was associated with two males. These cases argue strongly in favor of a quantitative response of the genital organs to the masculinizing influence from the male partners. Other multiple offspring were studied by RENDEL et al. (1962) (quintuplets, one female, two freemartins, two nearly normal females; erythrocyte and serum type chimerism); KANAGAWA et al. (1965c) (triplets, one male with two freemartins; chromosomally determined chimerism in leukocytes); HERSCHLER and FECHHEIMER (1966) (triplets, two males with one female; chromosomal chimerism in leukocytes); and BASRUR and STOLTZ (1966) (quintuplets, three males, two females; chromosomal chimerism of leukocytes with male cell preponderance). The last case, however, is of interest in that the single female survivor did not have the external features of a freemartin, despite the heavy (60%) male blood cell admixture. KANAGAWA et al. (1965c) similarly believe that there is no clearcut correspondence between the degree of blood chimerism and masculinization. This contrasts with the finding of RENDEL et al. (1962) and other cases previously mentioned where the two features were concordant.

The reason for these discrepancies, and many other reports not cited here, is not immediately apparent. Nor is the report of ovotestes in heifers of quintuplet calves (with normal external genitalia (OMURA and KATO, 1966) readily explained by the classical concept. Detailed descriptions are often lacking, however, and there is need for further succinct case reports in this area.

The classical means to establish the diagnosis of blood chimerism, of course, is that of blood grouping and, in a species in which blood types are as extensively studied as cattle, this is readily accomplished. In other animals, however, blood group data do not exist and other markers have become more convenient. As was mentioned in the preceding section, heterosexual cell admixture is best studied by bone marrow or lymphocyte chromosome study if the sex chromosomes are sufficiently different in structure. This is the case in cattle and several authors (KANAGAWA et al., 1965b; HERSCHLER et al., 1966) advocate the lymphocyte culture method as an easy way to identify freemartins at birth. It has been found that in all cases of heterosexual twins in which XY cells were identified in lymphocytes of the female partner the genitalia conformed to the freemartin pattern. Conversely, when no XY cells were present in the heifer's lymphocytes then normal development was certain. Moreover, the frequency of this latter event was of the same order of magnitude suggested from anatomical studies by KELLER and TANDLER (1916), LILLIE (1916), and LAZEAR et al. (1953). Namely, approximately 90% of heterosexual cattle twins share chorionic vessels; they can therefore be expected to be chimeras and the female a freemartin (see also ZIETZSCHMANN, 1931). HERSCHLER'S study has been extended by KANAGAWA and BASRUR (1968). These authors indicate not only that this technique is considerably easier and cheaper than blood grouping, but also a minor population is readily distinguished. Thus, in their thirteen freemartins the percentage of male cell admixture varied from 9 to 98%. This paper gives also valuable information on the rapidity of the decline in the culturability of cooled leukocytes. Treadwell and Cartwright (1968) found that in blood cells of bovine chimeras the replication pattern of the sex chromosomes, as determined by H_3-thymidine autoradiography, was no different than that of isosexual blood. This method has also been used to diagnose the twin origin of sporadic maldeveloped heifers. Thus, in the case described by Renzoni (1967) 111 XY and 10 XX cells were found in a severely malformed calf described in greater detail by Culzoni (1965). This method then should be considered as a valuable adjunct when one is faced with a sexual developmental anomaly in mammals which is, on first approach, not known to be the result of twinning.

Other markers that have been studied in cattle twins include transferrins (Datta and Stone, 1963) hemoglobin (Stormont et al., 1964) and sex chromatin (Moore et al., 1957). As expected, the latter methodology disclosed no evidence of cell exchange and, when hemoglobin genotypes A and B were admixed, both hemoglobins were found in the same proportions as the red cell admixture. The situation concerning transferrin types is more complicated. Earlier studies, which are reviewed by Datta and Stone (1963), indicated that transferrin types segregate in fraternal cattle twins and serve as a means of establishing dizygosity in the presence of seemingly identical blood types. Datta and Stone (1963) state that "using both transferrin and blood types, we found that the diagnosis (of dizygosity) was about 4% more efficient than using the blood type alone". Nevertheless, their study of 91 like-sex and 5 unlike-sex cattle twins yields a few sets with unlike staining intensity of the electrophoretic bands of this protein. The possibility is raised that the cells (? liver) which give rise to transferrin may very rarely also be chimeric in cattle twins, a point to which we need to return later.

Implicit in Owen's (1945) discovery of the permanence of red cell chimerism was the notion of immunological acceptance of this tissue graft. From this finding then originated a long series of studies which culminated in the concept of "acquired tolerance". In essence it is thought, and has been experimentally proven, that the admixture of a (usually self-replicating) foreign antigen early enough in embryonic life of an animal will lead to its permanent acceptance by the new host, i.e. it will not be rejected by immunologic means as is the case after the critical period. In line with this hypothesis Kanagawa et al. (1967) found the lymphocytic chimeric ratio constant over 15 months in seven animals. This critical period in the embryogenesis differs in mammals and, while it may coincide approximately with birth in some rodents, it occurs presumably on early embryonic stages for ruminants and primates, the only other species well studied (Silverstein, 1967). Experiments by Anderson et al. (1951), Billingham and Lampkin (1957), among others, showed that skin grafts among bovine fraternal twins, one a freemartin, enjoyed permanent survival. They also indicated, however, that no close relationship existed between the degree of masculinization of a freemartin and the degree of tolerance to the twin. Interestingly, in tetrazygous chimeric offspring the dam's skin had much prolonged transplant survival (70 vs. 14 days). A finding which is less frequently cited is the occasional rejection of such reciprocal skin grafts amongst blood chimeras, experiments which were repeated by STONE *et al.* (1965) in 21 pairs of cattle twins. They found that approximately one half of the skin grafts between marrow chimeras were rejected, albeit in a delayed response. Moreover, second set grafts were rejected more swiftly, in about half the time needed for the first rejection which is still longer than the controls. The timing of rejection or skin tolerance did not correlate well with the degree of blood chimerism, and whole body irradiation had no influence. NAYMAN *et al.* (1967) repeated studies of others on the survival of renal transplants in cattle twins. Although blood group chimerism was not formally established in their four subjects (they assumed on a statistical basis that chimerism existed), the type and slight delay of renal transplant rejection in these cases also suggested "split tolerance" to antigens.

These findings are not easily explained at the present time, even though some slight support has been published for the notion that the marrow admixture also diminishes (at least changes, STONE *et al.*, 1964) with time, both in cattle and man (*v. i.*). HERZOG (1969) observes a consistent change with age in blood chimeric cattle. What is pertinent in the present context, however, is the fact that these solid tissues of the twin are *not* regarded as "self" by the chimeric partner. In view of recent suggestions concerning the etiology of freemartinism these results may be of some importance.

2. Germ Cell Exchange

In 1962 OHNO and his colleagues made the remarkable discovery that two newborn male calves, which were cotwins to freemartins, possessed a large number of XX cells in their testes on direct cytologic preparations. The circumstance of this technique permitted them to exclude, for all intents and purposes, fibrous tissue as the source of these female cells and they suggested that the chimeric cells were germ cells which had "homed" to the twins' gonad via the circulation. It is important to note that their cytological preparations rule out the possible confusion arising from the frequent translocation event affecting bovine chromosomes. This phenomenon is often observed when one deals with this species and may give rise to confusion because from the completely acrocentric autosomal set of chromosomes metacentric elements which simulate X chromosomes may derive. Thus, HERSCHLER and FECHHEIMER (1966) describe it in the female leukocytes of a set of triplets; GUSTAVSSON (1966) finds such chromosomal fusion heterozygotes widely distributed amongst Swedish cattle; and NELSON-REES *et al.* (1967) report the considerable frequency of such events occurring in tissue culture of a variety of Bovidae. These artifactual interferences then were excluded. Moreover, in one case described, more female (34) than male (16) cells were identified in the newborn testis. The corresponding freemartin

Table 1. *Cytogenetic study of eight pairs of heterosexual newborn bovine twins, in which the females were freemartins. The placentas in all cases had broad anastomoses between the two fetal circulations. In only one case (No. 7) was a chimeric solid tissue cell identified (Fig. 1). Several other cells (Figs. 2—4) could easily have been mistaken for chimeric cells (see text)*

		Gonad		Fibrous tissue		Kidney		Lung		Skin	
		XY	XX	XY	XX	XY	XX	XY	XX	XY	XX
1	Male	con-taminated		con-taminated							
	Freemartin	0	116	0	446						
2	Male	111	0								
	Freemartin	0	137								
3	Male					59	0	22	0	20	0
	Freemartin					0	16	0	54	0	19
4	Male					103	0				
	Freemartin					0	16	0	86		
5	Male					100	0			42	0
	Freemartin					0	43	0	17	0	14
6	Male					32	0	27	0		
	Freemartin					0	19	0	58		
7	Male					1	191				
	Freemartin					con-taminated					
8	Male	247	0								
	Freemartin	0	45								
Totals		358	298	0	446	295	285	49	215	62	33

Grand total: 2,041.

gonads yielded only female cells although, as might be expected from the usual lack of germ cells, only very few cells were found in mitosis in these diminutive, fibrous organs. The authors suggested that, as in birds (Miller, 1938; Singh and Meyer, 1967) germ cells may reach the circulation and be distributed by the vascular system. The intrinsic mobility of early migrating avian germ cells and their attraction to the gonadal ridge has been described in numerous elegant studies (*e.g.* Dubois, 1967), however, for mammals the only accepted migratory path of primordial germ cells had been that described by Witschi (1948) and Mintz (1960), namely from the endoderm along the mesentery to the gonad. This alternate possibility, of migrating germ cells reaching the vascular compartment in mammals, perhaps regularly, raises at once the thought of better explaining extragonadal teratomas which are presumably derived from such precursors. Also, similar to birds and amphibia, it might be anticipated that germ cells of mammals are uncommitted and, irrespective of their chromosome complement, may develop into either spermatogonia or ova. That these immature, alkaline phosphatase positive germ

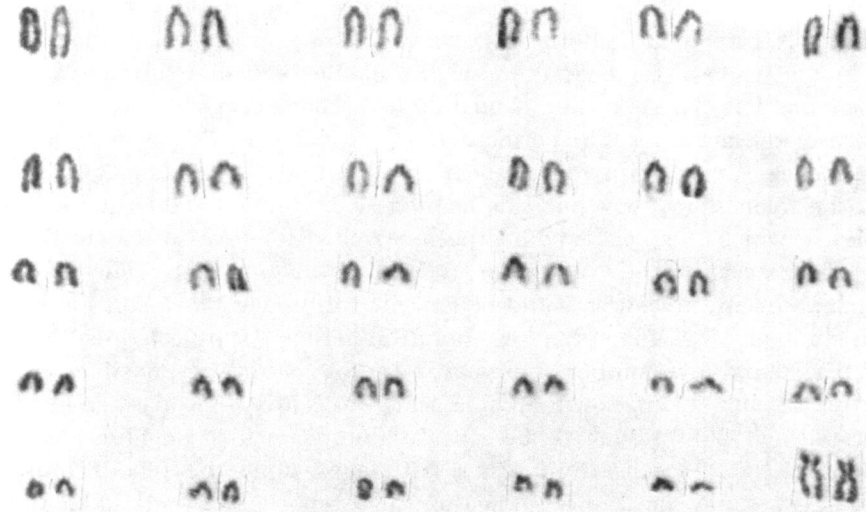

Fig. 1. Karyotype and metaphase of a presumed female bovine cell in a male. This kidney cell is the only one with a possible heterosexual chromosome complement of 2041 solid tissue cells cultured (see Table 1). It might represent a macrophage, but it must also be pointed out that the second X is not typical

cells really have access to the embryonic vascular bed has been shown directly in elegant anatomic studies by OHNO and GROPP (1965), GROPP and OHNO (1966), and later by JOST and PREPIN (1966). In these papers enzyme reacting cells were described directly within embryonic sinusoids and vessels, but the ultimate fate of the chimeric germ cells remains in dispute. OHNO et al. (1962) suggested the likelihood that a majority might vanish in neonatal life. It is therefore of interest to consider the report by HOFFMANN (1967a) who found what were interpreted as female cells in the testis of a 16 week old twin. This author prepared a tissue culture of the testis and analyzed 31 karyotypes of which 24 were normal male. Seven cells had 62 (!) chromosomes, two of which were metacentrics and these are, therefore, interpreted as XX cells. Unfortunately, the centric fusion of chromosomes with aneuploidy originating in aging cultures as discussed above (NELSON-REES et al., 1967) is not considered as a possible source of the metacentric elements in this case. Moreover, there is no good evidence that germ cells (or spermatogonia, as in this case) propagate in this type of tissue culture to yield mitoses as described. This case can then not be considered as giving conclusive evidence of germ cell survival. It is of parenthetic interest that the sex of the twin partner is unknown and blood chimerism was not studied. TEPLITZ et al. (1967) attacked the question more directly by studying the meiosis of the three adult chimeric bulls. The ratios of lymphocyte and spleen cell chimerism was similar in both cell populations while a much lower XX cell frequency was found in spermatogonial metaphases, ranging from 6—10% (as opposed to 28—43% somatic cells). In all testes some first diakinesis figures of meiosis I were observed in which no XY bivalent could be discerned. This means of determining an XX cell, by exclusion of the characteristic XY bivalent, is unfortunately the only present method. These authors conclude then that occasional XX germ cells mature in the male host to spermatogonia, to reach first meiotic stages. Perhaps they go on to form four X-bearing sperms with the genotype derived from the freemartin twin, but this has yet to be proven. They quote several studies in which this genotype has been searched for in vain among the progeny of chimeric bulls (STONE et al., 1964; DUNN et al., 1968). The frequency of such an event, however, would be expected to be very low, considering the small number of XX metaphases found. Whether "split tolerance" or the brief period and low number of circulating germ cells are responsible for these negative results is unknown at this time. Recently, however, WEISS and HOFFMANN (1969) present tissue culture findings which suggest a gradual diminution of XX cells from testes with age, while the blood chimerism remains constant. The same publication also reports the remarkable finding of XY cells in cultured freemartin gonads, which is contrary to most studies in the literature and our own findings (Table 1).

3. Vascular Fusion

The time of chorionic vascular fusion in multiple cattle pregnancy is not well known. In LILLIE'S (1917) numerous twins, chorionic overlapping was seen at 15 mm embryonic length but vessels had not yet fused; at 19 and 21 mm, however, fusion of vessels was observed. LILLIE estimates that at 25 mm the sex difference is established. Later studies differ somewhat. Thus, BISSONNETTE (1924) finds anastomoses established at 10 mm fetal length, and OHNO and GROPP (1965), likewise, find such early vascular fusion. In any event, it occurs earlier than the completion of germ cell migration. In an experimental study of superovulation in cows HAFEZ and RAJAKOSKI (1964) found that a common circulation was established sometimes as early as on the 30th day of pregnancy (fetal size about 10 mm) and BISSONNETTE (1928) describes established freemartinism already at 32 mm embryonic size. In a supplementary description of freemartins LILLIE (1923) had earlier found a 3.75 cm freemartin. These are then about the youngest specimens recorded and one must assume that vascular fusion with masculinization of the female twin takes place somewhere in the second month of pregnancy when the embryos measure between 10 and 30 mm in size. WILLIAMS et al. (1963) found that when twin calves were carried in the same uterine horn all (9 sets) showed blood chimerism. When, on the other hand, gestation took place in both horns, only 8 of 12 sets were chimeric. Thus, it appeared to these authors that the proximity of implantation site was of some importance, as is also the timing, when the expanding sacs make contact. Nevertheless, the reason for the frequent synchorial gestation with vascular fusion in cattle, and marmosets, as opposed to some other mammals with uterine crowding is not at all rationally explained.

4. The Current Controversy

Both, KELLER and TANDLER (1916) and LILLIE (1917) proposed that the etiologic mechanism causing the sterilization of the female freemartin might be of endocrine nature. Both groups envisaged that male embryonic testicular hormones may retard the female gonadal development and alter the ductal apparatus in a male direction. This plausible explanation has been taken over by most subsequent authors and its acceptance was enhanced by the quantitative findings in triplets, etc., previously referred to.

In subsequent studies this pathogenetic mechanism has been complicated by the following reports: WISLOCKI (1932, 1939) found typical chorionic vascular anastomoses between heterosexual marmoset monkey twins in which the female was not adversely affected. Chimerism has since been proven in these animals. Similarly, several human male/female blood chimeras developed normally. In these species then and in contrast to ruminants and pigs, blood chimerism established through chorionic parabiosis was not associated with freemartinism despite the fact that sexual differentiation is assumed to take place in a similar manner and through the aegis of sex hormones (JOST, 1953). Moreover, direct attempts at producing freemartinism by injecting androgens into early pregnant cows has failed. Female calves obtained after such injections were externally masculinized, but their internal genitalia did not show the typical freemartin features, *i.e.*, the reduction of mullerian ducts and retardation of ovarian development; indeed, these structures were entirely normal (JOST et al., 1963; JAINUDEEN and HAFEZ, 1965). Finally, while earlier studies seeking to identify testicular androgens in fetal bovine testes were negative (BENIRSCHKE and BLOCH, 1960) the employment of more modern techniques by STRUCK et al. (1968) showed both testosterone and Δ^4-androstenedione (3.17) in diminishing ratios (14 to 2.8) with advancing fetal age.

The chimerism of blood cells led FECHHEIMER et al. (1963) to advance the hypothesis that the intersexuality of freemartins "is caused not by a humoral agent produced by the male but (that it) may be a function of the sex chromosome mosaicism". In a subsequent paper (HERSCHLER and FECHHEIMER, 1967) these autors have further elaborated on this hypothesis. Studying the degree of masculinization of the freemartin they find a close correlation with the extent of blood chimerism and suggest that the presence of Y-bearing cells at the time of differentiation, rather than hormones, influence adversely the female gonadal development. They liken the process to that found in true hermaphrodites and to the experimental chimeras produced in mice. They also suggest that the reason for the lack of freemartinism in chimeric marmosets and man may be a delay in the timing of the chorionic fusion process. Several authors have subsequently supported this point of view without adding any evidence in its favor. Because we do not share this hypothesis the pros and cons are here briefly summarized and some new data presented.

Inasmuch as germ cell chimerism is detected as readily in marmoset male chimeras as in cattle and because the former female cotwins are not sterilized, we believe that germ cells cannot be held responsible for the sterilizing effect in cattle. It should also be pointed out that germ cell chimerism has *only* been searched for and detected in the males since the freemartin gonad is barren and because the technique of "sexing" ovarian germinal cells in marmosets is extremely difficult. GOODFELLOW *et al.* (1965) also suggest from the study of two heterosexual cattle twins (blood chimerism but no chimerism in solid tissues) that the condition is to be likened to true hermaphroditism. Their photograph of what is called an ovotestis is not convincing. In fact, CHAPIN (1917) and numerous other authors have demonstrated the great variability of freemartin gonads, ranging to nearly normal appearing testicular structures. To suggest, however, that this development ensues from only postulated cellular chimerism is not warranted. A few authors have taken the trouble of searching systematically for XY cells in the solid tissue of freemartins, including their gonads. Most have been completely negative. KANAGAWA *et al.* (1965c) studied two freemartins in triplets (thyroid, kidney, gonad, seminal vesicles, counting 50 metaphases of each tissue) and found only XX cells; conversely in the male twin only male cells were found, bone marrow being the exception. In a previous paper, however, KANAGAWA *et al.* (1965a) had reported their findings on 9 freemartins and 6 male cotwins. Aside from the expected blood chimerism they report a) no XY cells in solid tissues of three freemartins, and b) a small number in two others: (1) Lung 2 XY/22 XX; gonad 2 XY/136 XX; (2) Kidney 6 XY/101 XX; gonad 3 XY/192 XX. They depict one unquestionable XY metaphase from the gonadal culture of one freemartin. HANSEN (1967) found no chimerism in skin biopsies of one pair of heterosexual cattle. MAKINO *et al.* (1965) report tissue chimerism in two pairs, in kidney, gonad and lung, the XY population being very low. The same report appears in extended form later (MURAMATO *et al.*, 1965), again without photographic support. In three other male twins studied by HOFF-MANN (1967b) in which blood chimerism was confirmed, this author found a small percentage of female cells in testis, muscle, kidney and lung culture. In the freemartins only lymphocytes were studied. In a detailed morphological and cytogenetic study of freemartin sheep BRUERE and MACNAB (1968) found no XY cells in four cases in which large numbers of good metaphases were examined from cultures of muscle, kidney and gonad. In marmoset chimeras, likewise, we found no solid tissue chimerism, although an extensive study was made in this direction (BENIRSCHKE and BROWNHILL, 1962).

Because we consider this type of chimerism, that due to placental vascular anastomoses, as being fundamentally different from that due to fusion of blastocysts we examined in some detail eight pairs of newborn heterosexual cattle twins in which widely patent placental anastomoses were found connecting the two fetal circulations. The results of these tissue cultures are summarized in Table 1. As will be seen, in only one cell were we able to identify unequivocal solid tissue chimerism (Fig. 1). There were a number of instances, however, in which the centric fusion phenomenon described for older cultures by NELSON-REES *et al.* (1967) was observed, thus giving the

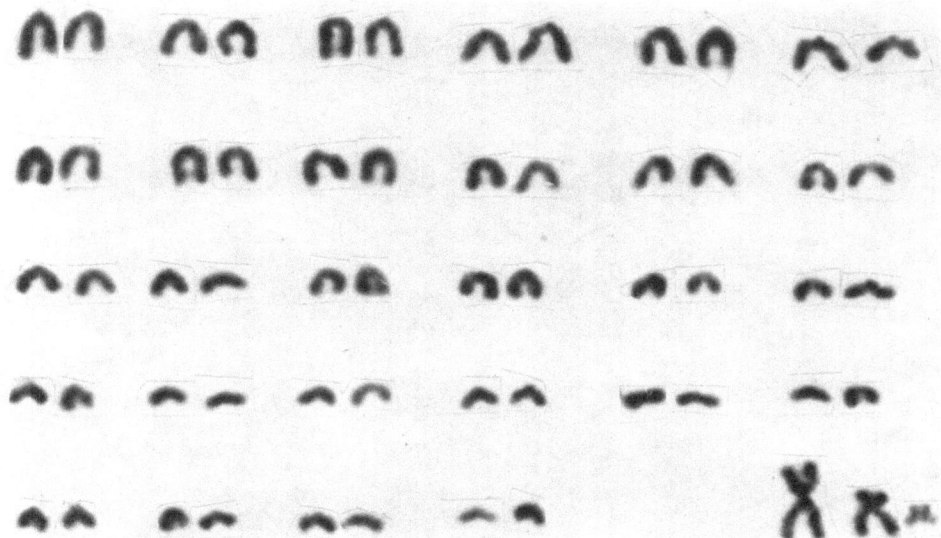

Fig. 2. Kidney cell from twin of freemartin (2n = 59). The last two elements are XY and normal. The third last element, a large metacentric, may simulate an X superficially. In fact, it is a translocation-fusion product of two acrocentrics

false impression of female cells (Fig. 2—4). The more crucial evidence of XY bearing cells in females was not seen.

We can thus not accept the theory that tissue admixture of XY cells could produce the genital malformations observed in freemartins. Nor is there any current support for GERNEKE'S (1967) speculation that "Y-chromosome enzymes" from hematopoietic tissues can be responsible for this effect. In any event, it seems to us that it is still necessary to explain the divergent effects of blood chimerism in ruminants as opposed to primates.

The hormonal aspects of this paradox are not fully explored as yet. LILLIE (1917) was very specific when he supported his theory of embryonic testicular secretions. He correlated the timing of visible gonadal differentiation with the postulated events. Specifically, interstitial testicular cells are present at a time when hormones are assumed to be present, as are chorionic anastomoses, in cattle as well as in marmosets. In order to further our understanding in this respect we postulated that primate placental tissue may remove effective gonadal androgens (at least lower their circulating levels) while this may not be the case in ruminants. Indeed, preparations from young marmoset monkeys' placentas did convert androgens to estrogens, while initial results with full-term unpurified cattle placental microsomes did not show such enzymic aromatization (RYAN et al., 1961). Since then the production of both testosterone and androstenedione have been identified in the testicular tissue of a wide variety of developing and very young embryos (BLOCH, 1967). This at least supports the notion that steroids may be involved in the process of genital differentiation. More importantly, AINSWORTH and RYAN (1966) have

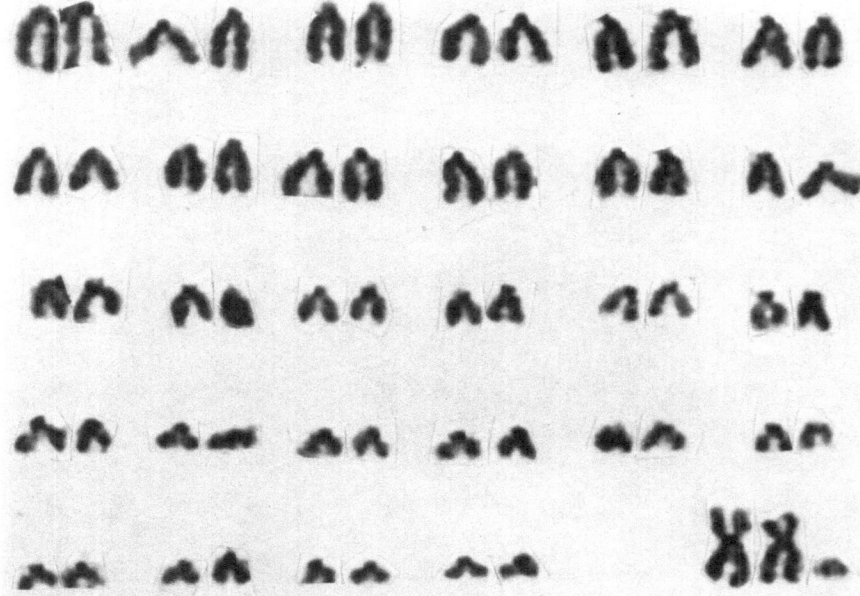

Fig. 3. Similar cell as in Fig. 2 from a different animal; not to be interpreted mistakenly
as XX. Y is not so characteristic as in Figs. 2 and 4

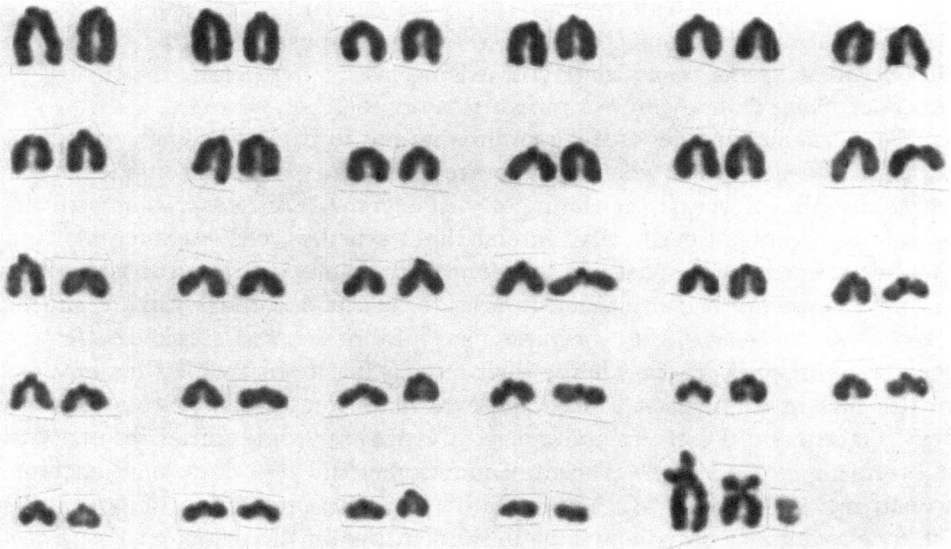

Fig. 4. Similar cell as in Figs. 2 and 3 from previous case. Different-sized acrocentrics
make up the large translocation element, hence, this cell is easier spotted as abnormal.
Moreover, the Y is typically metacentric

now demonstrated that highly purified bovine placental microsomes (as well as those from pig, horse and sheep) can indeed aromatize androstenedione *in vitro* and they conclude that the overall capacity of these mammalian placentas in this respect does not materially differ from human placentas. Although they are cautious to point out that these *in vitro* findings may not necessarily indicate the situation employed in the developing embryo and placenta, nevertheless, the indication is that the former hypothesis to "explain away" freemartinism is an oversimplification, if correct at all. There is then at the moment no plausible explanation why ruminants would produce free-martins while primates under seemingly identical embryological conditions do not. At least it does not appear to this author that any rational reason exists to discount hormonal factors at this time (see JOST, 1948, 1966). When steroid pathways and their quantitative aspects are explored more fully in these species and at early embryonic times, and when blood hormone studies on differentiating embryos can be undertaken, perhaps then a more rational explanation will be found. The controversy is also discussed by BERTRAND (1965); and WITSCHI (1965) has recently postulated a mechanism which demands further investigation. He suggests that through the chorionic anasto-moses a "medullary antagonist is carried into the female embryo and inhibits cortical development". He envisages this substance to arise from the testis but to differ from steroid hormones. Why the mullerian organs are made to regress in the freemartin while injected androgens fail to be effective in this respect is not explained; moreover, this explanation leaves unsettled the objection raised by the findings in marmosets and man.

5. Miscellaneous Observations; True Hermaphroditism; Cell Fusion

In a compilation of various intersex domestic animals McFEELY *et al.* (1967) report a cow with testes, uterus and male ductal structures whose peripheral blood was predominantly XY; no XX cells were found in the marrow, and lung fibroblasts were mostly XX cells. It was a single birth and from the anatomical and cytogenetic findings it is unlikely to have been a freemartin; more probably it is a fusion product of a type to be discussed below. The anatomical features were not unlike the bovine counterpart of the syndrome of testicular feminization, although the gonads differed in structure, and in that condition only XY cells have been found in various tissues (HEN-RICSON and AKESSON, 1967). It should be remembered that blood chimerism may rarely be found in a single-born animal. STORMONT (1954) documents such a case and discusses the possibility of an overlooked fetus papyraceus. Death of the cotwin is usually thought to follow, however, when one dies *in utero*. That this is neither true in twins nor in triplets is attested to by ROBERTS (1962) who discusses fetal mummification and quotes nine bovine cases in which fetus papyracei occurred alongside live fetuses. Thus blood chimerism may well occur in a single-born heifer whose fetus papyraceus cotwin was overlooked. Otherwise one needs to resort to other complicated and much less likely genetic events.

A true hermaphrodite cow with XX/XY chimerism of most tissues was reported by DUNN *et al.* (1968). This report attests to the complexity of the subject and the finding emphasizes the need for extensive studies and careful interpretation. This animal was externally male with empty scrotum; upon slaughter a small vagina was found, a seminal vesicle, uterus, right oviduct and ovary with follicles, left spermatic cord and ovotestis. Of 495 cells analyzed 12% were XY, the remainder XX:

Blood and marrow	95% XX	5% XY
Lymph node	88	12
Lung	100	
Muscle	100	
Uterus	100	
Kidney	71	29
Testis of ovotestis	80	20

The animal was a singleton and one of many types of possible zygotic fusion is the only rational way to explain these complex findings. This is discussed in detail by these authors and the case is contrasted to freemartinism in general.

A more complex chimera (60 XX; [61 XXY]; 90 XXY) is currently being studied by DUNN (personal communication, 1968).

STONE *et al.* (1964) have presented provocative blood group findings in bovine twins which suggest fusion of somatic cells *in vivo*. In a longitudinal study of the proportion of blood chimerism they find changes of the chimeric populations with time, usually in both twins in the same direction, which suggests to them mechanisms other than abrogation of tolerance. In an animal which possessed 90% of the cotwin's blood genotype it was seen that at age 8 years three blood types were found, one being a "hybrid type", as the authors like to call it. Since 96% of blood cells possessed this new type they consider it to have had a selective advantage over the parental type. Unfortunately, the alternative possibility of a previously existing (mummified) triplet could not be ruled out categorically. In a later report (STONE *et al.*, 1968) another possible example of this phenomenon was reported to have occurred in twins. In this instance it was thought to have been a transitory phenomenon, and presumably the hybrid population was less advantaged. The technical problems of such a study are formidable, nevertheless, the finding is of great theoretical importance to biology, not only for the study of twinning processes. One hopes, therefore, that further investigations will be conducted by cytologic means when appropriate markers, such as the translocation chromosome described by GUSTAVSSON (1966), can be employed in the recognition of fusion products.

6. Acardiac Twins

Less explored in cattle still is the phenomenon of the acardiac monster. This severe malformation of one of twins is not too uncommon in man and

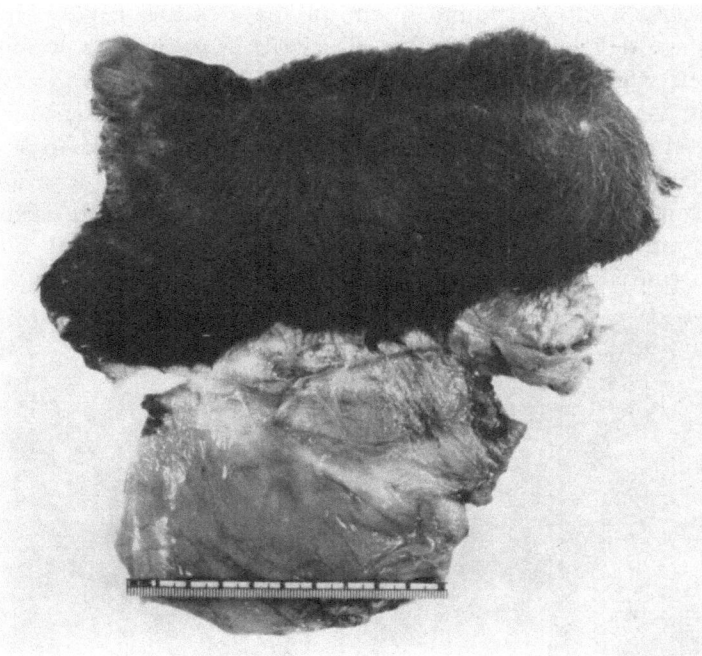

Fig. 5. Acardiac monster, twin to normal heifer. At top left is facial portion. The sac at the bottom is the portion of placenta which was attached to the normal partner's membranes. Ruler is 10 cm

its formal genesis has recently been reviewed in detail (BENIRSCHKE and DRISCOLL, 1967). For numerous reasons it is most likely that, in man, the condition arises only in one of monozygous twins when the nature of chorionic vascular connections is such that reversal of circulation in one twin is possible. In other words, with SCHATZ (1898) we believe that in early embryonic life the artery-to-artery plus vein-to-vein anastomoses regularly present allow for the reversal of blood flow in the twin which is being stunted as the result of this vascular event. Chimerism thus is only theoretical because identical genomes are involved. When SCHATZ reviewed the reports of the event in other species he noted already that acardiacs had been reported primarily in cattle. Since we have seen that monozygous twins in cattle are uncommon but that 90 % of fraternal twins have chorionic anastomoses, it may be suspected that heterosexual twins may be involved and chimerism will occasionally occur with acardiacs. Prior to the perfection of methodologies of sex determination by sex chromatin and chromosome techniques this facet could not be investigated. Thus, in SCHMINCKE's (1921) report of eleven acardiacs in cattle, two of goat, one each in sheep and pig, the sex of the acardiacs could not then be tested, nor can it in retrospect.

We have studied one such case in considerable detail but found no evidence of chimerism, neither by culture of lymphocytes nor by blood grouping. The

2*

monster (Figs. 5—6) was found in the placenta of a normally formed heifer who has since developed normally. The 600 g acardius was supplied by two large vessels which terminated in its mesentery. It had no genitalia but an enormously developed intestinal tract, a tongue and lip, the only other recognizable structures. Histologically, only lymph nodes and some bone marrow could be identified additionally in numerous sections. X-ray studies showed only two small bony structures, a cranial base and bipartite ischium, which are so diminutive, however, that presumably only a very small bone marrow population contributed to the circulating blood. Professor Wm. H. STONE of

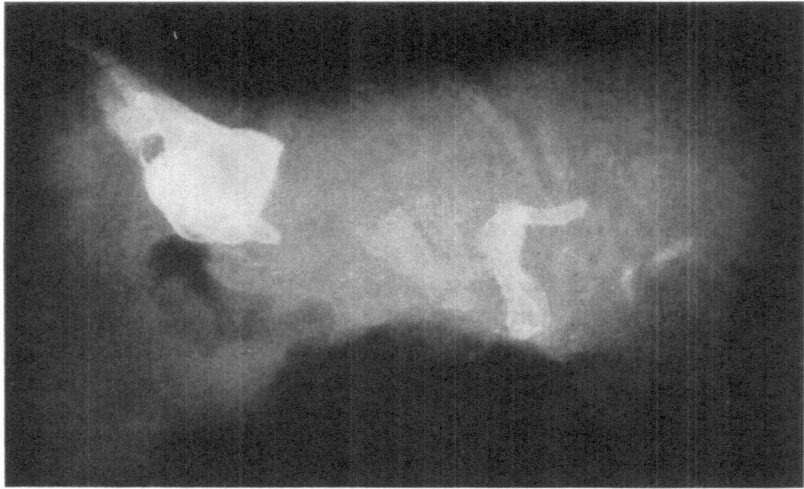

Fig. 6. Roentgenograph of specimen in Fig. 5. Only cranial base and portion of pelvis (right) are visible. These contained some bone marrow

Madison, Wisconsin kindly examined the blood groups on two separate occasions of the surviving heifer and found only one population of cells (lower level of detecting a chimeric population is about 5 %). Similarly, 25 metaphases prepared from two lymphocyte cultures of the survivor were normal XX. The possibilities are that a monozygous twin became an acardiac or, that the amount of marrow present in a presumably isosexual dizygous acardiac was insufficient to allow the detection of blood chimerism.

DUNN et al. (1967) had a similar case which was more revealing because they were able to culture two types of tissue of the acardiac in addition to the male cotwin's lymphocytes. In their monster also the intestinal tract was well developed, and from cultures of reticular and lymphoid tissues only XX cells (162) were obtained. The male cotwin's blood contained only XY cells (373). Here then surely fraternal twins were joined and the etiology of the anomaly can thus reasonably be inferred to have resulted from placental circulatory vagaries. In this case blood chimerism could also not be detected, presumably because no hematopoietic tissue was present in the monster. This could have vanished before birth or have been of such small proportion that, as in our case, no blood chimerism was evident. It will be of interest to see whether freemartinism will be observed in a situation when the sexes are of the opposite types than observed in this case. The closest comparable case is a description of a cow with parasitic limbs which showed freemartinism and blood XX/XY chimerism (McFEELY, 1969). Here, late fusion of twin blastocysts must be assumed although, usually, such double monsters have the same sex (ABT et al., 1962; FEHÉR and GYÜRÜ, 1966).

B. Bubalus and Syncerus

KELLER and TANDLER (1916) remarked that in the one case of male buffalo twins (one assumes from the context — p. 520 — this to be *Bubalus bubalis*) no anastomoses were found. In the water buffalo twinning seems to be very uncommon (FISCHER and ADENIL, 1956) although both monozygous and heterosexual twins have been described. In Egyptian buffaloes the rate is said to be 0.2%, in Indonesian swamp buffaloes it is only 0.0002% according to FISCHER (1964) and freemartinism has not apparently been described. This has been confirmed in a letter from W. R. COCKRILL who has extensive research experience with this species (COCKRILL, 1967). Perhaps even less is known concerning African buffaloes (*Syncerus*). In letters from GERNEKE in South Africa I am informed that twinning is not uncommon in the herd at Kruger National Park but no freemartinism has been reported and apparently the twin placentas have not yet been studied.

C. Sheep
1. Chimerism, Freemartinism

Fraternal twins are born to ewes much more commonly than to cows (ZIETZSCHMANN, 1931), however, freemartinism seems to be much less common. Perhaps it has not been looked for as vigorously as in cattle. LILLIE (1917) had observed chorionic fusion of bovine twin placentas but was unable to demonstrate vascular anastomoses. The first good description of a freemartin sheep, based on anatomical studies is usually credited to FRASER-ROBERTS and GREENWOOD (1928), but the sex of the cotwin was not recorded. ROTER-MUND (1930) describes a case of possibly common placental cotyledons in one of eleven twin pregnancies but the sexes are not clearly defined. A fairly typical case was described by EWEN and HUMMASON (1947), but not until STORMONT et al. (1963) described blood chimerism could the condition be proven to exist in sheep. These authors studied 26 pairs of sheep and found one case with freemartinism. From this experience they suggest an incidence of anastomoses in 5% of sheep twins, or an overall incidence of freemartinism in ewes of 0.8%. It is interesting that they feel this ewe would not have been suspected of being abnormal had they not undertaken the blood typing. YURCHENKO (1962) describes three sheep freemartins with severe masculinization, masculine behavior and he depicts clearly demonstrated chorionic anastomoses. Similarly, SLEE (1963) found placental anastomoses and demonstrates tolerance to skin switchgrafts in 3 pairs of twins of a study involving 7 twins, 14 triplets, 4 quadruplets and 1 quintuplet sets. He finds freemartinism also and from a detailed placental study of these litters he concludes that the frequency of placental anastomoses does not rise conclusively if more than two fetuses are present. ALEXANDER and WILLIAMS (1964) describe a larger artery-to-artery connection between a male and freemartin sheep fetus located in one uterine horn, a female triplet in the other horn being normal and having no anastomoses. GERNEKE (1967) demonstrated 41.5% XY/58.5% XY cells in bone marrow cells from an intersex sheep, whose tissue cultures from testis and kidney, however, yielded only XX cells. The most complete and convincing study comes from BRUERE (1967) and BRUERE and MACNAB (1968). In the former paper the author briefly describes six sheep freemartins shown to be XX/XY blood chimeric. He discusses the significant increase of aneuploidy in this population when compared with normal sheep. A detailed account of these animals is given in the second report. Five cases were known to be cotwins to rams; these and a sixth case were shown to be extensive blood chimeras. It is of interest that the extent of chimerism changed from culture to culture in the same animal; moreover, it did not correlate well with the degree of masculinization. Large numbers of metaphases from fibroblast cultures of muscle, kidney and gonad from four cases showed only XX cells. Judging from this report the condition may then not be so uncommon in sheep as is usually believed and many structural similarities to bovine freemartins emerge. What minor differences were found are readily explained by the authors.

Most recently, DAIN and TUCKER (1969) report five blood chimeric sheep twins with the females of the four heterosexual twins being freemartins. An additional female whose male co-twin was dead was a chimera by red cell antigen, hemoglobin type and chromosome studies.

2. Acardiac Twins

Parenthetically it may be mentioned that at least one typical acardiac monster has been described in sheep, associated with a normal female fetus (COLE and CRAFT, 1945).

D. Goat
1. Intersex Goats, Chimerism, Freemartinism

In this species freemartinism has been less frequently observed still, although twinning is not rare and intersex animals are very common. Indeed, the earliest description of "freemartins" (DAVIES, 1913) probably does not have any relationship to this topic but describes intersexed Toggenburg goats born as singletons. KELLER and TANDLER (1916) describe the frequent fusion of twin chorions in goats but they were unable to identify anastomoses. Later, KELLER (1920) writes that among many subsequent goat twins only one case with large anastomoses was observed in triplets with the freemartin malformation.

Anatomically the fetus was similar to those of cattle, although minor differences are noted. Cytogenetic studies on lymphocytes in 16 intersexed female goats by de GROUCHY *et al.* (1965) and 3 male pseudohermaphrodites by McFEELY *et al.* (1967) yielded only XX cells and no evidence of chimerism. These authors review other similar studies. A detailed analysis by SHORT *et al.* (1968) of a male with testes and uterus disclosed only XX cells in three tissues and these authors discuss in detail the complex problem of intersexuality in goats, other than chimerism (see also HAFEZ and JAINUDEEN, 1966). Anastomoses have been reported by PETSKOI (quoted by BIGGERS and McFEELY, 1966) but they occur apparently only rarely. ILBERY and WILLIAMS (1967) now report what must be considered to be an incontrovertible case of freemartinism in the goat. This animal was twin to a male and had extensive XX/XY lymphocyte and marrow chimerism, while tissue cultures of thymus, lymph node, skin and gonads yielded only female cells. Moreover, the anatomical findings were consistent with freemartinism although not appreciably different from other polled Saanen goats. The latter animals are thought to result from a single recessive gene which may be linked to the dominant gene for polledness, and the question arises whether some caprine freemartins may not have been mistaken for genetically polled Saanen goats on occasion. SOLLER *et al.* (1969) described recently their findings in 17 pseudohermaphroditic Saanen goats. Sixteen were XX but one, morphologically identical, was a 37 XX/59 XY blood chimera, a typical freemartin whose solid tissues were all XX. PADEH *et al.* (1965) describe the case of a single-born intersex Saanen with 60% XY/40% XX lymphocyte chimerism. This animal may represent a more complex fusion product (of blastocysts, or perhaps one due to dispermy, etc.) as the authors suggest, but is too incompletely studied to warrant further speculation.

E. Deer and Elk

Twins and also triplets are often observed in the North American white-tailed deer (*Odocoileus virginianus*), particularly in multiparous does. Occasionally one or more of the multiple offspring undergo mummification (MANSELL and CRINGAN, 1968). These authors describe a live fetus, associated with two atrophic stillbirths which were in a single chorion but whose sex is not given. In numerous twin deer studied by us we could not find either blood chimerism or vascular anastomoses in the placenta, although intimate chorionic fusion often exists (WURSTER and BENIRSCHKE, 1967). We have not heard of freemartins in this species and the development of antlers in does is almost certainly related to other factors. In elk (presumably *Cervus*) KURNOSOV (1962) describes small chorioallantoic anastomoses between two sets of seven twins studied. Both were isosexual and of presumed monozygous origin. The author concedes the possibility of the occurrence of freemartins in this species, in fact quotes an incompletely studied case from the past. Numerous other antelopes (*e.g.* Saiga antelope) have twins regularly or frequently. Whether chimerism exists in these awaits study.

F. Pig

1. Vascular Fusion; Freemartinism; Other Intersex States

Keller and Tandler (1916) report the frequent fusion of chorions in pigs but anastomoses were not detected in their preparations. Hughes (1929), on the other hand, describes freemartins in this species quite clearly. While side-to-side fusion of fetal sacs is common, the event of end-to-end chorio-allantoic vascular fusion seems to be rare. Evidently, this author believes that such vascular fusion must occur very early in these rare cases since in later development chorionic overlapping is the rule without parabiosis. She examined 500 pregnant uteri and concludes that a set of monochorionic twins occurs once in 30—40 uteri. By colored starch injection of vessels she finds AA and VV anastomoses in these cases, predominantly vein-to-vein communications. She describes seven obvious freemartins, four cases in particular detail. Contrary to cattle, a few oocytes were found in the ovaries. Johnston et al. (1958) discuss the frequent sex anomalies in pigs and describe a few intersexes which may well be freemartins, some of them are true hermaphrodites. This is before sex chromosomes could be studied with ease but undoubtedly some of these animals were chimeras and further studies in piglets would surely be rewarding. The interesting suggestion is made in this paper that a recessive gene might control the development of placental anastomoses. Makino et al. (1962) and Hard and Eisen (1965) were the first to study by leukocyte culture two intersex pigs. Both have only XX cells and the latter case is so extensively masculinized that it could not be considered a freemartin or a hermaphrodite.

2. Whole-Body-Chimerism

McFee et al. (1966) review all of these cases and similar ones reported by other authors (McFeely et al., 1967 add two more) and then they describe the first XX/XY chimera in a pig with 90% XX and 10% XY cells. Whether the animal is a freemartin cannot be ascertained since solid tissues were not studied; however, anatomically it differed from those reported by Hughes (1929). Another XX/XY leukocyte chimera is reported by Vogt (1968) which differed anatomically in that, contrary to the previous case, this animal had a uterus and one oviduct and also one good ovary. Six percent of its leukocytes were XY, the others XX which is similar to the previous case. Unfortunately, again no solid tissues were cultured and the question whether this is a freemartin or a whole-body-chimera must be left open. These observations point to the need for a more detailed study of such interesting cases in the future. That such whole-body-chimeras can be expected in this species can be assumed from McFeely's (1967) preliminary study of 88 swine blastocysts. A variety of chromosomal errors was found one of which was an XX diploid/XXX triploid chimera and it may well have arisen from fusion of two disparate blastocysts. A fusion of XX/XY fertilization products may thus occur in swine as it does in other species. In any event, in view of the frequency of swine intersex, the crowding of the uterus with closely spaced implantations, and the ease of karyotype analysis (only 38 easily paired chromosomes), this species seems a favorable one for the further study of blood- and whole-body-chimerism. Moreover, true hermaphroditism is common in pigs according to HAFEZ and JAINUDEEN (1966). An initial study of eight hermaphroditic pigs by GERNEKE (1967) disclosed only female cells but probably not enough cells were analyzed and derived from too few tissues in order to exclude the possibility of subtle chimerism.

IV. Perissodactyla
A. Horse
1. Twinning, Freemartinism

Multiple ovulation occurs frequently in the horse, in 14.5 % according to the large sample collected by OSBORNE (1966). Nevertheless, most twins do not develop since the twinning frequency is only 1—2 %, of which only a small proportion is born alive (JOHANSSON and RENDEL, 1968). The only cases of freemartinism known in horses are those described by FREUDENBERG (1960) and KELLER (1934). A typically malformed female foal was born twin to a male in the former case but neither the placenta nor chimerism were studied. A similar case had been described earlier by KELLER (1934) in heterosexual horse fetuses in which this author was also able to dissect the interplacental vascular anastomoses.

2. Other Intersex States

Intersex states are apparently less common in horses than in other domestic mammals, however, several cases are reviewed in BORNSTEIN'S (1967) paper, among them several true hermaphrodites. This author describes two intersexes, both with uteri and hypoplastic testes and variable external masculinization. In cultures of skin from both, and mullerian duct of one, only XX cells were found. While the identification of sex chromosomes in this species is not so easy as in the others here discussed, the karyotypes presented by this author are unequivocally female. The author points out that chimerism ("mosaicism") cannot be excluded in these cases and it is evident that further studies in horse intersexes are needed.

V. Carnivora
A. Dog

Relatively few cases of hermaphroditism have been described in the domestic dog. These are briefly cited by MURTI et al. (1966) who present two true hermaphrodites with bilateral ovotestes. Unfortunately, cytogenetic studies were not undertaken. HARE et al. (1966) refer to two cases of canine true hermaphroditism, one "determined to be female by the analysis of neutrophilic drumsticks" the other by sex chromosome studies of peripheral lymphocytes. Only XX cells were found but a population of XY cells could not be excluded. These authors also refer to the few inconclusive studies of the

rare canine pseudohermaphrodites (see also McFeely *et al.*, 1967). Two
canine intersexes were studied by Gerneke *et al.* (1968) who also review the
literature. Although both animals were interpreted as true hermaphrodites,
in the first animal leukocyte cultures yielded only XY cells and no Barr bodies
were found. In the second case Barr body count was suggestive of an XX/XY
chimerism but chromosomes were not studied.

More knowledge of these relationships in dogs is desirable since this species
is so frequently employed in experimental studies of transplantation and much
experience has been gained in dogs from irradiation or immunosuppression
experiments in conjunction with grafting.

We are currently studying an XX/XXY (? mosaic-chimeric) raccoon dog
(*Nyctereutes*) ascertained by routine skin biopsy for the comparative study
of chromosomes. Externally the animal is normal and histologically the
testis shows no unusual features. It has spermatogenesis but also typical Barr
bodies.

B. Mink

1. Blood Chimerism; Whole-Body-Chimerism

Two recent reports indicate that chimerism may occur commonly and that
close scrutiny of this species may be of interest, particularly because its
chromosome structure is so readily defined. Rapacz and Shackelford (1966)
report red blood cell chimerism in a pair of female littermates in which the
proportion of chimerism remained stationary over two years in one survivor.
The authors favor interplacental anastomoses as a mechanism in this case and
point out that their transplantation studies indicate that tolerance may be
frequent among mink littermates. Of course freemartinism could not have
been expected in this case. In the same year Nes (1966) reported a well studied
true chimera in mink. An apparently normal female was selected for breeding
because of its fur but had less pronounced heat than normal animals and she
was hostile. After mating vaginal bleeding occurred which led to its study. The
gonads were found to be ovotestes and ambisexual ductal differentiation was
found on dissection. Chromosomes were studied in cultures from liver, kidney,
lung and cornea. The former two tissues were diploid XX, the latter two were
chimeric with a 57% triploid XXY cell line. It is apparent that in this case the
hermaphroditism must be secondary to the chimeric cell lines but it should be
noted that this admixture was found in only two of four tissues. Thus, had
only liver cultures been available, no explanation for the intersex condition,
notably the presence of testicular tissue, would have been apparent. This
should be borne in mind when sweeping conclusions are drawn from scanty
studies in other intersex animals. Nes discusses the possibility that these two
cell lines may not have had the same growth potential and that one may have
overgrown the other (*in vivo* or *in vitro*). Moreover, an extensive consideration
of the various possible ways is presented by which this chimerism may have
been produced which so far has been found spontaneously in man, cattle,
pig and experimentally in rabbit.

C. Cat

1. Tricolored Males

A well-known developmental disturbance in cats associated with infertility is the male tortoiseshell cat, also referred to as tricolored, and calico males. The subject has been reviewed in great detail recently by JONES (1969) and it will thus suffice to summarize the salient features. From genetic studies it had been known that the coat colors orange and black are determined by allelic genes located on the X chromosome. Therefore, in order to have these two colors a cat must possess two X chromosomes, a condition not reconcilable in the past with maleness. THULINE and NORBY reported in 1961 two such cats with an XXY chromosome complement which, on first glance, neatly explained the phenomenon. Since then the picture has become more complicated because all subsequent six cases were chimeras and one wonders if enough cells were analyzed of the first two cases to exclude two or more cell lines. The cases are well summarized by JONES (1969) and represent the following admixtures: one XX diploid/XXY triploid; one XY/XXY; two XX/XY; one XX/XY/XXY/XXYY; one XY/XXY/XXYY.

These animals are of considerable interest from several points of view. *First*, it is of course astonishing that in so small a sample so many chimeras should be represented. It is here assumed that chimerism rather than mosaicism was the cause of the abnormality because this assumption requires the fewest abnormal events; indeed, some cases cannot otherwise be explained. JONES (1969) presents in lucid detail the various possible mechanisms by which the events can occur. This is also discussed in exemplary fashion by STERN (1968) and will be further elucidated when the human conditions are described. *Second* it is astonishing that no true hermaphrodites were found among these animals (*v. i.*). Most had atrophic testes and appeared thoroughly male; one animal had at least some spermatogenesis and was thus potentially fertile (MALOUF et al., 1967). *Third* one will note that the chimerism has only been described in this color variant and not in other cats. The reason, of course, is that the mosaic color provides an excellent marker and everyone knows that "male tortoiseshell cats don't exist", hence they come to attention. There is no reason to believe, however, that this type of cytogenetic — embryological error is confined to this strain of cats. In fact, one would expect it to occur in other cats as well but no survey has been made to ascertain it.

2. True Hermaphrodites

The only related case known to us and apparently occurring in an outbred cat is a true hermaphrodite seen in an eight month old "neuter" with odd behavior (THULINE, 1964). This cat had one cryptorchid testis, one ovary and one fallopian tube and one uterine horn. It was a solid white cat with one yellow and one blue eye whose lymphocyte and fibroblast cultures were diploid XX/XY. The author interprets this as the result of double fertilization. Whether the polyovular follicles occasionally found in cat ovaries (DEDERER,

1934) are causally related to this apparent frequency of chimerism in this species, also if these multiovular Graafian follicles are more common than in other animals awaits study. In any event, more detailed analyses seem warranted in cats with its well defined and easily analyzed karyotype.

Blood chimerism alone from chorionic fusion has apparently not been found in cats and other intersex states have been studied in detail on only few occasions (Hare *et al.*, 1966).

VI. Rodentia

A. Whole-Body-Chimerism in Mice

It is surprising that in spite of the extensive breeding and genetic surveillance of inbred lines of mice only one case of spontaneous chimerism has been recognized (Russell and Woodiel, 1966). This is an exemplary analysis of a large population of offspring which could be analyzed by genetic means. The XX/XX mouse was ascertained because of its yellow and black banded fur pattern and it had arisen, apparently spontaneously, in a closely supervised colony with known matings. Its eight littermates were normal. Cytogenetic studies from earlobe fibroblasts, taken from areas representing both colors, were normal, *i.e.* diploid; sex chromosomes are difficult to define in this species (Galton and Holt, 1965). A detailed analysis of the offspring of this mouse, in conjunction with its coat color leaves no doubt that the animal was an XX/XX whole-body-chimera and that the germ cells were also admixed. This study allows the conclusion that two sperm and two haploid maternal cells must have contributed in the formation of this exceptional animal. What the nature of the maternal cells which contributed is remains obscure, although the authors favor double fertilization following "immediate cleavage", *i.e.* formation of equal-sized cells at either meiotic division. Fusion of blastocysts cannot be excluded, as is the case in most other whole-body-chimeras. The event seems to be most exceptional in mice and neither placental vascular, let alone blastocystic fusion could be clearly achieved when McLaren and Michie (1959) literally stuffed the mouse uterus with blastocysts. This is all the more surprising since experimentally, after removing of the zona pellucida, fusion of mouse blastocysts is readily achieved. Perhaps in the experiments of McLaren and Michie (1959) striking genetic markers were not employed, or the result of possible blastocyst fusion was not studied in enough detail. Repetition of their experiments may be of interest now that chimerism has become a respectable entity.

B. Experimental Chimerism in Mice

Although this review concerns principally spontaneous chimerism, it is opportune to mention in passing how useful the study of experimentally induced chimerism in mice has been to our understanding of numerous biological phenomena. The hematopoietic and immunological consequences of chimerism produced after irradiation have been reviewed succinctly by

v. BEKKUM and DE VRIES (1967). The hematopoietic origin of macrophages has thus been shown for exudates and all kinds of inflammatory reactions by numerous investigators employing chromosomal markers in the marrow grafts (VIROLAINEN, 1968). Other investigators suggest that hematopoietic grafts are the source of fibroblasts and even hepatic cells, however, these are recent studies whose discussion is not immediately germane to the subject, except to say that twin blood chimeras, as we have seen, rarely if ever show solid tissue chimerism. The mouse with its translocation markers is a valuable tool to pursue these questions in detail.

Of even greater relevance to the present topic are the experiments by TARKOWSKI and by MINTZ. These authors have fused mouse blastocysts of different genetic background prior to the 32 cell stage by mechanical or enzymic (pronase) removal of the zona pellucida and approximation of the blastocysts *in vivo*; after fusion and transfer to a foster uterus a high percentage of the embryos develop. These experiments were reviewed recently by the principal authors TARKOWSKI (1965) and MINTZ (1965). When chromosome markers are employed in one strain, when color differences are used or, when accidentally blastocysts of different sex are fused, the chimeric state of the offspring can be ascertained by its variegated, composite nature. Thus, a baby may be mottled, it may be a true hermaphrodite, it may have different populations of cells, and embryos may develop from fused blastocysts even when one half is composed of a homozygous lethal gene combination which ordinarily kills the embryo at the morula stage. These experiments also showed that blastomeres are relatively undetermined, at least up to the 32 cell stage, and that extensive intermingling occurs still at that stage to produce the variegated effect. Recently, GARDNER (1968) was able to produce a similar mottled effect by injecting three disaggregated blastomeric cells into a 64 cell blastocyst.

C. True Hermaphroditism in Mice

In early work TARKOWSKI (1964) had noted an excess of males and three true hermaphrodites in these fusion products. These latter animals constituted proof that indeed chimerism was present, and that spontaneous hermaphroditism may equally be the result of chimerism. Those few cases described in rodents to have occurred spontaneously (mouse, rat, guinea pig, vole, golden hamster) are reviewed in detail by this author. He suggests that some chimeric (XX/XY) individuals develop into males to account for the unusual sex ratio and he reconciles this with what is known of the phenotype of other mammalian true hermaphrodites. Ovotestes develop, reasons TARKOWSKI, in those cases in which XX cells "form a compact" territory, while when the admixture is more diffuse, then testes form. The ductal differentiation (uterus, spermatic cord, etc.) is more difficult to predict but the inference is that "if testicular tissue does, in fact, elaborate a morphogenetic stimulus influencing the differentiation of XX gonadal tissue (as we assume it does from the freemartins) such a stimulus must be rather weak and act only near the site of its elaboration". In subsequent work (MYSTKOWSKA and TARKOWSKI, 1968) these questions were analyzed in greater detail and because they are relevant to a following section they will be reviewed briefly. Of 40 chimeras studied 28 (70%) were male, 8 (20%) female, and 4 (10%) hermaphroditic, thus confirming the original findings of a disturbed sex ratio. The type of progeny produced by three chimeras proved that intermingling of germ cells had also taken place. Two XX/XY male chimeras and a true hermaphrodite proved fertile, a possibly important finding with respect to human chimeras and hermaphrodites. However, these animals produced only spermatozoa which corresponded to the male genotype and in direct preparations of diakinesis figures no clear XX first meiotic divisions were found in the testes. As we have seen, this is contrary to the findings in blood chimeric marmosets and cattle and requires further study.

VII. Primates

A. Marmoset Monkeys

1. Anastomoses, Blood Chimerism, Tissue Chimerism

It had been known that several species of the South American marmosets, family Callithricidae, have twins or triplets almost regularly and HILL (1926) and HILL and HILL (1927) demonstrated that these twins were enclosed in a single chorion. Because two corpora lutea were found the embryos were considered dizygotic, the common chorion notwithstanding. WISLOCKI (1932) demonstrated the same type of placentation and anastomotic chorionic vessels but thought the twins monozygotic. In a larger study, however, WISLOCKI (1939) later corrected this mistake when he identified not only two corpora lutea but also twins of different sex in the single chorion. He considered then also the remarkable fact that, despite this similarity of placentation to that of cattle twins, it did not produce the freemartin effect. Indeed, since half of the females would be joined to males — there being a 50% chance of ♂/♀ twins, because all are dizygous — a freemartin effect would be detrimental to the species, WISLOCKI (1939) reasons. A presumed difference in timing and reciprocal effects of sex hormones were considered to be the reasons for the difference in developmental sequelae when compared with cattle. The observations by WISLOCKI and HILL, and a recent demonstration of very early chorionic fusion in *Leontocebus* (BENIRSCHKE and LAYTON, 1969) clearly indicate that delay of vascular fusion in marmoset twins cannot be held responsible for the lack of sterilization of its females. RYAN *et al.* (1961) suggested that different enzymatic handling of steroids by the primate placenta may explain the situation, a point which can no longer be held valid and which has been discussed above under the chapter heading of cattle.

That these anastomoses between marmoset twins lead to permanent blood chimerism has been demonstrated by the use of the sex chromosome differences in leukocytes cultures from blood (BENIRSCHKE *et al.*, 1962). In approximately one half adults, as expected, lymphocyte XX/XY chimerism was demonstrated which was of variable proportion and not unlike that found in cattle (BENIRSCHKE and BROWNHILL, 1962). Subsequent studies have fully confirmed these findings. Furthermore, this extensive XX/XY blood chimerism is compatible with the development of normal ovarian and mullerian structures and with fertility. It is unfortunate that blood groups have not been extensively studied in this family (WIENER et al., 1967) and they have not been used as yet for chimerism studies. GENGOZIAN et al. (1964) suggest that the drumstick marker of polymorphonuclear leukocytes may serve as

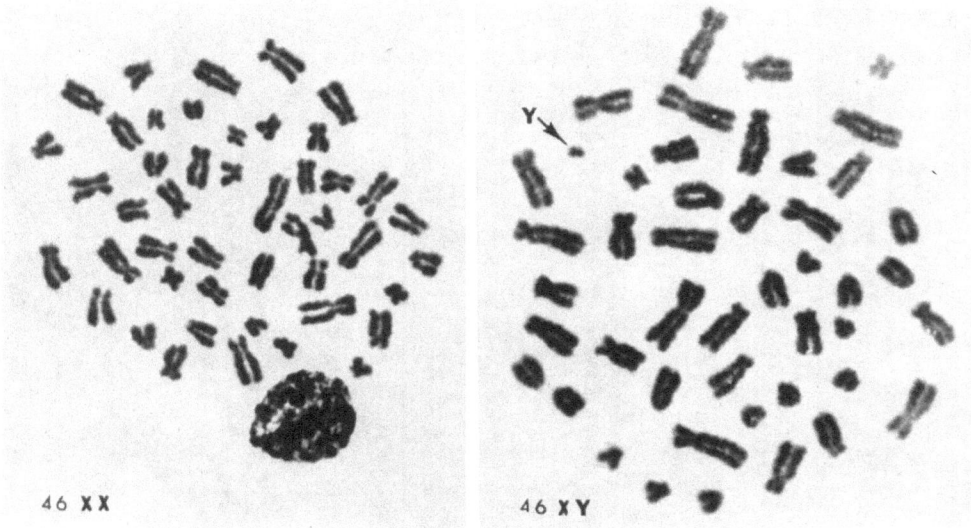

46 XX   46 XY

Fig. 7. Two metaphase plates from the bone marrow of a female "common" marmoset (*Callithrix jacchus*). The cell at left is of the female animal's own marrow, being XX. The cell at right declares its chimeric origin, from the twin brother, by possessing the characteristic small Y chromosome (at arrow)

a suitable marker of female cells in male chimeras. Exchange skin grafts between dizygous marmoset littermates have been uniformly successful, indicating the existence of acquired tolerance derived from the prenatal exchange of nucleated blood cells (PORTER and GENGOZIAN, 1968; PORTER, 1968).

Not all species of marmosets are equally useful in the study of sex chromosomal chimerism, but *Callithrix* and *Cebuella* have Y chromosomes of such small size that metaphases are easily scored by mere inspection (Fig. 7). This factor assumes importance when critical assessment of solid tissue chimerism becomes a problem. After the various claims of solid tissue chimerism in cattle blood chimeras were published (see above) we undertook a detailed study of a pair of *Callithrix jacchus* twins known to be blood chimeric (approximately 40% XY cells in each). Only excellent and complete metaphases of a first subculture of kidney cells were used for scoring (Table 2).

The two apparently chimeric cells of this culture are shown in Fig. 8. In previous studies (BENIRSCHKE and BROWNHILL, 1962) we found no such

Table 2. *Kidney cell cultures of a pair of blood chimeric marmoset monkeys (Callithrix jacchus) with one possible chimeric solid tissue cell in each (Fig. 8)*

		46XX	46XY	Total
M 58	Female	104	1	105
M 59	Male	1	175	176

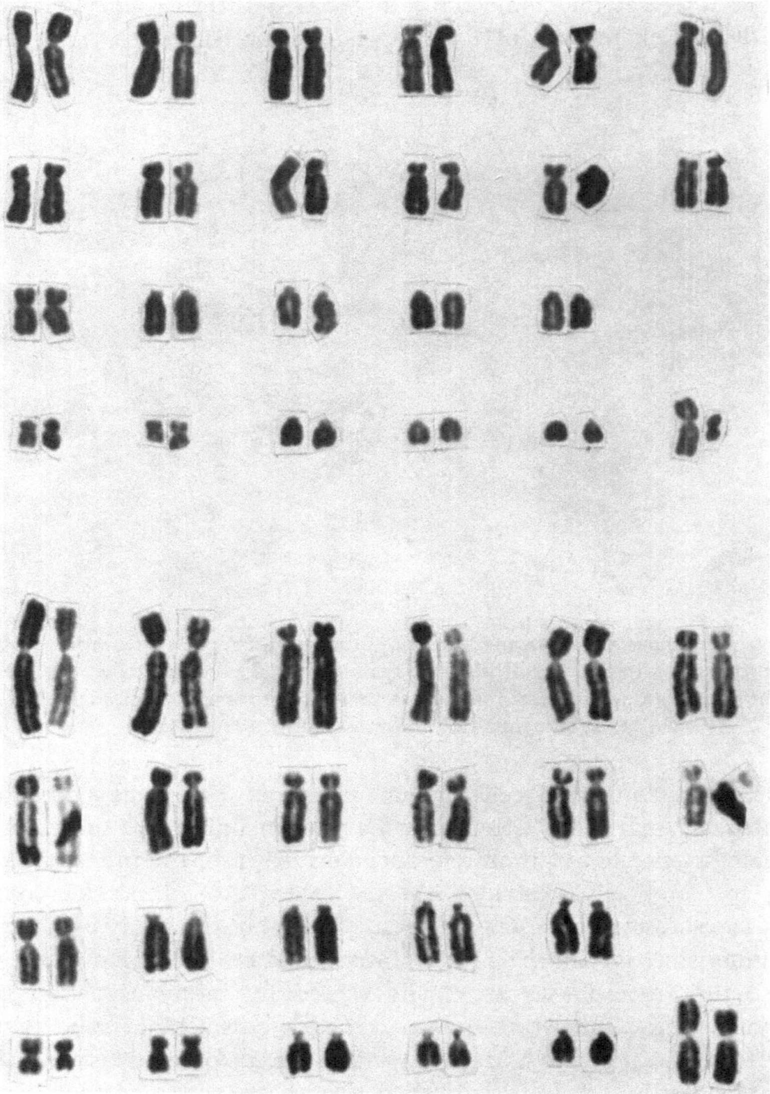

Fig. 8. Two karyotyped metaphases of kidney cell cultures in two blood chimeric "cotton-top" marmosets (*Saguinus [Oedipomidas] oedipus*). The top karyotype was present in the female culture and is interpreted to be XY. The bottom karyotype comes from a male and is interpreted to be XX. These are the only possibly chimeric solid tissue cells found in hundreds examined, in these, as many other animals (see Table 2). They may be macrophages

admixture in kidney and lung cells although it must be admitted that the number of cells scored then was much smaller and, in most cases, species with less favorable Y chromosomes were used. Thus, an occasional cell of solid tissues may be chimeric, both in cattle and marmosets. The question arises whether these are indeed renal, lung or fibroblastic cells or whether they are macrophages. It will be remembered that the latter two types of cells are thought to arise from experimentally transplanted marrow in mice and there would thus be no reason to preclude this as a possible explanation. We have not detected in marmoset monkeys the chromatid breaks and other abnormalities of chromosomes described by BASRUR and STOLTZ (1966) as frequently occurring in lymphocyte cultures of cattle chimeras. Furthermore, the question as to whether, with time, a shift in the chimeric population occurs has not been examined in marmosets.

2. Germ Cell Chimerism

As we have seen in the section on cattle above, in blood chimeric twins the presumptive evidence indicates an exchange of germ cells in embryonic life. Thus, newborn male animals were found to possess some XX metaphases in *direct* preparations of their testes, *i.e.* those not involving previous culture.

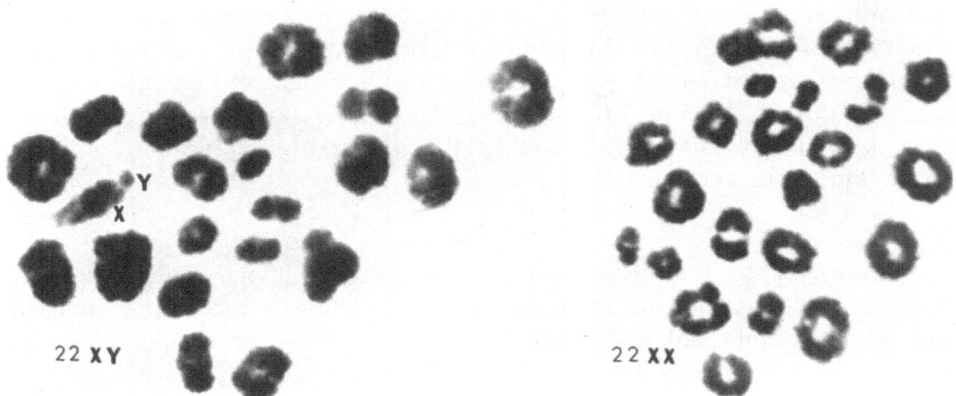

Fig. 9. Two cells of the testis of a mature, blood chimeric pigmy marmoset (*Cebuella pygmaea*). In contrast to the other species here discussed with 46 chromosomes, this monkey has 44 elements. Hence, at the first meiosis stage here depicted only 22 bivalents are found, the XY pair forming a typical rod-like arrangement (left). The cell at right lacks such an element, although it is complete. For this reason it is tentatively assumed to be an XX cell, the X bivalent being indistinguishable from autosomal bivalents. This represents germ cell chimerism. [From BENIRSCHKE and BROWNHILL, Cytogenetics 2, 335 (1963)]

In adult marmosets similar findings have been made (BENIRSCHKE and BROWNHILL, 1963). In order to ascertain whether these germ cells go on through maturation division and thus, potentially produce four X-bearing sperm, first meiotic division stages were analyzed. At diakinesis it is possible to distinguish the XY bivalent but the XX equivalent cannot be recognized.

A few well displayed first meiotic figures were indeed found in which no XY association is evident (Fig. 9). Therefore, it is presumed that meiosis may at least commence and that the germinal cells are subject to their environment, rather than to their genetic make-up because apparently female cells enter meiosis in the testis. The converse, the search for XY meioses in a chimeric ovary, is much more difficult and has not been undertaken successfully. Of relevance in this respect are the experimental studies of transplantation of fetal gonads into castrated male mouse kidney beds (TURNER and ASAKAWA, 1964). These authors find the formation of ovotestes to be induced in fetal mouse ovaries by the proximity of differentiating testes. They describe in these ovotestes the maturation of germ cells as far as to secondary spermato-cytes, but spermatozoa were not seen in these tubules nor in the normal testes. Of course, the final test of whether maturation of XX germ cells completes will be the demonstration that blood chimeric cattle, marmosets, or other species will bear offspring with the respective foreign genotype. This has so far been shown only for whole-body-chimeras as discussed above.

The so far most conclusive experimental attack of the puzzling phenomenon has been summarized by TURNER (1969). In studies of mice and rats injected various steroids only ductal changes could be induced, the gonads remained unaltered. Gonadal transplants at various ages, however, were interactive, and embryonic mouse ovaries could be made to differentiate into testis-like structures. The germ cells then differentiated to spermatids. Using millipore membranes as barriers, this investigator could conclude that the morpho-genetic factor is "chemical in nature", "does not attain effective concentra-tions in the general circulation", and that "gonadal sex determination is not a function of the germ cells".

B. Man

Various types of chimerism have been recognized in the extensive genetic studies now performed on exceptional human beings, particularly in twins and sexually abnormal individuals. To follow a more or less chronological sequence of their recognition this portion of the review will be divided into 1) maternal — fetal chimerism, 2) blood chimerism, 3) whole-body-chimerism, 4) the so-called heterokaryotic monozygous twins, and 5) the acardiac twins.

1. Maternal — Fetal Chimerism

It has long been known that, on occasion, maternal cells may pass from the mother to the developing fetus. By and large, such cells do not become permanently established in the baby. Best known is the transplacental meta-stasis of malignant melanomas from the mother to the placenta and thence to the fetus. HÖRMANN and LEMTIS (1965a) accept four melanoma and one sarcoma cases as well proven, although many other cases of melanoma are recorded to have metastasized to the placenta without reaching the fetus. A carcinoma is not reported to have reached the fetus. In a later publication (1965b) these authors assign the placental trophoblast an important protective role against tumor transgression. Four other cases should be added to their list. A well illustrated demonstration by HOLLAND (1949), one interesting case each by CAVELL (1963) and ARONSON (1963) in whom the fetal metastases involuted spontanteously in neonatal life, and a well documented and illustrated fatal case of BRODSKY et al. (1965). It is apparent then that this event is rare and one which could hardly be missed if it occurred more frequently. Similarly, malignant lymphomas, myeloma, and leukemia of the mother are very rarely, if ever, transmitted to the fetus via the placenta. This subject has been fully reviewed recently by us (BENIRSCHKE and DRISCOLL, 1967) and one gains the impression that the fetus has the immunologic capacity to reject these foreign tissues, should they arrive. For there can be no doubt that maternal cells are occasionally transported through the placenta. Such transfer has been traced in some instances with marked maternal cells (elliptocytes, sickle cells, chromated cells), although the evidence is by no means secure as the review will disclose.

Of pertinence to this review, however, is what evidence exists for the possibly permanent establishment of maternal lymphocytes (or bone marrow elements) via the transplacental route. Three independent studies have recently addressed themselves to this problem and it appears that, while maternal lymphocytes may occasionally traverse the placental barrier, only in one case did they establish themselves permanently. TURNER et al. (1966) found XX lymphocytes in two males of 100 neonates. Unfortunately, both were otherwise malformed and could not be further studied. In our own studies we found very few definite XX cells in the umbilical cord bloods of three normal male newborns, and this population of presumably maternal cells vanished within the first month of life (BENIRSCHKE and SULLIVAN, 1969). In a recent report by EL-ALFI and HARTHOUT (1969) a similar finding was made. A normally delivered male infant with hypospadias and bifid scrotum possessed 28 XY/20 XX lymphocyte chimerism. Five months later the XX clone had disappeared and of further interest is that maternal/fetal lymphocyte incubations proved immunologically compatible. The baby had no sex chromatin in buccal smears and there was no evidence of a vanished twin on placental study. It may be mentioned parenthetically here that, when intrauterine transfusions are given earlier in fetal life for the treatment of erythroblastosis, lymphocyte chimerism may be induced to last postnatally occasionally up to at least 16 months (HUTCHINSON et al., 1967), indicating that cell transfer near term through the placenta may indeed meet with fetal immunologic competence.

The results of studies in the rabbit by OEHME (1967) point in the same direction. Labelled leukocytes may reach the fetus but do not proliferate, and his findings in man suggest that this is true here as well.

The one exceptional case of presumed permanent maternal lymphocyte graft upon the fetus is the infant described by KADOWAKI et al. (1965). This male infant died at 16 months from what appeared to be the graft-versus-host reaction. The child is thought to have had the Swiss type of a gammaglobuline-

3*

mia with hypoplasia of the thymus. He had developed normally for one month but then developed repeated infections and the "runt syndrome". In three lymphocyte cultures he had between 27 and 40% XX cells while the bone marrow yielded only XY cells and no erythrocyte chimerism was detected. The most reasonable explanation would be that maternal lymphocytes were engrafted around the time of birth (? during labor) and gradually proliferated in the immunologically deficient newborn to produce this syndrome. A similar situation, produced neonatally by transfusions, but less well documented, has been reported by Hathaway et al. (1966) and it may well be that these circumstances occur more often than is currently appreciated.

Fetal cells traverse to the mother regularly, witness the trophoblast transport from the placenta to the maternal lung in most, if not all pregnancies. Moreover, fetal bleeding through the placenta occurs often, more frequently with obstetrical manipulations. Although fetal neoplasms have occasionally been reported to affect the placenta (leukemia, neuroblastoma), no seeding to the mother is known. If it were to take place, presumably it would be rejected as must be fetal lymphocytes, for permanent chimerism does not seem to develop in such cases. The one exception of course is the choriocarcinoma, a fetal (placental) tumor which seeds extensively and represents one form of chimerism. A discussion of this poorly understood problem goes beyond the central theme of this review and the reader is referred to our previous summary of current knowledge in this field (Benirschke and Driscoll, 1967).

2. Blood Chimerism

The initial report by Dunsford et al. (1953) of a human blood group chimera is remarkable in that it was discovered without knowledge of the woman having had a twin. Since then perhaps ten other blood chimeras have been described. These are summarized in Table 3 and it will be seen that the information on some of these individuals is sketchy, even doubtful. One recently described case (Sturgeon et al., 1969) has been deleted from this list because it does not represent as clear-cut a case of blood chimerism as the others here listed. The case illustrates well the difficulties experienced in attempting to accumulate proof for this condition.

Several interesting facts derive from this compilation of data. Thus, the admixture of chimeric cells varies greatly in these twins and the ratios are not the same in most pairs. Perhaps most remarkable are twins No. 2, 4 and 11 in which the admixture of one twin is considerable, in the other it is negligible or was not found. This suggests a one-way intrauterine exchange of precursor cells which is also seen in case 7 where both twins possess 85% of the female infant's cells. In this case both twins had nearly identical birth weights and their hemoglobins were similar, thus precluding a similarity to the "transfusion syndrome" of identical twins (Benirschke and Driscoll, 1967). In no case were placental anastomoses actually observed.

In several instances the female of heterosexual twins had normal sexual development, some even had several pregnancies. Thus, the freemartin effect of ruminants is not exhibited in man, in which respect the condition is similar to that of marmoset monkeys. Also, buccal smears and histologic study of the two skin grafts alone showed appropriate sex chromatin markers; only in case 5 is there possible chimerism of solid tissues, suggested by the weak H-saliva-antigen reaction.

So far as is known, all fraternal human twins have dichorionic placentation. The placentas may be extremely intimately fused, nevertheless, only two cases of interplacental anastomoses (these were in monozygous twins) have been well demonstrated, despite numerous detailed studies searching for this phenomenon (CAMERON, 1968). Other reports are less critical and have been discussed in detail previously (BENIRSCHKE and DRISCOLL, 1967). It can, therefore, be concluded that blood chimerism analogous to that of cattle and marmosets may be expected only very rarely in man. This is to be corroborated by the failure in two studies to detect this phenomenon by blood grouping of 58 additional dizygous pairs (DUNSFORD et al., 1953) and 77 additional dizygous pairs by BOOTH et al. (1957). Furthermore, UCHIDA et al. (1964) found no anastomoses in 409 dizygous pairs' placentas by injection although these were especially looked for.

The methods of detecting blood chimeras have been discussed in several of the papers listed in Table 3 and specifically by DAVIDSON et al. (1958) and WOODRUFF et al. (1962). It is relevant that blood grouping led to the recognition of most of these cases, either because a blood group 0 individual lacked anti-A or anti-B or, because upon blood grouping a certain percentage of cells remained unagglutinated with appropriate antibodies. Of interest then is to learn that by this sensitive technique the blood group ratios did not change over several months or years in several of these chimeras. Only case 1 showed a shift to a 70/30 ratio in favor of the patient's cells after she had two additional pregnancies (DUNSFORD and STACEY, 1957). This is reminiscent of some of the reports on cattle chimerism and is not fully understood at present. Partial abrogation of tolerance has been suggested to explain this phenomenon by these authors, perhaps induced by the pregnancies. STONE et al. (1964) it will be recalled, put forward more complex events for this phenomenon in cattle twins but it seems to this writer that a simpler mechanism might be considered. Thus, it is known that, with advancing age, some portion of the bone marrow space (e.g. femur) becomes occupied by fat. Not only is it likely that the foreign clones of marrow are irregularly distributed through the bone marrow space but also, we find variable admixtures by the chromosome technique when the marrow of femurs is compared with that of humeri in chimeric marmosets. Therefore, it may be that shifts in the ratios of a chimeric bone marrow population may occur with advancing age by fat replacement alone. It might also be mentioned that the first human chimera described developed for unknown reasons substantial amounts of anti-A, which reacted with foreign A and AB cells, but not with the patient's own chimeric population of A cells (DUNSFORD and STACEY, 1957).

Split tolerance to skin antigens of the female of twin 2 may have caused the delayed rejection of the skin graft while the blood admixture did not change (WOODRUFF and LENNOX, 1959). In two cases chimerism detected a

Table 3. *Summary of all human*

No.	Author date	Sex	Proportion of RBC %	Proportion of GPS	Age	Saliva
1	Dunsford *et al.* (1952)	F	61	0		no A
			39	A	25	
		M	?			?
2	Booth *et al.* (1957)	F	99	0	21	H
			1	A		
		M	14	0		
			86	A		A, H
3	Nicholas *et al.* (1957)	F	49	0		H, trace Le[a]
			51	A	29	
		M	39	0		no A, H
			61	A		strong Le[a]
4	Ueno *et al.* (1959)	F	68	0		A, H
			32	A	12	
		M	100	A		A, H (weak)
5	Velez-Orozco (1961)	F	5	A	Adult	?
			95	B		
		M	?			
6	Hartemann *et al.* (1963)	F	10	0	Newborns	?
			90	A		
		F	20	0		
			80	A		
		F	85	0		
			15	A		
7	Chown *et al.* (1963)	F	85	0	Newborns	0
			15	A		
		M	85	0		A
			15	A		
8	Hart *et al.* (1967)	M	99.8	0	18	H
			0.2	B		
		F	20	0		B, H
			80	B		
9		F	99	0	17	A, H
			1	A		
		F	99	0		
			1	A		H
10		M	99.7	A	20	?
			0.3	B		
11	Bias and Migeon (1967)	M	95	A	Newborns	?
			5	B		
		M	100	B		

blood chimeras published to date

Drumsticks on leukocytes	Lymphocyte culture	Other studies	Remarks
		See DUNSFORD and STACEY (1957)	Has had 2 pregnancies; chimeric for transferrin (DATTA and STONE, 1963). Male died age 3 months
Present	Skin grafts see WOODRUFF and LENNOX (1959)		Buccal smears correspond to sex
Present			
6/318			Has had 3 pregnancies
6/338			
?			Normal female sexual development at age 20 (Personal comm., 1963)
?			Five pregnancies
			Stillborn male twin
?			Trichorial placenta, very premature. Died at 4 hours. No anastomoses identified in the placenta
6.0%	70% XX 30% XY	See UCHIDA et al. (1964)	Dichorionic placenta, 34 weeks gestation
9.6%	78% XX 22% XY		
	37 XY 1 XX 32 XY 9 XX		
	153 XY TRI 21 11 XY 94 XY		

twin who died at age 3 months (case 1) or who was stillborn (case 5). In case 10 one can only assume that a twin had vanished *in utero* and was not recognized without making more problematic assumptions. Why the ratios observed in twin 8 should be reversed, so far as blood grouping and lymphocyte (chromosome marker) studies are concerned, is also unexplained. Finally, in contrast to the cases of monozygous twins with different chromosomes, the so-called heterokaryotic twins discussed below, the twins of case 11 must be considered dizygous because of their difference in blood groups. One can only assume that the eleven cells with 46 chromosomes found in the trisomic infant with mongolism derived from the normal cotwin, but this is unproven. Why no trisomic lymphocytes were found in the normal twin, for that matter why he has no blood group A red blood cells, is also unknown. In a way this case resembles the transitory blood chimerism in a set of twins described by Massimo *et al.* (1966). These authors observed a pair of dizygous, dichorionic twins (different blood groups) one of whom is a typical mongolian idiot, the other normal. The former was trisomic 21 on two lymphocyte cultures, the latter possessed 70% XY and 30% XY tri 21 lymphocytes on the thirteenth day of life. At age 5 months only 5% of cells had the trisomic structure; at 12 months no trisomic cells existed. The authors consider "a progressive loss of the reproductive capacity" of this chimeric population. Turpin *et al.* (1959) had previously reported a very similar instance. One of dizygous girl twins had a 5% red blood cell admixture at age 4 months which had disappeared by 6 months of age. The chimeric twin accepted switchgrafts for 16 days, as opposed to 12 days of the nonchimeric twin, and the authors assume a gradual elimination of the chimeric population by immunologic mechanisms.

The many problems raised by various authors indicate how valuable such chimeric twins may become in answering basic biologic questions in reproduction, embryology and immunology. It is also evident, however, that it will be necessary in the future to have alongside the clinical and genetic findings of such twins the results of a detailed morphologic study of the placental vascular relationship before we can hope to interpret the complex findings.

3. Whole-Body-Chimerism and True Hermaphroditism

It is no longer possible to review adequately the literature on these topics in man. Since the advent of modern cytogenetic techniques there has been a profusion of reports, some of which are so incomplete that they will not be considered in this context. The principal difficulty in careful scrutiny of this voluminous literature is that, from available data, a meaningful distinction between mosaicism and chimerism is impossible in most case reports.

When two different populations of cells are found in cytogenetic studies, theoretically it should be possible from the concurrent study of other genetic markers (blood groups, hemoglobins, enzymes, pigments, etc.) to make a reasonable deduction whether one or more zygotes produced the admixture.

In only few cases have such studies been undertaken and has critical proof for chimerism been supplied. In a majority, these studies were either not feasible, as in abortuses, or they were not carried out. In the latter instances then often complex modes of genesis, such as multiple nondisjunction, are offered as explanation for the findings. This should not be necessary in the future as more genetic markers are now available for study.

In other instances, such as in the numerous reports of true hermaphroditism with only XX cells, this cytogenetic finding often perhaps reflects an inadequate search for other clones, and an attempt is rarely made to seek other markers which might give evidence of chimerism. Hence, this large field of human mosaics and possible chimeras is in a confused state and only some specifically pertinent cases will be cited here as illustrations. In particular, I will draw attention to those six case studies in which multiple zygotic origin seems incontrovertible in an effort to stimulate search for what may be a more common developmental error than is presently believed.

Ascertainment because of ambiguous sexual development has favored the reporting of sex chromosome mosaics and chimeras. For this reason then, a report by Brøgger and Gundersen (1968) of a five year old boy with typical Down's syndrome is of particular interest. Double fertilization is suggested as the possible origin of a lymphocyte population with about 80 % normal and 20 % trisomic G cells. The patient also had two antigenically different populations of red blood cells with like proportions, but skin culture yielded 100 % trisomic cells. No mention is made of a twin and these authors do not consider blood chimerism between dizygous twins (one perhaps a fetus papyraceous) in their pathogenetic considerations.

Double fertilization seems perhaps more plausible in abortion specimens in which diploid and polyploid lines are admixed, as for instance in a specimen with populations of cells containing 2n/4n ploidies reported by Thiede and Salm (1964). While other studies on spontaneous human abortions have often uncovered polyploid conceptuses (Carr, 1969), the findings by Schlegel and his colleagues (1966) of 2n/3n, and two cases of 2n/4n abortuses raise the possibility that such errors may also occur postzygotically; for it was their observation that these anomalies were associated with peculiar proliferative and presumably polyploid events in the amnion. In any event, the cases do not prove chimerism convincingly.

Some children with an admixture of diploid and triploid or tetraploid cells have survived infancy on occasion. These are reviewed by Giraud (1968) and a case by Kohn et al. (1967) should be added to their list of five children; severe developmental defects were associated with the cytogenetic error. The 2n/4n admixture was limited to the leukocytes in Kohn's case and it was a stable ratio during the seven months of study. Skin and lung cultures, however, were always diploid. In all other five cases the skin participated in the 2n/3n cell admixture. In several instances, however, simple blood group studies did not disclose two populations of red cells. The patient with 48 XXYY/71 XXXYY described by Schmid and Vischer (1967) is cited as indicative of mosaicism, as opposed to chimerism, because of the unusual sex chromosome constitution of the two cell lines. It is envisaged that an XYY sperm fertilized a normal ovum; from this 48 (XXYY) zygote, daughter cells derived, one of which fused with the haploid second polar body to yield a clone with 71 (XXXYY) chromosomes.

It is evident then that from these diploid/polyploid case reports in man no conclusive evidence in favor of chimerism emerges, as appealing as such a hypothesis might be on first glance. The fact that, as we will see, this is not invariably so warrants caution in interpreting the six cases just cited. In fact, if the hypothesis is correct that is used to explain the complex case of SCHMID and VISCHER (1967), then fusion of at least one additional segregation product is involved. Here, the definition of "chimerism" becomes a difficult problem over which no uniformly acceptable nomenclature decision has been made. The interested reader is referred to statements by STEWART (1968) and FORD (1969), in which diverse types of chimerism are considered also with respect to their potential use in genetic mapping. The latter author includes this particular case as an instance of chimerism.

As has been alluded to, cytogenetic studies of true hermaphrodites have commonly uncovered only normal female karyotypes. Inasmuch as it is generally assumed that a Y chromosome is necessary for the induction of testicular tissue, a formal explanation of the different types of true hermaphroditism is difficult. Furthermore, the great variability of the external genitalia, ductal structures and gonads defies a simple solution.

McDANIEL et al. (1968) estimate that more than 120 true hermaphrodites have been reported and their case, with positive buccal smears and an XX lymphocyte constitution is representative of many case reports. Six cases with similar cytogenetic findings are presented by JONES et al. (1965) in which cultures even from testes were XX. They present a good review, including the cases with different stem lines. Most recently KOONTZ et al. (1969) report three XX cases in which only leukocytes were studied. At present the main obstacle for the satisfactory pathogenetic explanation of true hermaphroditism seems to be that "hidden mosaicism" (SARTO et al., 1969) is difficult to rule out, even when searched for. In this respect BRØGGER and AAGENAES (1965) have provided the most interesting example. In their patient with true hermaphroditism cultures from bone marrow, lymphocytes, skin and left testis yielded only XX cells (214, of which 36 were karyotyped). Not satisfied with these results, they took a second testis biopsy and this time discovered a substantial number of normal XY cells. Here then the hidden clone was detected by perseverance only and one needs to wonder about the identity of less adequately scrutinized cases. What is of particular interest in this case, interpreted here as a probable chimera, is the fact that an XY clone was detected only in the testis biopsy and, consequently, blood grouping study disclosed no chimerism. A very similar case was described by LEJEUNE et al. (1966) with a small clone of XY cells in one gonad. BRØGGER and AAGENAES (1965) review previous reports of chimeric/mosaic cases, including the

XX/XXY/XXYYY patient reported by FRACCARO *et al.* (1962) who considered it "plausible that all human intersexes are chromosomal mosaics" and who thought that postzygotic nondisjunction had given rise to this complex admixture. Numerous other similar cases can be cited, all suffering from the same syndrome and in almost all it is impossible to make a clear-cut decision as to mosaicism *vs.* chimerism.

Unfortunately then, these interesting subjects have been of little help in furnishing new data concerning primary gonadal sex differentiation; in an *Editorial* (Lancet, 1967) the various complex assumptions made about this problem are adequately discussed. A final point worth mentioning here is that evidence is accumulating that mosaic cell lines may have different survival value. Thus, TAYLOR (1968) finds in a group of children with mosaic Down's syndrome an *in vivo* selection of one clone with advancing age. If a similar phenomenon of selection holds for chimeric cells then complete elimination of say an XY clone in a true hermaphrodite with only XX cells can be envisaged and could be difficult to ever ascertain. Similar reasoning was employed by TAYLOR (1968) for the single case report of an euploid child with Down's syndrome.

The three cases of true hermaphroditism in which the diagnosis of chimerism appears to be securely founded are summarized in Table 4. In these patients the chimeric nature of the admixture was supported by cytogenetic findings of two populations in blood as well as solid tissue cultures (thus ruling out blood chimerism), and by the finding of admixed populations of other genetic markers (serologic or cellular). In addition, three patients are listed who, while fulfilling the other criteria of chimerism and two suffering maldevelopment, do not show true hermaphroditism. These six cases are the only ones for which whole-body-chimerism may be assumed to be reasonably critically established. In many others with XX/XY admixture chimerism *may be* the pathogenetic mechanism but it has not been convincingly proven. Indeed, some were extensively studied for the presence of double genetic markers other than XX/XY chromosomes and none were detected (MANUEL *et al.*, 1965; BAIN and SCOTT, 1965; DEMINATTI and MAILLARD, 1967; MARINE and JACKSON, 1968). This leaves out a vast number of cases with reported admixtures of cytogenetically different cell lines (*e.g.* XX/XY; XO/XX/XY) and with true hermaphroditism in which other markers could not be studied. In a few instances the assumption of chimerism is specifically excluded, as in case 1 of SARTO *et al.* (1969) whose XX/XXYr patient is believed to derive from an XXYr zygote with postzygotic loss, in some clones of cells, of the Y ring chromosome.

This sketchy review then provides evidence that a) whole body chimerism does occasionally exist in man, and b) that it is usually ascertained when malformations of one type or another lead to a very extensive analysis of the patient. There is no *a priori* reason why the type of isosexual chimerism as described for a mouse by RUSSELL and WOODIEL (1966) may not also be found in man nor, that once more intensive investigations are performed on

Table 4. *Summary of most human whole-body-chimeras,*

	Clinical condition	Lymphocyte culture	Fibroblast culture	Gonad culture
1	Ovary; ovotestis; enlarged clitoris	XX/XY	XX/XY	Ovary XX Ovotestis XX/XY Clitoris XX/XY
2	Ovary; ovotestis; enlarged clitoris	XX/XY	XX/XY	—
3	Hypospadias; bifid scrotum; ovary; descended ? testis	XX/XY	XX/XY dark skin more XX	Ovary XX
4	Normal blood donor; normal testes; gynecomastia	XX/XY Many tetra-ploids	XX/XY light skin only XY Many tetra-ploids	—
5	Hypospadias; congenital heart disease; abnormal testes	XX/XY	Inferred XX clone from buccal smear	—
6	Hypospadias; "triploid anomaly"; testes	2n XX/3n XXY	XX/XXY in skin, liver, fascia	Testis XX/XXY

the patients in whom only cell admixture is found cytogenetically, these will not also be shown to be products of irregular, multiple fertilization. To pursue such a study is difficult and the various and divergent genetic consequences of such events as dispermy, suppression of polar body, etc. must be clearly understood. These are discussed in considerable detail by Jones (1969) and by Ford (1969). Since critical studies of early zygotic errors are not yet available in man, and because none of the cases so far described allows a definitive conclusion, it is premature to discuss the likelihood of one type of abnormal event or the other as leading to whole-body-chimerism in man.

From the available data (Table 4) one is led to believe that two sperms were involved in every case of human chimerism. In several instances fertilization of an ovum and a polar body is assumed rather than the involvement of two normal ova. This is perhaps not completely warranted, and of particular interest then is the finding of a history of dizygotic twinning in the mother of case No. 5 and the presence of a macerated twin in No. 6. Perhaps this is further justification for the term "geminism" for these chimeras, coined by Bruce Chown (Corey et al., 1967). In any event, the potential for twinning by either double ovulation or abnormal segregation in two of six cases is striking and should be borne in mind in future studies.

recognized largely because of intersexuality

Other evidence of chimerism	Other unusual findings	Suggested explanation	Author
2 populations of red cells	Heterochromia of iris	2 sperms 2 oval nuclei	GARTLER *et al.* (1962)
? Haptoglobin mixture	—	2 sperms 2 oval nuclei	GROUCHY *et al.* (1964)
2 populations of red cells; ? haptoglobin mixture; phosphoglugomutase mixture	Pigment mottling with striking laterality	2 sperms 2 oval nuclei	COREY *et al.* (1967)
2 populations of red cells; including sickling; Lewis secretor genotype mixture	Pigment mottling; predominantly male cells. XX clone assumed to derive from polar body fertilization	2 sperms ovum and polar body	ZUELZER *et al.* (1964)
2 populations of red cells	Maternal family history of 2 dizygous twin pairs	2 sperms 2 identical oval nuclei ? polar body	MYHRE *et al.* (1965)
2 populations of red cells	Triploid line smaller; heterochromia of iris; macerated twin with separate placenta	2 sperms 2 ova or polar body	LEJEUNE *et al.* (1967)

Finally, and most relevant to the current controversy concerning the development of the freemartin syndrome discussed above, these six cases provide evidence that a) general XX/XY chimerism is compatible with normal ovarian differentiation, and b) tissue cultures from gonads generally yield cultures with XY cell preponderance in testes and XX cells in ovaries. Indeed, strong XY representation in the overall chimeric constitution favors testicular differentiation. Thus, it seems likely that the gonadal territory, XY or XX, decides the fate of an undifferentiated gonad.

4. Heterokaryotic Monozygous Twins (a Type of Mosaicism)

This error of development perhaps does not properly fit into a discussion of chimerism, as is also true of the next heading; however, from their study much can be inferred that has direct reference to whole-body-chimerism, and it is for this reason that the topics are briefly discussed.

It is axiomatic, of course, that monozygotic, single-ovum-derived twins should have the same sex, chromosome number and phenotype. They should be truly "identical". Numerous environmental influences affect their development before birth, however, and discordant anomalies in monozygous twins have often been described, some of which can be traced to untoward intra-

Table 5. *Summary of all published cases of monozygous twins differing in karyotype, the so-called heterokaryotic monozygous twins*

No.	Authors	Sex	Phenotype	Cytogenetic findings		Diagnosis of monozygosity by	Placenta	Remarks
				lymphocytes	solid tissues			
1	Beukering and Vervoorn (1956)	? ? died	Normal Down's syndrome	— —	— —	Placenta	DiMo	See also Fanconi (1962)
2	Fanconi (1956)	F F	Down's syndrome Normal	— —	— —	Blood groups, likeness study		
3	Turpin et al. (1961)	F M	Turner's syndrome Normal	100% XY 2 XO/18 XY	100% XO skin and fascia 100% XY skin and fascia	Blood groups, serotypes, saliva, switchgrafts, dermatoglyphics, placenta	Mono-chorial	See Lejeune and Turpin (1961), and Turpin (1967)
4	Wolff et al. (1962)	M died M	Down's syndrome Normal	— 2 tri 21/102 normal	Tri 21 skin Normal skin	Blood groups, serotypes, saliva, dermatoglyphics, placenta	DiMo	See Lejeune et al. (1962), Turpin (1967), Mirror imagery of dermatoglyphics
5	Mikkelsen et al. (1963)	F F died	Normal Turner's syndrome	17 XO/31 XX 15 XO/33 XX	30 XO/35 XX skin 24 XO/4 XX skin	Blood groups, placenta	DiMo	

#	Author	Sex	Phenotype	Karyotype	Chromatin/skin	Evidence	Placenta	Remarks
6	BENIRSCHKE and SULLIVAN (1965)	F died	Turner's syndrome, anomalies	—	Chromatin negative	No blood group chimerism, placenta	DiMo	The deceased twin had many anomalies, including streak ovaries, arrhinencephaly and webbing of the neck
		F	Normal, pulmonic stenosis	5 XO/115 XX				
7	DEKABAN (1965)	F	Down's syndrome	132 XX trisomic 21	44 XX trisomic marrow 10 XX trisomic skin	Blood groups, dermatoglyphics, serotypes	—	The abnormal infant has, in addition to trisomy 21, one small extra chromosome
		F	Normal	27 XX	—			
8	EDWARDS et al. (1966)	F	Turner's syndrome, mild	9 XY/8 XO	? 1 XY/59 XO skin	Blood groups, serotypes, dermatoglyphics	—	Heterochromasia of eyes of male
		M	Normal	? 1 XY/37 XO	143 XO skin			
9		F	Turner's syndrome	28 XO/65 XX	—	Blood groups, serotypes, dermatoglyphics	"Single" ? DiDi	
		F	Normal	21 XO/95 XX	—			
10	SHINE and CORNEY (1966)	F died	Turner's syndrome, anomalies	—	Chromatin negative	Blood groups, dermatoglyphics	"Single"	
		F	Normal	100% XX				
11	RUSSELL et al. (1966)	F	Turner's syndrome	31 XO	128 XO skin	Blood groups, serotypes, dermatoglyphics, partial mirror imagery	"Single"	Multiple discordant anomalies of genitalia. Twin 2 has one testis
		F	Turner's syndrome	3 XY/75 XO	9 XY/159 XO skin 17 XY/171 XO gonads, tube			

DiMo = Diamnionic, monochorionic placenta; DiDi = Diamnionic, dichorionic placenta.

uterine influences. In a like manner the twinning process may be coupled with postzygotic chromosomal errors. The majority of aneuploid syndromes (*e.g.* Down's syndrome, Klinefelter's syndrome) has been assumed to result from faulty gametogenesis, but the abundance of chromosomal mosaics now detected in man, particularly those associated with abnormal sex development, gives ample evidence for the frequent occurrence also of postzygotic nondisjunction of chromosomes. Thus, the existence of "identical" twins differing in chromosome number and even in sexual phenotype becomes explicable. The published cases with acceptable evidence are summarized in Table 5 for which the descriptive title "heterokaryotic monozygous twins" (LEJEUNE *et al.*, 1962) has been used. These twins form but one part of the biologic continuum which is assumed for the general subject here under discussion.

Most monozygous twins have identical karyotypes as might be expected (see WOLFF *et al.*, 1962; NIELSEN, 1967) but it is astonishing that in a relatively short time these eleven discordant sets have been reported. These findings have led to the question whether the events of aneuploidy and twinning may be causally related which cannot be answered at this time, but it is pertinent to reiterate that much can be learned from the complete study of these exceptional cases. When the type of placentation is known in particular, then some conclusions can be drawn as to the timing of the twinning event (BENIRSCHKE and DRISCOLL, 1967). In at least five cases of Table 5, the fact that monochorial placentation was found indicates that twinning occurred relatively late in embryonic development. This is further supported by the partial mirror imagery in two cases, and by the complex somatic mosaicism of genotypes. Furthermore, because of the presence of interfetal anastomoses in most monochorial twins one may expect different admixtures of blood cell mosaicism in these twins when compared with the mosaicism of somatic tissues. This has been the case when all these studies were undertaken, as Table 5 indicates.

To separate these complex events clearly from chimerism in an individual case may indeed be most difficult, particularly when the parental blood groups are very similar. Nevertheless, the theoretic importance of the distinction is emphasized. These cases will eventually aid materially in our understanding of the mechanism of normal and abnormal sex differentiation; some of these aspects have been discussed in lucid detail by EDWARDS *et al.* (1966). The cytologic events leading to this admixture are detailed by TURPIN (1967) and, to some extent, in an editorial comment of the paper by RUSSELL *et al.* (1966).

In heterokaryotic monozygous twins then, an admixture of cells with different chromosomal types exists which simulates that of chimerism. Because it occurs in two individuals which originate from one fertilized ovum, however, the event is best construed as a complex type of mosaicism in which various tissues are differently affected. The degree of admixture can be understood when one takes into consideration the timing of the twinning event and the possibility that in some cases interfetal placental anastomoses further influence the cellular admixture in a manner not unlike that known from blood chimerism. The failure to identify two blood groups in these twins generally allows differentiation from the state of chimerism as here defined.

5. The Acardiac Twins

In man, there is every reason to believe that acardiacs arise only as one of monozygous twins and for this reason their discussion under the subject heading of chimerism is also less appropriate. We concur with SCHATZ (1898) that acardiacs result from fortuitous large interplacental anastomoses in twins. Since these exist, for all intents and purposes, only among monochorial and hence monozygous twins in man, they should possess identical genomes; chimerism cannot exist. The situation is different for ruminants, as was described previously in the report by DUNN *et al.* (1967) of heterosexual twins in cattle, one of whom was acardiac. This finding is taken to be a beautiful confirmation of the etiologic contribution of the placental anastomoses (see also SIMONDS and GOWEN, 1925).

In man, acardiac monsters have all been of the same sex as the normal twin (BENIRSCHKE, 1959), and in the cytogenetic studies we have done on three such individuals we found them to be normal and the same as those of the normal cotwin (BENIRSCHKE and DRISCOLL, 1967). This has been confirmed in a case report by TURPIN *et al.* (1967). On the other hand, aneuploidy has been reported in such a monster by RASHAD and KERR (1966, see also KERR and RASHAD, 1966), whose fibrous tissue culture yielded mostly 47 chromosomes. Lymphocyte culture of the normal twin, as in other cases (*e.g.* FUJIKURA and WELLINGS, 1964; two of our own) were normal. In other words, whatever the clone of abnormal cells in the monster, the normal twin did not share in it. These authors liken their findings to the heterokaryotic monozygous twins discussed above and consider it possible that the aneuploidy was responsible for the malformation. In our view it is more likely that the chronic hypoxic intrauterine existence of the acardiac may well be responsible for abnormal events in tissue culture, an opinion also shared by TURPIN *et al.* (1967).

VIII. Concluding Remarks

As this extensive review has shown, spontaneous chimerism occurs in many mammals that have been studied closely. Perhaps it is an event that exists more commonly than is evident from the published data. It presents in many different forms, involving only small portions of the body or almost all tissues as the "geminisms" of whole-body-chimeras. It is an abnormal event of development that is often difficult to prove, at least it is often difficult to set apart from mosaicism. Its pathogenesis is poorly understood although currently much insight is gained from blastocyst fusion studies in mice with respect to pathogenesis and its effect upon general embryonic development.

The condition has important theoretical and practical importance. Through its understanding the fields of immunology, sex differentiation and general

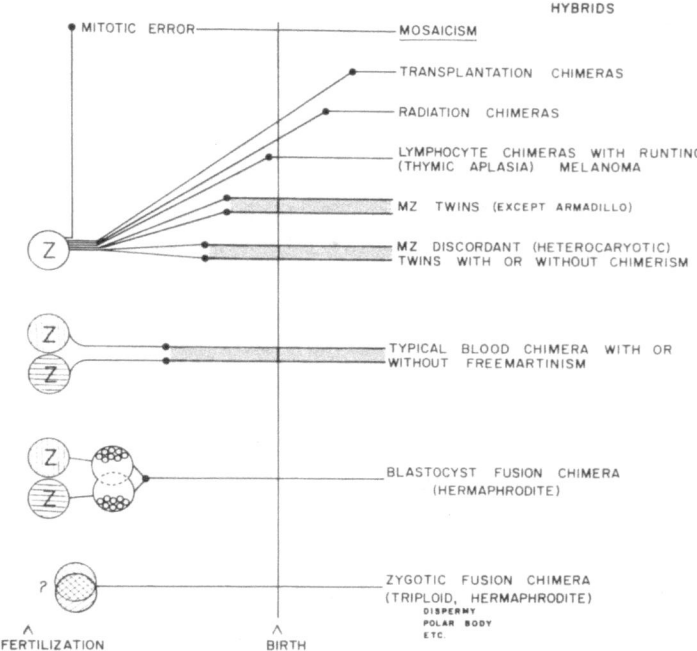

Fig. 10. In this schematic representation the point of view is taken that a biological continuum exists between the various forms of genic admixtures. These types are largely determined by the timing of the adverse event. Z zygote at left at the time of fertilization. Confluence of genotypes is indicated by black dot and placed on the scale of fetal development when the event is believed to occur. Shaded areas represent placental blood vessel communications only. Dizygous twins occupy the lower, monozygous twins the upper part of the diagram

embryology have benefited greatly in the past and every indication exists that its detailed study will clarify puzzling aspects of fertilization and prenatal development in the future. The broader perspectives of the phenomenon are analyzed in the searching monograph by STERN (1968) that is warmly recommended to the reader.

At the end of many considerations of chimerism an attempt is often made to arrive at a useful classification of these abnormal events (COTTERMAN, 1958; FORD, 1969; COREY and MILLER, 1966). In general, however, these schemes do not place the varied types of chimerism described in these pages into an overall biologic perspective and it is for this reason that Fig. 10 was constructed with the generous help of Drs. GROPP and MARIN-PADILLA. It attempts to depict our point of view, namely that no rigid boundaries exist between various types of twins, chimeras and mosaics. Rather, these processes are judged as events on the scale of a biological continuum where it is principally the timing that determines which particular state will be the outcome of an adverse embryonic event. Similar thoughts have been expressed by SCHWALBE (1907) in his discussion on the classification of twins. His ideas are aptly paraphrased by v. VERSCHUER (1927): "Schwalbe ist schon 1907 so weit gegangen, eine vollständige Reihe aufzustellen von eineiigen Zwillingen, ja sogar von den zweieiigen Zwillingen an bis zur Mißgeburt", a statement that is readily applicable to the subject of this discussion.

Acknowledgement. I am most grateful to many loyal colleagues for their collaboration, and the critical discussion of many aspects of this review. These include Mrs. V. BABCOCK, K. IMREDY, Drs. A. GROPP, M. MARIN-PADILLA, M. M. SULLIVAN, D. WURSTER, Mr. R. J. LOW and Miss M. WISE.

References

ABT, D. A., CROWSHAW, J. E., HARE, W. C. D.: Monocephalus dipygus parasiticus and other anomalies in a calf. J. Amer. vet. med. Ass. 141, 1068—1072 (1962).

AINSWORTH, L., RYAN, K. J.: Steroid hormone transformations by endocrine organs from pregnant mammals. I. Estrogen biosynthesis by mammalian placental preparations *in vitro*. Endocrinology 79, 875—883 (1966).

ALEXANDER, G., WILLIAMS, D.: Ovine freemartins. Nature (Lond.) 201, 1296—1298 (1964).

ANDERSON, D., BILLINGHAM, R. E., LAMPKIN, G. H., MEDAWAR, P. B.: The use of skin grafting to distinguish between monozygotic and dizygotic twins in cattle. Heredity 5, 379—397 (1961).

ARONSON, S.: A case of transplacental tumor metastasis. Acta paediat. (Uppsala) 52, 123—124 (1963).

BAIN, A. D., SCOTT, J. S.: Mixed gonadal dysgenesis with XX/XY mosaicism. The evidence for the occurrence of fertilisation by two spermatozoa in man. Lancet 1965 I, 1035—1039.

BALLANTYNE, J. W.: The history and etymology of the freemartin. Brit. med. J. 1910 I, 1125—1126.

BASRUR, P. K., STOLTZ, D. R.: Chromosome studies in bovine quintuplets. Chromosoma (Berl.) 19, 176—187 (1966).

BEKKUM, D. W. VAN, VRIES, M. J. DE: Radiation chimeras. London: Logos Press 1967.

BENIRSCHKE, K.: Nuclear sex of holoacardii amorphi. Obstet. and Gynec. 14, 72—78 (1959).

— Mosaicism and chimerism. McGraw Hill Yearbook of Science and Technology, p. 248—251 (1967).

— ANDERSON, J., BROWNHILL, L. E.: Marrow chimerism in marmosets. Science 138, 513—515 (1962).

— BLOCH, E.: Failure to demonstrate C_{19}-steroids in bovine testes. Acta endocr. (Kbh.) 34, 65—68 (1960).

— BROWNHILL, L. E.: Further observations on marrow chimerism in marmosets. Cytogenetics 1, 245—257 (1962).

— — Heterosexual cells in testes of chimeric monkeys. Cytogenetics 2, 331—341 (1963).

— DRISCOLL, S. G.: The pathology of the human placenta. Berlin-Heidelberg-New York: Springer 1967.

— LAYTON, WM.: An early twin blastocyst of the golden lion marmoset, *Leontocebus rosalia*. Folia primatol. 10, 131—138 (1969).

— SULLIVAN, M. M.: Chromosomally discordant monozygous twins. Hum. Chromosomes Newsletter 15, 3 (1965).

— — The human placenta in relationship to the development of chimerism. In: The foeto-placental unit, p. 37—44. Amsterdam: Excerpta Medica Foundation 1969.

BERTRAND, M.: Le freemartinisme. Rev. méd. Vét. 66, 575—599 (1965).

Beukering, J. A. v., Vervoorn, J. D.: A case of uniovular twins of which one child was normal and the other had the syndrome of mongolism. Acta genet. med. (Roma) **5**, 113—114 (1956).

Bias, W. B., Migeon, B. R.: Blood group chimaerism with Down's syndrome. Lancet **1967 II**, 257.

Biggers, J. D., McFeely, R. A.: Intersexuality in domestic mammals. In: Advances in Reproductive Physiology. London: Logos Press 1966.

Billingham, R. E., Lampkin, G. H.: Further studies in tissue homotransplantation in cattle. J. Embryol. exp. Morph. **5**, 351—367 (1957).

Bissonnette, T. H.: The development of the reproductive ducts and canals in the freemartin with comparison of the normal. Amer. J. Anat. **33**, 267—345 (1924).

— Notes on a 32 mm freemartin. Biol. Bull. **54**, 238—253 (1928).

Bloch, E.: The conversion of 7-^{3}H-pregnenolone and 4-^{14}C-progesterone to testosterone and androstenedione by mammalian fetal testes *in vitro*. Steroids **9**, 415—430 (1967).

Booth, P. B., Plaut, G., James, J. D., Ikin, E. W., Moores, P., Sanger, R., Race, R. R.: Blood chimerism in a pair of twins. Brit. med. J. **1957 I**, 1456—1458.

Bornstein, S.: The genetic sex of two intersexual horses and some notes on the karyotype of normal horses. Acta vet. scand. **8**, 291—300 (1967).

Brehm, A. E.: Die Fische. In: Brehms Tierleben, Bd. 8. Pechnel-Loesche, 3. Ausg. Leipzig: Bibliographisches Institut 1892.

British Medical Journal: Letters to the editors, pp. 47, 87, 93, 141 (1887).

Brodsky, I., Baren, M., Kahn, S. B., Lewis, G., Tellem, M.: Metastatic malignant melanoma from mother to fetus. Cancer (Philad.) **18**, 1048—1054 (1965).

Brøgger, A., Aagenaes, Ö.: The human Y chromosome and the etiology of true hermaphroditism. With the report of a case with XX/XY sex chromosome mosaicism. Hereditas (Lund) **53**, 231—246 (1965).

— Gundersen, S. K.: Double fertilisation in Down's syndrome. Lancet **1966 I**, 1270—1271.

Bruere, A. N.: Evidence of age aneuploidy in the chromosomes of the sheep. Nature (Lond.) **215**, 658—659 (1967).

— MacNab, J.: A cytogenetical investigation of six intersex sheep, shown to be freemartins. Res. Vet. Sci. **9**, 170—180 (1968).

Buyse, A.: A case of extreme sex-modification in an adult bovine free-martin. Anat. Rec. **66**, 43—58 (1936).

Cameron, A. H.: The Birmingham twin survey. Proc. roy. Soc. Med. **61**, 229—234 (1968).

Carr, D. H.: Lethal chromosome errors. In: Comparative mammalian cytogenetics (K. Benirschke, ed.), Berlin-Heidelberg-New York: Springer 1969.

Cavell, B.: Transplacental metastasis of malignant melanoma. Report of a case. Acta paediat. (Uppsala), Suppl. **146**, 37—40 (1963).

Chapin, C. L.: A microscopic study of the reproductive system of foetal free-martins. J. exp. Zool. **23**, 453—582 (1917).

Chown, B., Lewis, M., Bowman, J. M.: A pair of newborn human blood chimeric twins. Transfusion **3**, 494—495 (1963).

Chu, E. H. Y., Thuline, H. C., Norby, D. E.: Triploid-diploid chimerism in a male tortoiseshell cat. Cytogenetics **3**, 1—18 (1964).

Cockrill, W. R.: The water buffalo. Sci. Amer. **217**, 118—125 (1967).

Cole, L. J., Craft, W. A.: An acephalic lamb monster in sheep. J. Hered. **36**, 29—32 (1945).

Corey, M. J., Miller, J. R.: A proposed classification of genetically determined mosaicism in man. J. med. Genet. **3**, 230—236 (1966).

— — MacLean, J. R., Chown, B.: A case of XX/XY mosaicism. Amer. J. hum. Genet. **19**, 378—387 (1967).

COTTERMAN, C. W.: Erythrocyte antigen mosaicism. J. cell. comp. Physiol. **52**, 69—95 (1958).

CULZONI, V.: Osservazioni sulla morfologia esterna e sul comportamento di soggetti intersessuati nei suini e nei bovini. Atti Soc. ital. Sci. vet. **19**, 337—340 (1965).

DAIN, A. R., TUCKER, E. M.: Chromosome and blood-group studies of sheep twin chimaeras. J. Physiol. (Lond.) **200**, 37p—38p (1969).

DATTA, S. P., STONE, W. H.: Transferrins of cattle twins. Proc. Soc. exp. Biol. (N.Y.) **113**, 756—759 (1963).

DAVIDSON, W. M., FOWLER, J. F., SMITH, D. R.: Sexing the neutrophil leukocytes in natural and artificial blood chimeras. Brit. J. Haematol. **4**, 231—238 (1958).

DAVIES, C. J.: Caprine free martins. Vet. J. **20**, 62—70 (1913).

DEDERER, P. H.: Polyovular follicles in the cat. Anat. Rec. **60**, 391—403 (1934).

DEKABAN, A.: Twins, probably monozygotic: one mongoloid with 48 chromosomes, the other normal. Cytogenetics **4**, 227—239 (1965).

DEMINATTI, M., MAILLARD, E.: Etude d'un cas d'hermaphrodisme humain a caryotype 46, XY/46, XX. C. R. Acad. Sci. (Paris) **265**, 365—368 (1967).

DUBOIS, R.: Sur l'origine et l'amoeboidisme des cellules germinales de l'embryon de poulet, en culture *in vitro* et leur localisation dans le germe non incubé. C. R. Acad. Sci. (Paris) **265**, 497—500 (1967).

DUNN, H. O., KENNEY, R. M., LEIN, D. H.: XX/XY chimerism in a bovine true hermaphrodite: An insight into the understanding of freemartinism. Cytogenetics **7**, 390—402 (1968).

— — STONE, W. H., BENDEL, S.: Cytogenetic and reproductive studies of XX/XY chimeric twin bulls. VIe Congr. Reprod. Insem. Artif. Paris, p. 139, 1968.

— LEIN, D. H., KENNEY, R. M.: The cytological sex of a bovine anidian (amorphous) twin monster. Cytogenetics **6**, 412—419 (1967).

DUNSFORD, I., BOWLEY, C. C., HUTCHISON, A. M., THOMPSON, J. S., SANGER, R., RACE, R. R.: A human blood group chimera. Brit. med. J. **1952** II, 81.

— STACEY, S. M.: Partial breakdown of acquired tolerance to the A antigen. Vox Sang. **2**, 414—417 (1957).

Editorial: True hermaphroditism. Lancet **1967** I, 149—150.

EDWARDS, J. H., DENT, T., KAHN, J.: Monozygotic twins of different sex. J. med. Genet. **3**, 117—123 (1966).

EL-ALFI, O. S., HATHOUT, H.: Maternofetal transfusion: immunologic and cytogenetic evidence. Amer. J. Obstet. Gynec. **103**, 599—600 (1969).

EWEN, A. H., HUMMASON, F. A.: An ovine freemartin. J. Hered. **38**, 149—152 (1947).

FANCONI, G.: Weitere Fälle von wahrscheinlich eineiigen Zwillingen von denen der eine gesund ist, der andere einen Mongolismus zeigt. Helv. paediat. Acta **17**, 490—491 (1962).

FECHHEIMER, N. S., HERSCHLER, M. S., GILMORE, L. O.: Sex chromosome mosaicism in unlike sexed cattle twins. In: Genetics Today (S. J. Geerts, ed.), vol. I, p. 265. Oxford: Pergamon Press 1963.

FEHÉR, G., GYÜRÜ, F.: Doppelmißbildungen beim Rind. Acta vet. Acad. Sci. hung. **16**, 83—106 (1966).

FISCHER, H.: Water buffalo twins. Maha Magazine **21**, 43 (1964).

— ADENIL, C.: A new case of buffalo twins in the island of Sumba. Hemera zoa **63**, 446—449 (1956).

FORBES, T. R.: The origin of *freemartin*. Bull. Hist. Med. **20**, 461—466 (1946).

FORD, C. E.: Mosaics and chimeras. Brit. med. Bull. **25**, 104—109 (1969).

FRACCARO, M., TAYLOR, A. I., BODIAN, M., NEWNS, G. H.: A human intersex ("true hermaphrodite") with XX/XXY/XXYYY sex chromosomes. Cytogenetics **1**, 104—112 (1962).

FRASER-ROBERTS, J. A., GREENWOOD, A. W.: An extreme freemartin and a freemartin-like condition in sheep. J. Anat. (Lond.) **63**, 87—94 (1928).

Freudenberg, F.: Intersexuelle Genitalmißbildung beim Stutenfohlen eines zwei-geschlechtlichen Zwillingspaares. Dtsch. tierärztl. Wschr. **67**, 214—216 (1960).

Fujikura, T., Wellings, S. R.: A teratoma-like mass on the placenta of a mal-formed infant. Amer. J. Obstet. Gynec. **89**, 824—825 (1964).

Galton, M., Holt, S. F.: Asynchronous replication of the mouse sex chromosomes. Exp. Cell Res. **37**, 111—116 (1965).

Gardner, R. L.: Mouse chimaeras obtained by injection of cells into the blastocyst. Nature (Lond.) **220**, 596—597 (1968).

Gartler, S. M., Waxman, S. H., Giblett, E.: An XX/XY human hermaphrodite resulting from double fertilization. Proc. nat. Acad. Sci. (Wash.) **48**, 332—335 (1962). [Also Proc. Soc. exp. Biol. (N.Y.) **110**, 722—724 (1962); Amer. J. hum. Genet. **15**, 62—68 (1963).]

Gengozian, N., Batson, J. S., Eide, P.: Hematologic and cytogenetic evidence for hematopoietic chimerism in the marmoset, *Tamarinus nigricollis*. Cytogenetics **3**, 384—393 (1964).

Gerneke, W. H.: Cytogenetic investigations on normal and malformed animals, with special reference to intersexes. Onderstepoort J. vet. Res. **34**, 19—300 (1967).

— deBoom, H. P. A., Heinichen, I. G.: Two canine intersexes. J. S. Afr. vet. med. Ass. **39**, 56—59 (1968).

Giraud, F.: La triploidie chez l'homme. Gaz. méd. Fr. **75**, 979—992 (1968).

Goodfellow, S. A., Strong, S. J., Stewart, J. S. S.: Bovine freemartins and true hermaphroditism. Lancet **1965 I**, 1040—1041.

Gropp, A., Ohno, S.: The presence of a common embryonic blastema for ovarian and testicular parenchymal (follicular, interstitial and tubular) cells in cattle, *Bos taurus*. Z. Zellforsch. **74**, 505—528 (1966).

Grouchy, J. de, Lauvergne, J. J., Ricordeau, G.: Etudes cytogénétiques chez 16 chèvres intersexuées. C. R. Acad. Sci. (Paris) **260**, 2932—2935 (1965).

— Moullec, J., Salmon, Ch., Josso, N., Frezal, J., Lamy, M.: Hermaphrodisme avec caryotype XX/XY. Etude génétique d'un cas. Ann. Génét. **7**, 25—30 (1964). [Also J. clin. Endocr. **25**, 114—126 (1965).]

Gustavsson, I.: Chromosome abnormality in cattle. Nature (Lond.) **211**, 865—866 (1966).

Hafez, E. S. E., Jainudeen, M. R.: Intersexuality in farm animals. Anim. Breed., Abstr. **34**, 1—15 (1966).

— Rajakoski, E.: Placental and fetal development during multiple bovine preg-nancy. Anatomical and physiological studies. Anat. Rec. **150**, 303—316 (1964).

— — Anderson, P. B., Frost, O. L., Smith, G.: Problems of gonadotropin-induced multiple pregnancy in beef cattle. Amer. J. vet. Res. **25**, 1074—1079 (1964).

Hansen, K. M.: Kønskromosomer hos en tyrekvie, p. 207—218. Ann. Report Roy. Vet. Agricult. Coll., Copenhagen (1967).

Hard, W. C., Eisen, J. D.: A phenotypic male swine with a female karyotype. J. Hered. **46**, 255—258 (1965).

Hare, W. C. D., Weber, W. T., McFeely, R. A., Yang, T. J.: Cytogenetics in the dog and cat. J. small Anim. Pract. **7**, 575—592 (1966).

Hart, M. v. d., Loghem, J. J. v.: Blood group chimerism. Vox Sang. **12**, 161—172 (1967).

Hartemann, J., Peters, A., Dellestable, P., Duprez, A., Touat, E.: Les trans-fusions foeto-foetales lors des grossesses biovulaires existentelles? Gynéc. et Obstét. **62**, 663—668 (1963).

Hathaway, Wm. E., Brangle, R. W., Nelson, T. L., Roeckel, I. E.: Aplastic anemia and alymphocytosis in an infant with hypogammaglobulinemia: Graft-versus-host reaction? J. Pediat. **68**, 713—722 (1966).

Henricson, B., Akesson, A.: Two heifers with gonadal dysgenesis and the sex chromosomal constitution XY. Acta vet. scand. **8**, 262—272 (1967).

HERSCHLER, M. S., FECHHEIMER, N. S.: Centric fusion of chromosomes in a set of bovine triplets. Cytogenetics 5, 307—312 (1966).

— — The role of sex chromosome chimerism in altering sexual development of mammals. Cytogenetics 6, 204—212 (1967).

— — GILMORE, L. O.: Identification of freemartins by chromosomal analysis. J. Dairy Sci. 49, 113—114 (1966).

HERZOG, A.: Chromosomenanomalien bei Haustieren. Gießener Beitr. Erbpath. Zuchthyg. 1, 7—17 (1969).

HILL, J. P.: Demonstration of the Embryologia Varia (development of *Hapale jacchus*). J. Anat. (Lond.) 60, 486—487 (1926).

— HILL, C. J.: An early blastocyst of *Hapale* (demonstration). C. R. Ass. Anat. (22nd reunion, London) p. 264 (1927).

HÖRMANN, G., LEMTIS, H.: Zur Frage der diaplazentaren Metastasierung maligner Blastome der Mutter. Z. Geburtsh. Gynäk. 164, 1—8 (1965a).

— — Abwehrleistungen der "Einheit Fetus und Plazenta" gegenüber hämatogen verschleppten Zellverbänden maligner Blastome der Mutter. Z. Geburtsh. Gynäk. 164, 129—142 (1965b).

HOFFMANN, R.: Chromosomenanomalie der Hodenzellen eines kryptorchiden Kalbes (60(XY)/62(XX)-Chimerismus). Berl. Münch. tierärztl. Wschr. 80, 390—391 (1967a).

— Methodik und Theorie der Chromosomenanalyse beim Haustier. Zugleich ein Beitrag zur Erklärung der Zwickenbildung. Vet.-Inaug.-Diss. Munich 1967b.

HOLLAND, E.: A case of transplacental metastasis of malignant melanoma from mother to foetus. J. Obstet. Gynaec. Brit. Emp. 56, 529—538 (1949).

HUGHES, W.: The freemartin condition in swine. Anat. Rec. 41, 213—245 (1929).

HUTCHINSON, D. L., MAXWELL, N. G., TURNER, J. H.: Advantages of maternal erythrocytes for fetal transfusion. Amer. J. Obstet. Gynec. 99, 702—708 (1967).

ILBERY, P. L. T., WILLIAMS, D.: Evidence of the freemartin condition in the goat. Cytogenetics 6, 276—285 (1967).

JAINUDEEN, M. R., HAFEZ, E. S. E.: Attempts to induce bovine freemartinism experimentally. J. Reprod. Fertil. 10, 281—283 (1965).

JOHANSSON, I., RENDEL, J.: Genetics and Animal Breeding. San Francisco: W. H. Freeman & Co. 1968.

JOHNSTON, E. F., ZELLER, J. H., CANTWELL, G.: Sex anomalies in swine. J. Hered. 49, 255—261 (1958).

JONES, H. W., FERGUSON-SMITH, M. A., HELLER, R. H.: Pathologic and cytogenetic findings in true hermaphroditism. Report of 6 cases and a review of 23 cases from the literature. Obstet. and Gynec. 25, 435—447 (1965).

JONES, T. C.: Anomalies of sex chromosomes in tortoiseshell male cats. In: Comparative mammalian cytogenetics (K. BENIRSCHKE, ed.). Berlin-Heidelberg-New York: Springer 1969.

JOST, A.: Le controle hormonal de la differenciation du sexe. Biol. Rev. 23, 201—236 (1948).

— Problems of fetal endocrinology, the gonadal and hypophyseal hormones. Recent Progr. Hormone Res. 8, 379—418 (1953).

— Steroids and sex differentiation of the mammalian foetus. Excerpta Medica, International Congress Ser. No 132, 74—81 (1966).

— CHODKIEWICZ, M., MAULÉON, P.: Intersexualité du foetus de veau produite par des androgènes. Comparaison entre l'hormone foetale responsable du freemartinisme et l'hormone testiculaire adulte. C. R. Acad. Sci. (Paris) 256, 274—276 (1963).

— PREPIN, J.: Données sur la migration des cellules germinales primordiales du foetus de veau. Arch. Anat. micr. Morph. exp. 55, 161—186 (1966).

56   K. Benirschke:

Kadowaki, J., Thompson, R. I., Zuelzer, W. W., Woolley, P. V., Brough, A. J.,
  Gruber, D.: XX/XY lymphoid chimaerism in congenital immunological deficiency
  syndrome with thymic alymphoplasia. Lancet 1965 II, 1152—1155.
Kanagawa, H., Basrur, P. K.: The leukocyte culture method in the diagnosis of
  freemartinism. Canad. J. comp. Med. 32, 583—586 (1968).
— Kawata, K., Ishikawa, T.: Chromosome studies on heterosexual twins in cattle.
  II. Significance of sex-chromosome chimerism (XX/XY) in early diagnosis of
  freemartin. Jap. J. vet. Res. 13, 43—49 (1965 b).
— — — Inoue, T.: Chromosome studies on heterosexual twins in cattle. IV. Long-
  term observations of sexchromosome chimera ratio in cultured leukocytes. Jap.
  J. vet. Res. 15, 31—36 (1967).
— Kawata, K., Ishikawa, T., Muramoto, J.: Chromosome studies on heterosexual
  twins in cattle. I. Sex chromosome chimerism (XX/XY). Jap. J. vet. Res. 13,
  33—41 (1965 a).
— — — Muramoto, J., Ohno, H.: Sexchromosome chimerism (XX/XY) in
  heterosexual bovine triplets. Jap. J. vet. Res. 13, 121—126 (1965 c).
Keller, K.: Zur Frage der sterilen Zwillingskälber. Wien. tierärztl. Mschr. 7,
  146—162 (1920).
— Über das Verhalten des Chorions bei der Zwillingsträchtigkeit des Pferdes. Wien.
  tierärztl. Mschr. 21, 453—456 (1934).
— Tandler, J.: Über das Verhalten der Eihäute bei der Zwillingsträchtigkeit des
  Rindes. Wien. tierärztl. Mschr. 3, 513—527 (1916).
Kerr, M. G., Rashad, M. N.: Autosomal trisomy in a discordant monozygotic
  twin. Nature (Lond.) 212, 726—727 (1966).
Kohn, G., Mayall, B. H., Miller, M. E., Mellman, W. J.: Tetraploiddiploid-
  mosaicism in a surviving infant. Pediat. Res. 1, 461—469 (1967).
Koontz, W. W., Young, R. B., Tucker, H. St. G., Prout, G. R.: True hermaph-
  roditism; a report of 3 cases. J. Urol. (Baltimore) 101, 102—105 (1969).
Kurnosov, K. M.: Interfetal placental connections of the elk in embryonic parabiosis. Proc. Akad. Nauk. SSR Doklady, Biol. Sect. 142, 92—94 (1962).
Lazear, E. J., Ferguson, L. C., Ely, F.: The frequency of in utero vascular anastomosis in bovine twins as determined by blood typing. J. Dairy Sci. 36, 597—598
  (1953).
Lejeune, J., Berger, R., Rethore, M.-O., Vialatte, J., Salmon, Ch.: Sur un
  cas d'hermaphrodisme XX/XY. Ann. Génét. 9, 171—173 (1966).
— Lafourcade, J., Schärer, K., deWolff, E., Salmon, Ch., Haines, M., Tur-
  pin, R.: Monozygotisme hétérocaryote, normal et jumeau trisomique 21. C. R.
  Acad. Sci. (Paris) 254, 4404—4406 (1962).
— Salmon, Ch., Berger, R., Rethore, M.-O., Rossier, A., Job, J. C.: Chimère
  46 XX/69 XXY. Ann. Génét. 10, 188—192 (1967).
— Turpin, R.: Détection chromosomique d'une mosaique artificelle humaine. C. R.
  Acad. Sci. (Paris) 252, 3148—3150 (1961).
Lillie, F. R.: The theory of the free-martin. Science 43, 611—613 (1916).
— The free martin; a study of the action of sex hormones in the foetal life of cattle.
  J. exp. Zool. 23, 371—452 (1917).
— Supplementary notes on twins in cattle. Biol. Bull. 44, 48—78 (1923).
Makino, S., Muramoto, J., Ishikawa, T.: Notes on XX/XY mosaicism in cells of
  various tissues of heterosexual twins of cattle. Proc. Jap. Acad. 41, 414—418
  (1965).
— Sasaki, M. M., Sofuni, T., Ishikawa, T.: Chromosome condition of an intersex
  swine. Proc. Jap. Acad. 38, 686—689 (1962).
Malouf, N., Benirschke, K., Hoefnagel, D.: XX/XY chimerism in a tricolored
  male cat. Cytogenetics 6, 228—241 (1967).

MANSELL, W. D.. CRINGAN, A. T.: A further instance of fetal atrophy in white-tailed deer. Canad. J. Zool. **46**, 33—34 (1968).

MANUEL, M. A., ALLIE, A., JACKSON, W. P. U.: A true hermaphrodite with XX/XY chromosome mosaicism. S. Afr. med. J. **39**, 411—414 (1965).

MARINE, N., JACKSON, W. P. U.: 3 hermaphrodites with XX/XY mosaicism. 3rd Int. Congr. Endocr. Excerpta Med. Found. Int. Congr. Series No **157**, 185—186 (1968).

MASSIMO, L., GEMME, G., VIANELLO, M. G., VERRI, B.: Studio di una coppia di gemelli dizigotici di cui uno mongoloide con trisomia 21, e l'altro normale con chimerismo transitorio di cellule con trisomia 21. Acta Genet. med. (Roma) **15**, 208—211 (1966).

MCDANIEL, E. C., NADEL, M., WOOLVERTON, W. C.: True hermaphrodite with bilaterally descended ovotestes. J. Urol. (Baltimore) **100**, 77—81 (1968).

MCFEE, A. F., KNIGHT, M., BANNER, M. W.: An intersex pig with XX/XY leuco-cyte mosaicism. Canad. J. Genet. Cytol. **8**, 502—505 (1966).

MCFEELY, R. A.: Chromosome abnormalities in early embryos of the pig. J. Reprod. Fertil. **13**, 579—581 (1967).

— Aneuploid, polyploidy and structural rearrangement of chromosomes in mammals other than man. In: Comparative mammalian cytogenetics. Berlin-Heidelberg-New York: Springer 1969.

— HARE, W. C. D., BIGGERS, J. D.: Chromosome studies in 14 cases of intersex in domestic mammals. Cytogenetics **6**, 242—253 (1967).

MCLAREN, A., MICHIE, D.: Experimental studies on placental fusion in mice. J. exp. Zool. **141**, 47—73 (1959).

MIKKELSEN, M. FRØLAND, A., ELLEBJERG, J.: XO/XY mosaicism in a pair of presumably monozygotic twins with different phenotypes. Cytogenetics **2**, 86—98 (1963).

MILLER, R. A.: Spermatogenesis in a sex-reversed female and in normal males of the domestic fowl, *Gallus domesticus*. Anat. Rec. **70**, 155—189 (1938).

MINTZ, B.: Embryological phases of mammalian gametogenesis. J. cell. comp. Physiol. **56** (Suppl. 1), 31—47 (1960).

— Experimental genetic mosaicism in the mouse. In: Preimplantation stages of pregnancy. Boston: Little, Brown & Co. 1965.

MOORE, K. L., GRAHAM, M. A., BARR, M. L.: The sex chromatin of the bovine freemartin. J. exp. Zool. **135**, 101—125 (1957).

MURAMOTO, J., ISHIKAWA, T., KANAGAWA, H.: XX/XY cell chimerism in hetero-sexual bovine twins. Nucleus **8**, 25—32 (1965).

MURTI, G. S., GILBERT, D. L., BORGMANN, A. R.: Canine intersex states. J. Amer. vet. med. Ass. **149**, 1183—1185 (1966).

MYHRE, A., MEYER, T., OPITZ, J. M., RACE, R. R., SANGER, R., GREENWALT, T. J.: Two populations of erythrocytes associated with XX/XY mosaicism. Trans-fusion **5**, 501—505 (1965).

MYSTKOWSKA, E. T., TARKOWSKI, A. K.: Observations on CBA-p/CBA-T$_6$T$_6$ mouse chimeras. J. Embryol. exp. Morph. **20**, 33—52 (1968).

NAYMAN, J., DATTA, S. P., DE BOER, W. G. R. M.: Renal transplantation in cattle twins. Nature (Lond.) **215**, 741—742 (1967).

NELSON-REES, W. A., KNIAZEFF, A. J., DARBY, N. B. Jr.: Debut and accumulation of centric fusion products: An index to age of certain cell lines. Cytogenetics **6**, 436—450 (1967).

NES, N.: Diploid-triploid chimerism in a true hermaphrodite mink (*Mustela vison*). Hereditas (Lund) **56**, 159—170 (1966).

NICHOLAS, J. W., JENKINS, W. J., MARSH, W. L.: Human blood chimeras: A study of surviving twins. Brit. med. J. **1957** I, 1458—1460.

NIELSEN, J.: Inheritance in monozygotic twins. Lancet **1967** II, 717—718.

Oehme, J.: Das Schicksal der transplacentar übergetretenen mütterlichen Lympho-cyten im Organismus des Kindes. Mschr. Kinderheilk. 115, 148—150 (1967).

Ohno, S., Gropp, A.: Embryological basis for germ cell chimerism in mammals. Cytogenetics 4, 251—261 (1965).

— Trujillo, J. M., Stenius, C., Christian, L. C., Teplitz, R. L.: Possible germ cell chimeras among newborn dizygotic twin calves (Bos taurus). Cytogenetics 1, 258—265 (1962).

Omura, Y., Kato, B.: Freemartins as quintuplets calved by a dairy cow [in Japanese]. J. Jap. vet. med. Ass. 19, 12—14 (1966). Quoted by Basrur and Stoltz (1966).

Osborne, V. E.: An analysis of the pattern of ovulation as it occurs in the annual reproductive cycle of the mare in Australia. Aust. vet. J. 42, 149—154 (1966).

Owen, R. D.: Immunogenetic consequences of vascular anastomoses between bovine twins. Science 102, 400—401 (1945).

— Erythrocyte mosaics among bovine twins and quadruplets. Genetics 31, 227 (1946).

— Davis, H. P., Morgan, R. F.: Quintuplet calves and erythrocyte mosaicism. J. Hered. 37, 291—297 (1946).

Padeh, B., Wysoki, M., Ayalon, N., Soller, M.: An XX/XY hermaphrodite in the goat. Israel J. med. Sci. 1, 1008—1012 (1965).

Porter, R. P.: Chimerism and immunologic tolerance: A consequence of fraternal twinning in the marmoset. Dissertation Abstract 29, 601 (No. 479B) (1968).

— Gengozian, N.: Immunologic tolerance of grafted skin exchanged between marmoset dizygotic co-twins. Fed. Proc. 27, 505 (1968).

Price, D.: A historical review of embryology and intersexuality. Fact and fancy. Leiden: E. J. Brill 1967.

Rapacz, J., Shackelford, R. M.: Erythrocyte antigen mosaicism in domestic mink. J. Hered. 57, 19—22 (1966).

Rashad, M. N., Kerr, M. G.: Observations on the so-called holoacardius amorphus. J. Anat. (Lond.) 100, 425—426 (1966).

Rendel, J., Gahne, B., Maijala, K.: A set of five-egg cattle quintuplets with complicated chimerism. Hereditas (Lund.) 48, 201—214 (1962).

Renzoni, A.: Blood cell chimerism in a calf (Bos taurus). Mamm. Chromosomes Newsletter 8, 225—226 (1967).

Roberts, S. J.: The enigma of fetal mummification. J. Amer. vet. med. Ass. 140, 691—698 (1962).

Romer, A. S.: Vertebrate Paleontology, 3rd ed. Chicago: University of Chicago Press 1966.

Rotermund, H.: Über Zwillingsfruchtsäcke kleiner Wiederkäuer. Gegenbaurs morph. Jb. 64, 178—222 (1930).

Russell, A., Moschos, A., Butler, L. J., Abraham, J. M.: Gonadal dysgenesis and its unilateral variant with testis in monozygous twins: related to discordance in sex chromosomal status. J. clin. Endocr. 26, 1282—1292 (1966). [Editorial Comment: Obstet. gynec. Surv. 22, 631 (1967).]

Russell, L. B., Woodiel, F. N.: A spontaneous mouse chimera formed from separate fertilization of two meiotic products of oogenesis. Cytogenetics 5, 106—119 (1966).

Ryan, K. J., Benirschke, K., Smith, O. W.: Conversion of androstenedione-4-C^{14} to estrone by the marmoset placenta. Endocrinology 69, 613—618 (1961).

Sarto, G. E., Opitz, J. M., Inhorn, S. L.: Considerations of sex chromosome ab-normalities in man. In: Comparative mammalian cytogenetics (K. Benirschke, ed.), Berlin-Heidelberg-New York: Springer 1969.

Schatz, F.: Die Acardii und ihre Verwandten. Berlin: Hirschwald 1898.

Schlegel, R. J., Neu, R. L., Leao, J. C., Farias, E., Aspillaga, M. J., Gardner, L. I.: Observations on the chromosomal, cytological and anatomical characteristics of 75 human conceptuses. Including euploid, triploid XXX, triploid XYY and mosaic triploid XXY/diploid XY cases. Cytogenetics 5, 430—446 (1966).

SCHMID, W., VISCHER, D.: A malformed boy with double aneuploidy and diploid-triploid mosaicism 48, XXYY/71, XXXYY. Cytogenetics 6, 145—155 (1967).

SCHMINCKE, A.: Vergleichende Untersuchungen über die Anlage des Skelettsystems in tierischen Mißbildungen mit einem Beitrag zur makro- und mikroskopischen Anatomie derselben. (Hemiacardius acephalus von Schwein, Holoacardius amorphus vom Rind). Virchows Arch. path. Anat. 230, 564—607 (1921).

SCHWALBE, E.: Die Morphologie der Mißbildungen des Menschen und der Tiere. II. Die Doppelbildungen, S. 111—113. Jena: Gustav Fischer 1907.

SHINE, I. B., CORNEY, G.: Turner's syndrome in monozygotic twins. J. med. Genet. 3, 124—128 (1966).

SHORT, R. V., HAMERTON, J. L., GRIEVES, S. A., POLLARD, C. E.: An intersex goat with a bilaterally asymmetrical reproductive tract. J. Reprod. Fertil. 16, 283—291 (1968).

SILVERSTEIN, A. M.: Ontogenesis of the immune response. In: Comparative aspects of reproduction. Berlin-Heidelberg-New York: Springer 1967.

SIMONDS, J. P., GOWEN, G. A.: Fetus amorphus. Surg. Gynec. Obstet. 41, 171—179 (1925).

SINGH, R. P., MEYER, D. B.: Primordial germ cells in blood smears from chick embryos. Science 156, 1503—1504 (1967).

SLEE, J.: Immunological tolerance between litter-mates in sheep. Nature (Lond.) 200, 654—656 (1963).

SOLLER, M., PADEH, B., WYSOKI, M., AYALON, N.: Cytogenetics of Saanen goats showing abnormal development of the reproductive tract associated with the dominant gene for polledness. Cytogenetics 8, 51—67 (1969).

STERN, C.: Genetic mosaics and other essays. Cambridge: Harvard University Press 1968.

STEWART, J. S. S.: Chimerism and genetic mapping. Genet. Res. 12, 91—93 (1968).

STONE, W. H., FRIEDMAN, J., FREGIN, A.: Possible somatic cell mating in twin cattle with erythrocyte mosaicism. Proc. nat. Acad. Sci. (Wash.) 51, 1036—1044 (1964).

— CRAGLE, R. G., BENDEL, S., CAULTON, J.: A possible second case of somatic cell mating in twin cattle with erythrocyte chimerism. Genetics 60, 73—79 (1968).

— — SWANSON, E. W., BROWN, D. G.: Skin grafts: delayed rejection between pairs of cattle twins showing erythrocyte chimerism. Science 148, 1335—1336 (1965).

STORMONT, C.: Erythrocyte mosaicism in a heifer recorded as singleborn. J. Anim. Sci. 13, 94—98 (1954).

— MORRIS, B. G., SUZUKI, Y.: Mosaic hemoglobin types in a pair of cattle twins. Science 145, 600—601 (1964).

— WEIR, W. C., LANE, L. L.: Erythrocyte mosaicism in a pair of sheep twins. Science 118, 695—696 (1953).

STRUCK, H., KARG, H., JORK, H.: Thin-layer chromatographic determination of testosterone and Δ^4-androstene-3,17-dione from bovine foetal testicular tissue. J. Chromat. 36, 74—83 (1968).

STURGEON, P., McQUISTON, D. T., SPARKES, R., SOLOMON, J., BARNETT, E. V.: Atypical immunological tolerance in a human blood group chimera. Blood 33, 507—526 (1969).

TANDLER, J., KELLER, K.: Über das Verhalten des Chorions bei verschiedengeschlechtlicher Zwillingsgravidität des Rindes und über die Morphologie des Genitales der weiblichen Tiere, welche einer solchen Gravidität entstammen. Dtsch. tierärztl. Wschr. 10, 148—149 (1911).

TARKOWSKI, A. K.: Mouse chimeras developed from fused eggs. Nature (Lond.) 190, 857—860 (1961).

TARKOWSKI, A. K.: True hermaphroditism in chimaeric mice. J. Embryol. exp. Morph. **12**, 735—757 (1964).

— Embryonic and postnatal development of mouse chimeras. In: Preimplantation Stages of Pregnancy. Boston: Little, Brown & Co. 1965.

TAYLOR, A. I.: Cell selection *in vivo* in normal/G trisomic mosaics. Nature (Lond.) **219**, 1028—1030 (1968).

TEPLITZ, R. L., MOON, Y. S., BASRUR, P. K.: Further studies of chimerism in heterosexual cattle twins. Chromosoma (Berl.) **22**, 202—209 (1967).

THIEDE, H. A., SALM, S. B.: Chromosome studies on human spontaneous abortions. Amer. J. Obstet. Gynec. **90**, 205—215 (1969).

THULINE, H. C.: Male tortoiseshells, chimerism, and true hermaphroditism. J. Cat Genet. **4**, 2—3 (1964).

— NORBY, D. E.: Spontaneous occurrence of chromosome abnormality in cats. Science **134**, 554—555 (1961).

TREADWELL, M., CARTWRIGHT, T. C.: Sex chromosome replication patterns in bovine chimeras. J. Anim. Sci. **27**, 1127 (1968).

TURNER, C. D.: Experimental reversal of germ cells. Embryologia (Nagoya) **10**, 206—230 (1969).

— ASAKAWA, H.: Experimental reversal of germ cells in ovaries of fetal mice. Science **143**, 1344—1345 (1964).

TURNER, J. H., LI, C. C., WALD, N., BORGES, W.: Preliminary reports on a continuing study of chromosome patterns in a general neonatal population. In: Research methodology and needs in perinatal studies. Springfield: Ch. C. Thomas 1966.

TURPIN, R.: Gémellités monozygotes et aberrations chromosomiques (monozygotisme hétérocaryote). In: De l'Embryologie Expérimentale à la Biologie Moléculaire (E. WOLFF, ed.), p. 97—114. Paris: Dunod 1967.

— BOCQUET, L., GRASSET, J.: Etude d'un couple monozygote: Fille normale — monstre acardique féminin. Considérations anatomopathologiques et cytogénétiques. Ann. Génét. **10**, 107—113 (1967).

— LEJEUNE, J., LAFOURCADE, J., CHIGOT, P. L., SALMON, CH.: Présomption de monozygotisme en dépit d'un dimorphisme sexuel: sujet masculin XY et sujet neutre haplo X. C. R. Acad. Sci. (Paris) **252**, 2945—2946 (1961).

— SALMON, C., CRUVEILLER, J.: A propos des chimères humaines. Présence temporaire d'une double population d'hématies chez l'un des jumeaux d'un couple dizygote. Rev. franc. Étud. clin. biol. **4**, 809—811 (1959).

UCHIDA, I. A., WANG, H. C., RAY, M.: Dizygotic twins with XX/XY chimerism. Nature (Lond.) **204**, 191 (1964).

UENO, S., ZUZUKI, K., YAMAZAWA, K.: Human chimerism in one of a pair of twins. Acta genet. (Basel) **9**, 47—53 (1959).

VELEZ-OROZCO, A. C.: Estudio de una quimera. Bol. Inst. Estud. méd. biol. (Méx.) **19**, 41—50 (1961).

VERSCHUER, O. v.: Die vererbungsbiologische Zwillingsforschung. Ergebn. inn. Med. Kinderheilk. **31**, 35 (1927).

VIROLAINEN, M.: Hematopoietic origin of macrophages as studied by chromosome markers in mice. J. exp. Med. **127**, 943—952 (1968).

VOGT, D. W.: Sex chromosome mosaicism in a swine intersex. J. Hered. **59**, 166—167 (1968).

WEISS, E., HOFFMANN, R.: Eliminierung der XX-Zellen im Hoden heterosexueller Rinderzwillinge mit XX/XY-Chimerismus. Cytogenetics **8**, 68—73 (1969).

WIENER, A. S., MOOR-JANKOWSKI, J., GORDON, E. B.: Marmosets as laboratory animals. V. Blood groups of marmosets. Lab. Anim. Care **17**, 71—75 (1967).

WILLIAMS, G., GORDON, I., EDWARDS, J.: Observations on the frequency of fused foetal circulations in twin-bearing cattle. Brit. vet. J. **119**, 467—472 (1963).

Winkler, H.: Über Propfbastarde und pflanzliche Chimaeren. Ber. dtsch. bot. Ges. **25**, 568—576 (1907).

Wislocki, G. B.: Placentation in the marmoset (*Oedipomidas geoffroyi*) with remarks on twinning in monkeys. Anat. Rec. **52**, 381—400 (1932).

— Observations on twinning in marmosets. Amer. J. Anat. **64**, 445—483 (1939).

Witschi, E.: Migration of the germ cells of human embryos from the yolk sac to the primitive gonadal folds. Contr. Embryol. Carneg. Instn **32**, 67—80 (1948).

— Hormones and embryonic induction. Arch. Anat. micr. Morph. exp. **54**, 601—611 (1965).

Wolff, E. de, Schärer, K., Lejeune, J.: Contribution à l'étude des jumeaux mongoliens. Un cas de monozygotisme hétérocaryote. Helv. paediat. Acta **17**, 301—328 (1962).

Woodruff, M. F. A., Fox, M., Buckton, K. A., Jacobs, P. A.: The recognition of human blood chimaeras. Lancet **1962** I, 192—194.

— Lennox, B.: Reciprocal skin grafts in a pair of twins showing blood chimaerism. Lancet **1959** II, 476—478.

Wurster, D. H., Benirschke, K.: Chromosome studies in some deer, the springbok, and the pronghorn, with notes on placentation in deer. Cytologia (Tokyo) **32**, 273—285 (1967).

Yurchenko, V. T.: Cases of freemartinism in Karakul ewes as a consequence of vascular parabiosis in heterosexual twins. Dokl. Akad. Nauk SSSR, Biol. Sci. **146**, 254—256 (1962).

Zietzschmann, O.: Über einfache und Zwillingsfruchtsäcke der Wiederkäuer. Zugleich ein Beitrag zur Frage der eineiigen Zwillinge. Z. mikr.-anat. Forsch. **27**, 243—268 (1931).

Zuelzer, W. W., Beattie, K. M., Reisman, L. E.: Generalized unbalanced mosaicism attributable to dispermy and probable fertilization of a polar body. Amer. J. hum. Genet. **16**, 38—51 (1964). [Also Transfusion **4**, 77—86 (1964).]

Department of Pathology, College of Medicine, State University of New York, Downstate Medical Center, Brooklyn, New York 11203 and The Department of Biostatistics, Montefiore Hospital, Bronx, New York 10467. U.S.A.

Quantitative Autoradiography: Statistical Study of the Variance, Error and Sensitivity of the Labeling Index (Thymidine-H3 and DNA Synthesis)*

Patrick J. Fitzgerald, M. D., and Bernard Carol, M. S., M. A.

With 7 Figures

Table of Contents

* Aided by Research Grant AM 05556 from the National Institute of Health, U.S. Public Health Service.

Introduction

The introduction of tritium as a radioactive marker for intracellular auto-radiographic localization of labeled precursors from the laboratory of one of us (FITZGERALD et al., 1951) has been followed by its extensive use in many cellular metabolic studies (MAUER, 1965; SCHULTZE et al., 1965). This has been particularly so in the study of deoxyribonucleic acid (DNA) metabolism after the introduction of tritium labeled thymidine (TAYLOR et al., 1957; VERLEY et al., 1957) and the concept of the DNA synthetic (S) period (HOWARD and PELC, 1953).

As have many other investigators we have made extensive use of the percent of radioactively labeled cell nuclei in autoradiograms after the injection of thymidine-H[3] (the labeling index) as an indicator of DNA synthesis (LEBLOND and WALKER, 1956) (BASERGA, 1968). In our studies of the rat pancreas acinar cell only a small percent of the nuclei was labeled and the distribution of the radioactively labeled nuclei was not uniform (FITZGERALD, 1960, 1963) (FITZGERALD and VINIJCHAIKUL, 1959) (FITZGERALD et al., 1963a, 1963b, 1968a). We found that different persons counting the same autoradiogram obtained different labeling indices. These observations led us to examine our sampling and counting techniques (FITZGERALD et al., 1968b) (CAROL and FITZGERALD, 1968).

Our report consists of 3 sections: (1) a description and discussion of a microscopic field selection technique to insure some randomness in selecting the microscopic field in the autoradiogram to be counted; (2) possible additional applications of the field selection technique in cytometry; and (3) an analysis of variance of factors involved in the determination of the labeling index (3 A) and estimations of the error and sensitivity of the labeling index as used in pancreas experiments (3 B).

1. The Random Field Selection Technique

One important aspect of the counting procedure is the selection of the microscopic field. So-called random sampling as described by most authors, obviously, is not a true random sampling. The closest approach to true randomization is some method similar to the Chalkley (1943) or the Weibel (1963a, 1963b) techniques. Even with the former, systematic error conceivably could occur with eccentric wear of the microscopic ocular so that a constant bias towards a part of the field to be examined would occur. There also persists with the Chalkley method the problem of selecting the microscopic fields. With the techniques described by Weibel reliance upon fields selected completely at random may give rise to a fortuitous cluster of skewed values, not a sample of average fields, especially if the sample number is limited. The limited, crenalated up-over-down-over-up method employed by many authors for microscopic field selection may be adequate for some studies with a high labeling index but it may also be inadequate for low indices with focal variation. Another precaution is worth mentioning; if a counter views the autoradiogram while selecting the field to be counted, he may, unconsciously, tend to focus on fields with a greater number of labeled nuclei.

Using the vernier markings of an ordinary graduated mechanical stage of a light microscope and a series of random numbers we developed a method of selecting a sample of widely and randomly distributed microscopic fields in autoradiograms which we found, empirically, reduced considerably the range of values obtained by the crenalated method (Fitzgerald and Vinijchaikul, 1959).

The autoradiogram, positioned in a mechanical stage, is moved while being viewed at low magnification so that the outermost lateral boundary of the tissue of the autoradiogram is brought into the center of the microscopic field and the vernier number of the movement of the mechanical stage is recorded (Fig. 1). The opposite lateral boundary of the tissue is similarly placed in the field of the microscope and its vernier number is recorded. The vernier numbers setting the superior and inferior boundaries of the tissue are determined and recorded. A rectangle is drawn on a score sheet and the margins are numbered with the vernier numbers delineating the lateral, superior and inferior tissue boundaries, i.e., the lateral border numbers form the horizontal margins and the vernier numbers indicating superior and inferior tissue borders are the vertical margins (Fig. 2). (The inversion of the image is ignored.)

Consecutive whole numbers that fall within the vernier numbers marking the margins of the horizontal sides of the rectangle are written on the sides. Similarly, consecutive whole numbers that fall between the vernier numbers marking the superior and inferior tissue boundaries are written on both vertical margins. A decimal point is placed to the right of each number (Fig. 2).

From a table of random numbers a sequence of random numbers is drawn and these are added successively to the right of the decimal point of each whole number of the score sheet along *one* horizontal and *one* vertical side

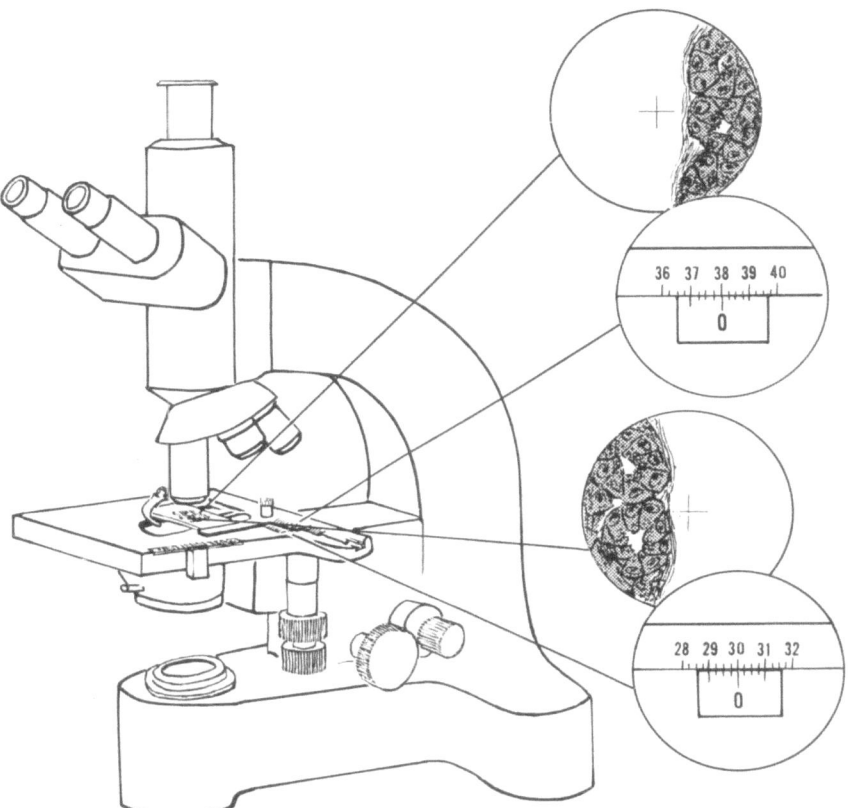

Fig. 1. The determination of tissue boundaries of the pancreas tissue in the autoradiogram. Autoradiogram is moved into the field of the microscope by the movement of the mechanical stage so that the outer-most lateral boundary is near the center of the microscopic field. The vernier number of the lateral movement of the mechanical stage is noted and recorded (e.g. 38). The opposite lateral boundary of the tissue is similarly determined by moving the autoradiogram to the center of the field and then noting the vernier number of this margin (e.g. 30). Superior and inferior tissue boundaries would be determined by moving the autoradiogram by the forward-backward movement of the mechanical stage (giving 12 and 6, respectively)

of the rectangle. The same random numbers are added to the right of the decimal point of the corresponding whole vernier numbers of the opposite margin. The vernier whole number and the random number make up a combination number (Fig. 2).

Lines are drawn on the score sheet connecting each combination number of a margin to the corresponding combination number of the opposite margin. A grid of points is thereby set up where the lines cross to indicate the microscopic fields to be selected and examined. To select the microscopic field in the autoradiogram the counter, without looking through the microscope, moves the autoradiograms by the mechanical stage to the selected field through the use of the combination vernier and random number coordinates of the grid

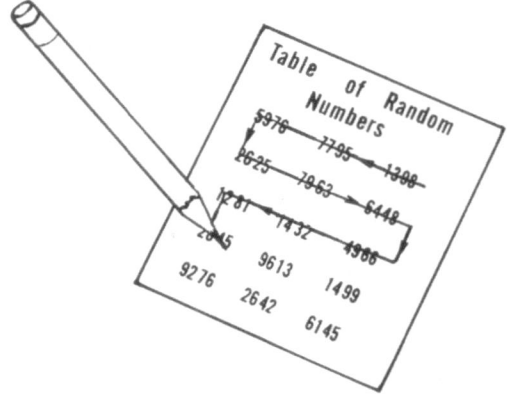

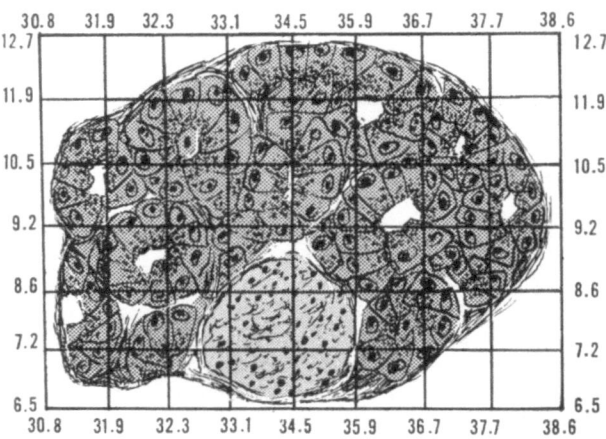

Fig. 2. Construction of a rectangle on a score sheet using as margins the mechanical stage vernier numbers which marked the tissue boundaries, i.e., 30 and 38 for the lateral margins (forming the horizontal sides of the rectangle) and 12 and 6, for the superior and inferior margins, respectively (to give the vertical sides). Tissue outlines are drawn on the score sheet for orientation; the small circular zone at the bottom represents an islet of Langerhans. The whole vernier numbers between the lateral margin vernier numbers 38 and 30 are written on the horizontal sides of the rectangle and the whole vernier numbers between 12 and 6, the superior and inferior margin vernier numbers, are written on the vertical sides of the rectangle. A decimal point is added to the right of each number. A sequence of numbers is taken from a table of random numbers and they are added consecutively to the whole vernier numbers of *one* of the lateral and to *one* of the superior-inferior sides of the rectangle. The same random numbers are added to the corresponding whole numbers of the opposite margin. A whole vernier number and a random number make up a combination number. All combination numbers of each margin are connected by straight lines to the corresponding combination number of the opposite margin. The intersections of these lines give a grid of points which indicate the microscopic fields to be examined. The specimen is positioned at a grid point by means of the vertical and horizontal combination numbers and the mechanical stage

point. He then systematically moves from field to field, examining all microscopic fields corresponding to the grid points. *For statistical purposes all fields must be examined and all specimens present in these fields counted.*

The counting of the number of labeled and unlabeled acinar nuclei in the microscopic field is done at about 1,000—1,250 times magnification with the oil immersion objective. The counter may recount the autoradiogram by using the same whole numbers of the rectangle but substituting a new random number to the right of the decimal point of each whole number of one horizontal and one vertical side of the rectangle. The new random number is used with the corresponding vernier number of the opposite margin. A "counting with replacement" technique is used so that occasionally a whole number might receive the same random number in the second count as in the first one.

The number of labeled nuclei counted is recorded as a numerator and the total number of nuclei, labeled and unlabeled, counted is written as the denominator for each field counted and the fraction is written at its corresponding grid point in the rectangle of the score sheet.

Discussion

If a labeled cell type were uniformly distributed, or if the labeled cells made up a high percentage of the cells present in a specimen there would be little need for a field selection technique. In our autoradiograms only a relatively small percent of the cell nuclei was labeled, the labeled nuclei were focally distributed and in some autoradiograms of experimental tissues the labeled cells made up only a very small fraction of the total cell population. In the normal adult rat pancreas the labeling index of acinar cell nuclei is only 0.5 % (FITZGERALD et al., 1968a). Under such circumstances fields selected by non-randomizing methods might be misleading, particularly if a small number of cells were examined. This might also be true even if the samples were selected at random. The wider the sampling the more representative should the results be. Our field selection technique has the merit of sampling throughout the whole autoradiogram.

The whole number divisions of the vernier of the mechanical stage alone might be used as coordinates for grid points since one would not ordinarily expect there to be a systematic relationship between the vernier markings of a mechanical stage and a cellular or extracellular distribution of substances in tissue. It is conceivable that an oriented structure, e.g. parallel muscle fibers, might have some phasic relationship with the vernier markings. The re-positioning of the specimen at a different angle to the mechanical stage by the cytologist might decrease or nullify such an obvious relationship (ERÄNKÖ, 1955). However, the addition of a random number to the vernier number reduces the possibility of such an occurrence, or one less obvious to the cytologist.

WEIBEL used similar principles to obtain random samples of gross specimens of lung (WEIBEL, 1963a, 1963b) and suggested using the integer settings of the mechanical stage vernier to select microscopic fields for study. He mentioned that random numbering could be used in selecting the microscopic field, but stated that "... this proved too cumbersome to be justified at this stage" (WEIBEL, 1963b). Empirically, we had found that with our field selection technique the spread of values was less and the average labeling index was lower (FITZGERALD, 1963) than when other methods were used (FITZGERALD and VINIJCHAIKUL, 1959). With our pathologic material of focal concentrations of regenerating cells we prefer to take the small number of samples dictated by logistical considerations from widely spread points rather than relying on the same number of samples taken completely at random. In this way we may avoid the bias of a possible clustering of foci of extremes of labeling.

Continued experience with the method has confirmed its convenience and its reduction of labeling index variation (FITZGERALD et al., 1968a).

The use of a score sheet with the fraction of the number of labeled nuclei over the total number of nuclei counted placed in the position of the corresponding microscopic field often made more apparent relationships between labeling and cytologic or cytopathologic features.

With the conventional use of oil immersion viewing and an ocular lens with a narrow field, the movement of the mechanical stage by a whole number division of the stage vernier covers about 10 microscopic fields. Because of some inaccuracy in positioning tenth divisions between vernier numbers the possibility exist of an occasional overlap of microscopic fields. Bias should not occur if the error is random in test and control measurements. Small magnifying lenses built into the stationary indicators of the mechanical stage could permit greater accuracy and precision in the positioning of the autoradiogram.

The principle of random sampling is equally pertinent to the original selection of tissue for autoradiographic examination unless uniformity of the process has been demonstrated. WEIBEL's method for the selection of tissue blocks (WEIBEL, 1963a, 1963b) should reduce error unless there were few samples and large focal variations. In normal rats we have taken samples of normal tissue from the splenic, gastric, duodenal and parabiliary segments (RICHARDS et al., 1964) of the pancreas and found no significant differences between the average labeling indices of the segments when multiple tissue specimens in each segment were counted. However, there often were large differences from microscopic field to microscopic field within the same autoradiogram and some differences between autoradiograms of different tissues taken from the same segment. In pathologic lesions of the pancreas even more variation was encountered (FITZGERALD et al., 1968a).

The cytologist could be aided in his work by recent scientific advances. With a computer it is possible to generate triples of random numbers falling within the prescribed boundaries of the tissue. Automatic positioning of the cytological specimen at the selected grid points is possible. The vernier numbers defining the tissue boundaries could be set either by the cytologist or by a scanning device. The mechanical stage with the slide holding the autoradiogram would be positioned by a driving mechanism controlled by the computer program containing the random numbers. The driving mechanism would give finer precision in the positioning the autoradiogram at grid points than with manual movements.

The principles of the field selection technique suggested here might be applied to some problems in cytology where light, ultraviolet, fluorescent, interference or electron microscopy is used with a graduated device for the positioning of the specimen.

2. Relative Areas of Distinctive Tissue Zones

In a study of acinar cell labeling of the pancreas after experimental procedures the results of the counting of one autoradiogram by multiple counters were varied (Table 1). In the autoradiogram there was a separate lobule of pancreas with acinar atrophy and cellular degeneration adjacent to lobules of normal pancreas (Fig. 3). In the abnormal lobule there was a much higher percent of radioactively labeled nuclei (Fig. 4A) than in the lobules of normal tissue (Fig. 4B).

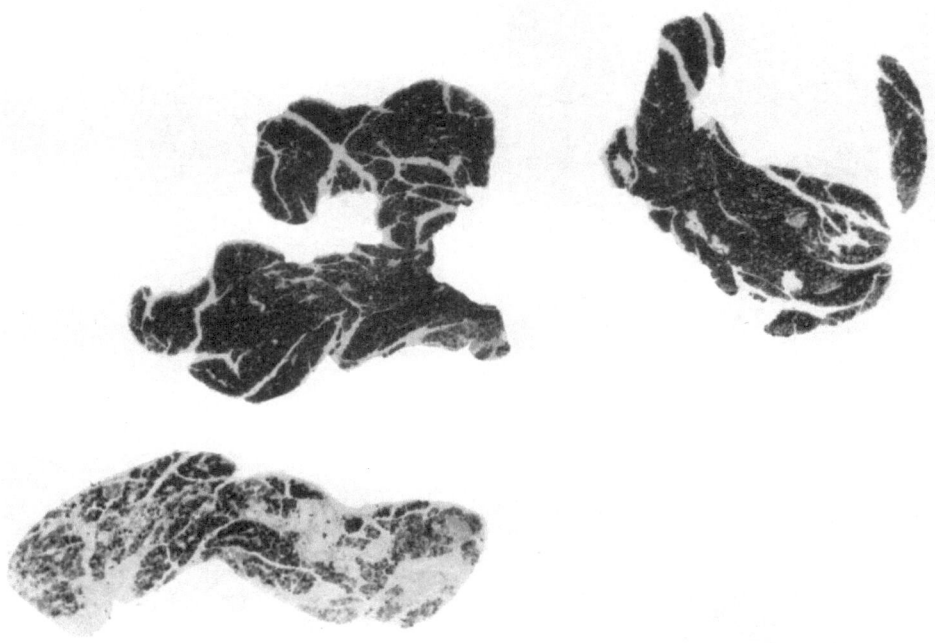

Fig. 3. Low magnification of an autoradiogram of rat pancreas. Animal had the major duct of the splenic pancreas segment ligated 7 days prior to sacrifice. Tissue section taken from splenic segment shows mixture of normal and abnormal lobules. Two lobules of normal tissue present in center and right. Lobule at lower left shows ischemic degenerative changes, indicated by lighter staining than adjacent normal lobules, atrophy and disappearance of many acini. Hematoxylin and eosin staining. × 20

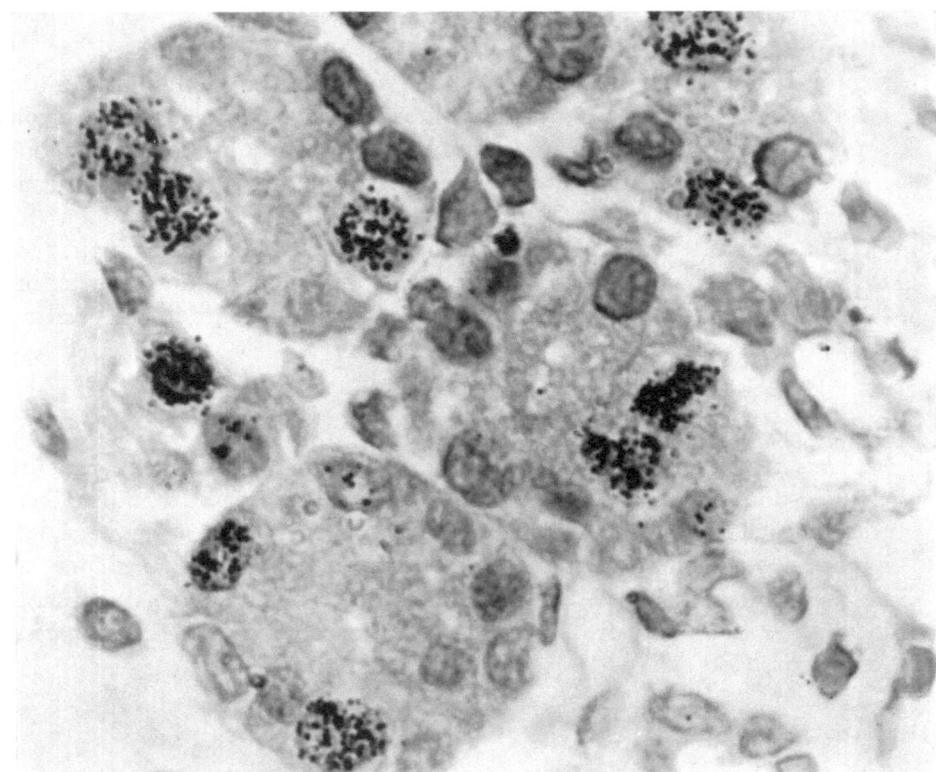

Fig. 4 A

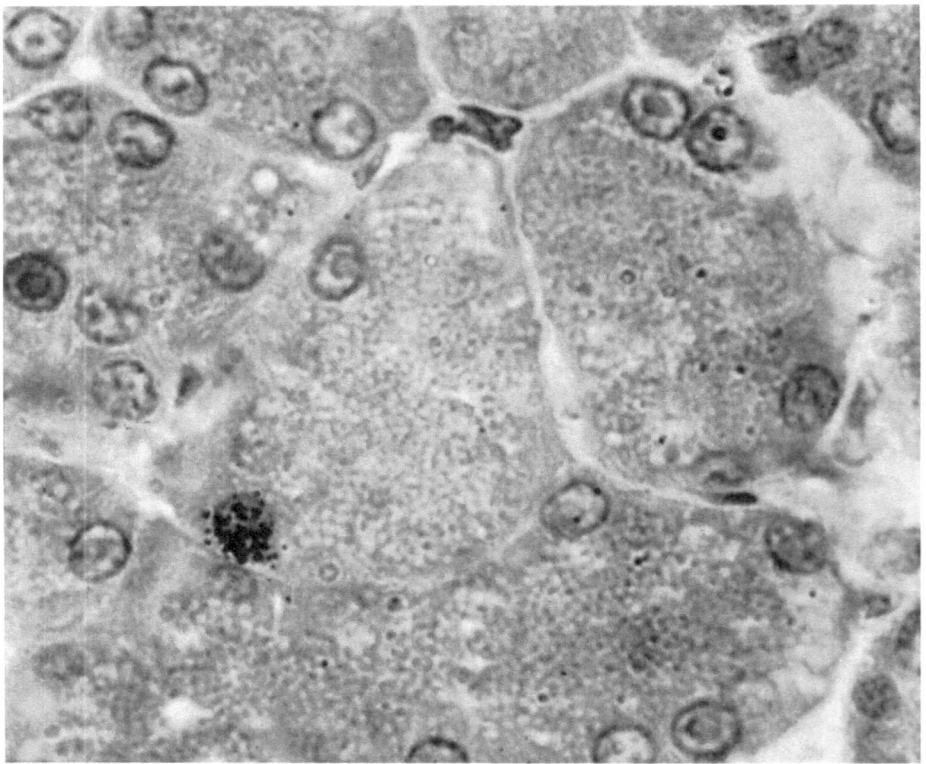

Fig. 4 B

It occurred to us that under appropriate circumstances where there are two distinctive zones of tissue with a large difference between their labeling indices, it would be possible to calculate the relative percent of total tissue area occupied by each zone. For if the labeling index of the degenerative tissue and that of the normal pancreas were representative of their respective zones then the labeling index of the whole pancreas tissue, comprising both the normal and the degenerate zones, would be the sum of the products of the labeling index of each zone multiplied by the percent of total area occupied by the zone. Conversely, if accurate labeling indices of the 3 zones (normal, degenerate and the labeling index of the total pancreas tissue) were known, one might calculate the relative percents of the whole pancreas tissue occupied by the normal and degenerative zones. This would not be true if the labeling indices were equal, in cases in which extremely marked differences in the relative sizes of the zones occurred, or where the concentration of nuclei in the different zones differed greatly.

Methods and Materials

In the animal (No. 164) from which the tissue for the autoradiogram was taken there was operative ligation of a duct leading to the splenic segment of the pancreas 7 days prior to sacrifice. The tissue for the autoradiogram was taken from the involved splenic segment of pancreas (Figs. 3 and 4).

Medical students were employed to count labeled nuclei in autoradiograms after a period of training (see below). In a study of the variance of the labeling index technique (FITZGERALD et al., 1968b) each of five counters had originally determined the labeling index of the acinar cell nuclei in the whole pancreas tissue of the autoradiogram by the field selection technique. They therefore sampled widely in both normal and degenerated zones. Later, the counters were then shown the isolated tissue zone of degenerate pancreas and the adjacent zone of normal pancreas. The two tissue were readily distinguishable (Fig. 3). The counters were told to determine the labeling index of the normal and degeneration zones separately.

A test of significance (SCHEFFÉ. 1959) was used to determine whether there were mean differences between the labeling indices of the zones. Whether counter variability was greater than zero, or not, was also tested. A similar test was made on the interaction between counter and area. The design was a 2 way, mixed one with zone as a fixed factor and counter as a random factor. Zone had two levels and counter had five levels.

Fig. 4A and B. Microscopic fields of autoradiograms of Fig. 3 at higher magnification. Thymidine-H^3 given 1 hour prior to sacrifice. Hematoxylin and eosin staining. A. Zone of atrophy and degeneration. Acini and acinar cells smaller than normal (compare with B). Labeling of many acinar cell nuclei with H^3. × 1040. B. Acinar tissue in lobule of normal pancreas. Normal cytologic structure. One acinar cell nucleus shows evidence of radioactivity. In the normal pancreas usually only one nucleus out of 200 is labeled (0.5% labeling index) under the circumstances of the experiment. × 1040

As a basis for estimating the validity of our method of calculating relative area we measured the relative areas of the normal and degenerative zones by conventional methods. The pancreas tissue in the autoradiogram was photographed at low magnification and enlarged photographs of the tissue were made (Fig. 3). By use of a planimeter the areas of the degenerate, normal and whole tissue zones were determined, independently, twice by each of two observers and averaged. The percent of total tissue area occupied by the different zones was calculated and the results of the two observers were averaged. From photographic enlargements of the whole pancreas tissue the degenerate and normal zones were cut out and each zone weighed to tenths of a milligram twice, independently, by the two observers. Each person expressed the weight of the zones as an average percent of the combined weight of all of the zones and the results of both observers were averaged.

Results

The average labeling index of the 5 original counts of the whole pancreas tissue was 4.3 % (Table 1). The average labeling index of the normal tissue was

Table 1. *Data of labeling indices of different zones and analysis of variances on the data*
Counting data of different zones of pancreas (No. 164b)

Counter	Whole pancreas	Normal pancreas	Degenerating pancreas
A	$\dfrac{62}{1,027} = 5.8\%$ [a]	$\dfrac{2}{1,015} = 0.2\%$	$\dfrac{184}{1,101} = 16.7\%$
B	$\dfrac{50}{1,027} = 4.9\%$	$\dfrac{4}{1,038} = 0.4\%$	$\dfrac{149}{960} = 15.5\%$
C	$\dfrac{34}{957} = 3.6\%$	$\dfrac{10}{1,369} = 0.7\%$	$\dfrac{145}{920} = 15.8\%$
D	$\dfrac{53}{1,032} = 5.2\%$	$\dfrac{12}{1,045} = 1.2\%$	$\dfrac{92}{1,280} = 7.2\%$
E	$\dfrac{27}{1,356} = 2.0\%$	$\dfrac{8}{1,263} = 0.6\%$	$\dfrac{81}{1,042} = 7.8\%$
	Average = 4.3%	Average = 0.6%	Average = 12.6%

Analysis of variance (mixed model): counter, random factor; zone fixed factor [b]

Source	Symbol	Degrees of freedom	Sum of squares	Mean squares	Tested to	F value	P value
Counter	INTER	4	6.6	1.7	1	1.7	>0.1
Zone	Z	1	227.3	227.3	INTER$\times Z$	48.9	<0.001
Counter-zone	INTER$\times Z$	4	18.5	4.7	1	4.7	<0.001
Total		9	252.4				

[a] Numerator of the fraction = number of radioactively labeled acinar cell nuclei; the denominator = total number of cells, labeled and unlabeled, counted; percent = nuclear labeling index.

[b] The exact test of average difference (FISHER, 1954) between the labeling indices of the normal and degenerating pancreas zones equalling zero confirmed the approximate analysis of variance test.

0.6% and that of the degenerating pancreas 12.6%. The relationship could be represented by:

$$1(4.3) = X(0.6) + (1-X)(12.6)$$

where 1 = the relative area of the whole pancreas tissue, X = the relative area of the normal pancreas zone and $1-X$ = the relative area of the degenerate zone. Solving for X gives 69% for the relative area of normal zone and 31% for the relative area of the zone of degeneration.

A simpler relationship may be expressed by considering the whole tissue to be made up of two zones, zone 1 and 2 (zone 2 = whole tissue zone — zone 1):

(Relative area of zone 1) (labeling index of zone 1) + (1-relative area of zone 1) (labeling index zone 2) = (Relative area of whole tissue) (labeling index of whole tissue).

This could be further simplified to:

(Relative area, zone 1) [(labeling index, zone 1) — (labeling index, zone 2)] = (Relative area of whole tissue) (labeling index of whole tissue) — (labeling index of zone 2).

Relative area, zone 1 =

$$\frac{\text{(relative area of whole tissue) (labeling index whole tissue)} - \text{(labeling index, zone 2)}}{\text{(labeling index, zone 1)} - \text{(labeling index, zone 2)}}.$$

Since the relative area of whole tissue $= 1$ then.

$$\text{Relative area zone 1} = \frac{\text{(labeling index whole tissue)} - \text{(labeling index, zone 2)}}{\text{(labeling index, zone 1)} - \text{(labeling index, zone 2)}}.$$

Substituting the labeling indices.

$$\text{Relative area zone 1} = \frac{4.3 - 0.6}{12.6 - 0.6} = \frac{3.7}{12} = 31\%.$$

The planimetric method of determining relative areas gave 31% for the zone of degeneration. The photographic cut-out technique gave a value of 34% of the total tissue area for the degenerative zone.

The difference in labeling indices between the normal area and the degenerating area was very highly significant ($p<0.001$) using the exact test for the fixed factor in a mixed model (one random factor, one fixed factor) (Table 1).

The average difference among counters (SCHEFFÉ, 1959) was not significant (p. >0.10). The interactions between counters and zones were very highly significant ($p<0.0001$).

Discussion

From our planimetric measurements and the weighing of the two tissue zones cut from a photograph the estimate of relative area by use of the labeling indices appears reasonably valid. The considerable difference between the average labeling indices of the two different zones probably was a factor in increasing the accuracy of the estimation of relative areas as was the averaging of the labeling indices of the 5 counters.

If cytologically distinctive foci of cells or processes occurred throughout the whole tissue (e.g. cancer, degenerations, etc.), if the concentration of nuclei were similar in the distinctive zones, if accurate zonal labeling indices were determined and if there was a considerable difference in labeling indices between zones, then our method would require only a simple computation to determine the relative areas of two zones. The more diffusely the distinctive zone extended throughout the tissue the more accurate would be the estimate of its area.

It would be possible to obtain estimates of relative volumes of different zones if one knew the size and shape of zones, the thickness of tissue sections and some other relationships (CHALKLEY et al., 1949) (HENNIG, 1956) (HENNIG and MEYER-ARENDT, 1963).

The procedure of relative area determination could be generalized to include more than two distinct types of tissue zones by counting two zones or more together in order to achieve as many equations as there were unknowns.

In biological specimens focal accumulation or decrease of cellular organelles, isotopes, granules or other substances occur often. Concentration — the amount per unit area or per unit volume — may give an additional important dimension to some studies. If the average nuclear volumes and the number of nuclei per unit area in the two zones were about the same, and if the nuclei were distributed diffusely throughout both zones (very large assumptions), the ratio of the labeling indices would indicate the relative concentrations of radioactivity in each zone. Thus the ratio of $\frac{12.6}{0.6} = 21$ indicates the relative concentrations of radioactivity and the radioactive precursor in the degenerate and normal zones. The relative total amount of radioactivity in each zone would be approximately 90 % in the degenerate tissue and about 10 % in the normal. Although the error of such an estimate would be quite large, at least it would indicate the wide variation often found between tissue areas in pathologic lesions. Such consideration as the above might be of significance in the assessment not only of DNA synthesis in normal and regenerating cells but also on the effect of tritium radiation on these two types of tissue.

Intercounter variance was not significant, but interaction between zone and counter was highly significant (Table 1). Examination of the autoradiographic score sheets and their corresponding microscopic fields in the autoradiograms showed that counters D and E with two lowest indices of the degenerative zone happened to sample multiple areas at the periphery of the degeneration zone where there was no labeling of acinar nuclei. Counters A, B and C with higher values for the degenerative tissue did not sample the non-labeled peripheral parts of the degenerative zone. This may explain, partially, the significance of the counter-zone interaction.

Since the original labeling indices of the whole pancreas tissue obtained by the 5 counters ranged from 2.0 % to 5.8 %, and the labeling indices of the degenerative and normal tissue zones counted separately, averaged 12.6 % and 0.5 %, respectively, each counter, therefore, must have sampled fields in both the normal and degenerate zones.

These findings point up the differences that may be present at cytologic levels between adjacent cells and tissues, particularly in pathologic lesions. They also illustrate some of the merits and limitations of the random field selection technique.

3. Analysis of Variance and Estimates of Error of the Labeling Index

A. Analysis of Variance

Empirically, it would appear that autoradiographic studies of pathologic processes require the counting of many autoradiograms. In studies of DNA synthesis during pancreas degeneration and regeneration using autoradiography and thymidine-H³ we obtained large numbers of autoradiograms for counting. From sample autoradiograms of one of these studies (FITZGERALD, 1963; FITZGERALD *et al.*, 1963) an analysis of variance was performed to determine the relative importance of some of the components in producing the total variance of the experiment (SCHEFFÉ, 1959).

Methods

From experiments in which liver or pancreas operations were performed and DNA synthesis of the rat pancreas acinar cell was studied after thymidine-H³ administration (FITZGERALD, 1963) (FITZGERALD *et al.*, 1963) we selected by a randomization technique sample autoradiograms for analysis. The labeling index was calculated from counts made by multiple counters using the random field selection technique (FITZGERALD *et al.*, 1968b). The variance and the percents of total variance caused by animal, counter, duplicate count, duplicate autoradiogram and possible interactions were derived (SCHEFFÉ, 1959).

From 180 male Wistar rats of an experiment involving 3 groups (normal animals, animals with a liver operation and those subjected to a pancreas segment artery or duct ligation) a total of 15 animals, 5 from each group, was selected.

Thymidine-H³, 0.36 c/mM (Schwarz Bioresearch, Orangeburg, New York), 0.25 µc/g of total body weight, was injected intraperitoneally, 1 hour prior to sacrifice. Our autoradiograms were prepared from tissue taken from the splenic segment of the pancreas.

Medical students who had completed their second year course in Pathology were employed at an hourly rate of compensation to determine the labeling index. They received a period of training in labeling index determinations of autoradiograms of normal and abnormal pancreas tissue after the injection of thymidine-H³. They were limited to the counting of a small number of slides weekly. Although, it was known that they varied considerably in ability and temperament (some were not retained because of their lack of consistency) their results were included in the analysis to indicate the range amongst counters. They counted slides without knowledge of experimental conditions but they did learn that the slides were being counted as part of a study of the technique.

To determine the variation among counters each counter determined the labeling index of an autoradiogram of each of the animals of Problems I and II (see below) and each of the 5 animals of the 3 groups in Problem III. The variance between counters was called intercounter variance.

Some weeks to months after each counter had counted the autoradiograms of pancreas-operated animals he recounted them. Each counter also made duplicate counts of the duplicate autoradiograms of Problem I. Variance between a counter's original and duplicate counts was called intracounter variance. Also included in this component was residual random error.

Additional histologic sections were cut for autoradiograms from the same block of pancreatic tissue from two animals. The duplicate autoradiogram was counted and recounted by all counters.

Statistical Methods

In order to meet the requirements of equal residual variance in a analysis of variance components (SCHEFFÉ, 1959), an approximate procedure was used. It involved scaling indices by their estimated standard deviations, i.e. obtaining:

$$\frac{\dfrac{LN}{TN}}{\sqrt{\dfrac{\dfrac{LN}{TN}\left(1-\dfrac{LN}{TN}\right)}{TN}}}.$$

Analysis of variance tests compared mean squares due to hypotheses against "tested to" mean squares with the same expectation assuming the hypothesis of a particular component being zero. Intracounter components in Problem I and interactions in Problem II, were tested against 1 or the sum of squares was compared to chi squares since the variance within categories was transformed to approximately 1. The analysis was also done with a transformation of numerators so that the numerators were comparable with the numerator that had the lowest denominator in the particular study. Each such scaled numerator was transformed into its square root. The second method served to corroborate the first.

The mathematical model expressed the total variance of an observation in terms of components of variance plus a residual random error term. All these components were independent of each other. Their relative magnitudes with respect to the total determined the percentages of total variance.

Analysis of Variance of Animal, Counter, Autoradiogram and Duplicate Count (Table 2)

Problem I

In order to examine duplicate counts of original and duplicate autoradiograms the two autoradiograms from each of 2 animals which had been subjected to pancreas splenic segment operations were counted by all five counters and later recounted. The analysis of variance performed (SCHEFFÉ, 1959), was a 4-way, random factor design by: (1) animal; (2) counter (intercounter); (3) autoradiogram-nested-in-animal and (4) duplicate count-nested-in-auto-radiogram-and-in-counter (intracounter). Percentages of total variance were derived from the various components. Differences between counters could also be examined.

Problem II

For analysis between counters and duplicate counts, and animal variation 4 animals which had been subjected to a pancreas operation each provided an autoradiogram of the operated segment and each autoradiogram was counted twice by the 5 counters. A 3-way random factor design analysis of variance (SCHEFFÉ, 1959) was performed by: (1) animal; (2) counter (intercounter): and (3) duplicate count-nested-in-animal-and-in-counter (intracounter).

Problem III

Five autoradiograms of normal pancreas (A), 5 autoradiograms from liver operations (B), and 5 autoradiograms from pancreas-operated animals (C) were counted by each of the 5 counters. The percents of intercounter and animal variance for each group were calculated. The variance components caused by intercounter, animal, and intercounter-animal interaction were tested for significant differences from zero (SCHEFFÉ, 1959).

All analyses involving computer calculation of sums of squares were performed on an International Business Machine Corporation (IBM) computer, No. 1620, Model II and some, in addition, were independently confirmed by a commercial concern (CEIR) using an IBM computer, No. 7090.

Results

In all our analyses animal variance was the highest of all components of variance — from 45 to 88 % of total variance (Table 2). Animal variance ranged from significant to very highly significant. Intracounter variance was highly significant in one study and not significant in another. Intercounter effect was varied, being highly significant to not significant. Duplicate autoradiograms did not give significant differences. Intercounter animal interactions were also varied, ranging from non-significant to significant. Residual variance varied from 6 % to 33 % of total variance (FITZGERALD et al., 1968b).

Discussion

In spite of the small number of samples used the variance components and percents of variance obtained probably indicate the relative rank of components in contributing to variability.

The relatively high animal variance throughout all parts of the study was somewhat surprising as was the relatively low intercounter and intracounter

Table 2. *Summary of analyses of variance from previous publication where original data for analyses presented* (Fitzgerald et al., 1968b)

Source of variation	Symbol	Tested to	Variance component	Percent of total variance	p value
Problem I					
Animal	AN	AU +INTER × AN −INTER × AU	14.6	87.5	<0.026
Autoradiogram (within animal)	AU	INTER × AU	—	0.0	>0.50
Intercounter	INTER	INTER × AU	0.1	0.8	>0.10
Intercounter-animal	INTER × AN	INTER × AU	—	0.0	>0.85
Intercounter-autoradiogram	INTER × AU	INTRA	—	0.0	>0.40
Intracounter (count within intercounter and within auto-radiogram)	INTRA	1	0.9	5.6	<0.005
Residual	RES	—	1.0	6.0	—
Total	—	—	16.7	100.0	—
Problem II					
Animal	AN	INTER × AN	1.8	58.6	<0.001
Intercounter	INTER	INTER × AN	0.1	3.3	>0.25
Intercounter-animal	INTER × AN	INTRA	0.2	5.0	>0.25
Intracounter (count within animal and within intercounter)	INTRA	1	—	0.0	>0.90
Residual	RES	—	1.0	33.1	—
Total	—	—	3.0	100.0	—
Problem III *Control*					
Animal	AN	INTER × AN	1.5	45.3	<0.001
Intercounter	INTER	INTER × AN	0.9	25.1	<0.005
Intercounter-animal interaction	INTER × AN	1	—	0.0	>0.70
Residual	RES	—	1.0	29.6	—
Total	—	—	3.4	100.0	—
Problem III *Liver operation*					
Animal	AN	INTER × AN	4.3	72.4	<0.001
Intercounter	INTER	INTER × AN	0.6	10.7	<0.01

Table 2 (continued)

Source of variation	Symbol	Tested to	Variance compo- nent	Percent of total variance	p value
Intercounter- animal interaction	INTER × AN	1	—	0.0	>0.50
Residual	RES	—	1.0	16.9	—
Total	—	—	5.9	100	—

Problem III
Pancreas operation

Animal	AN	INTER × AN	5.6	73.1	<0.001
Intercounter	INTER	INTER × AN	0.04	0.7	>0.25
Intercounter- animal interaction	INTER × AN	1	1.0	13.1	<0.02
Residual	RES	—	1.0	13.1	—
Total	—	—	7.7	100.0	—

variations. Increasing the number of animals would be the most efficient method of decreasing variation relative to other components. It may be that the field selection technique had reduced the sampling technique variation in the autoradiograms so that animal variance thereby became more prominent.

It was also unexpected, in view of some large differences in individual labeling index determinations, to find that intercounter and intracounter variances were not consistently significant and that they made up, in general, such a small percent of the total variance. Conservatively, we attempt to obtain two counters for our studies. It also decreases the likelihood of employing a counter who consistently counts low or high in relation to other counters.

Our results suggest that the autoradiographic technique itself is not a significant source of variance.

B. Estimates of Error—MPRE and S Tables

1. Maximum Possible Relative Error (MPRE)

To our knowledge no overall estimate of the error of the labeling index determination has been made. For the estimate of error we have chosen to define error in terms of the sample average (SA). We have employed a concept which we call maximum possible relative error (MPRE), i.e., error relative to the SA. Tables of MPRE were devised for different combinations of the numbers of animals, the number of counters and the number of nuclei counted per count.

Methods

Experimental design, materials and methods have been indicated in section 3 A. A different analysis of variance from that of section 3 A was used for our estimates of error.

The variable under study was the labeling index and in all our calculations the numerator and denominator were considered to be random Poisson numbers.

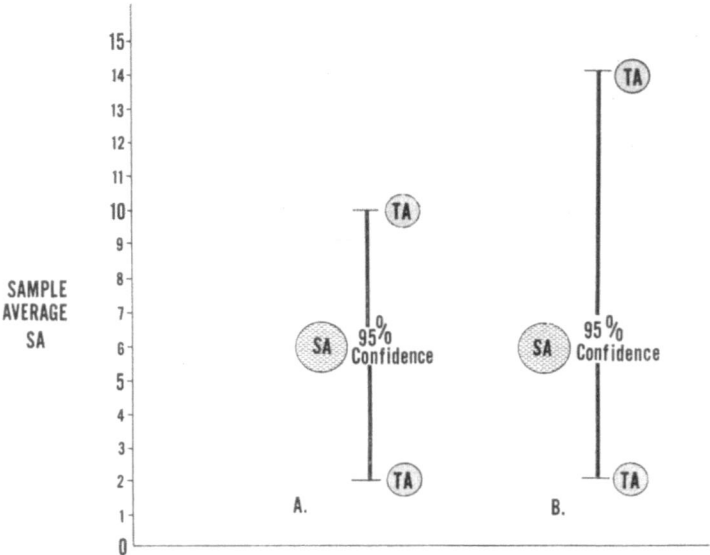

Fig. 5. Schematic diagram of maximum possible relative error (MPRE) concept. Error is expressed in relation to the sample average (SA) and the 95 % confidence bounds. The true average (TA) is placed for illustrative purposes at the furthest possible distance away from the sample average (within a 95 % bound), i.e., at the confidence bounds.

$$\text{MPRE (\%)} = \frac{\text{TA—SA}}{\text{SA}}.$$

In example A the MPRE $= \frac{10-6}{6} = 67\%$. In example B (a rare case when the confidence bounds are not equal; the one furthest distant from the SA is chosen) the MPRE $= \frac{14-6}{6} = 134\%$

The concept of maximum possible relative error (MPRE) utilizes the 95 % confidence bound (Cramér, 1946) a statistical value which indicates, 95 % of the time, the circumscribed limits around the sample average (SA) within which the true average (TA) will be found (Fig. 5). The SA of the labeling indices was determined by dividing the sum of all the numerators by the sum of all of the denominators of the labeling indices of all the animals in a group sacrificed on the same day. The MPRE estimates the farthest distance away from the SA, with 95 % confidence, that the TA might be found, expressing the distance away from the SA as a percent of the SA:

$$\text{MPRE} = \frac{\text{TA} - \text{SA}}{\text{SA}} \times 100.$$

Where the confidence bounds are equidistant from the SA (Fig. 5 A) the MPRE would occur when the TA is at either confidence bound (in Fig. 5 A, giving an MPRE of 67 %). In the rare case where the confidence bounds are unequally distant from the SA the confidence bound more distant from the SA is used (in Fig. 5 B giving an MPRE of 134 %).

In applying our data to the determination of the numerator, TA-SA, with 95 % confidence, we used 1.96 times the large sample standard error of a ratio.

Each of the above variances and the covariance consists of components of variance or covariance caused by factors such as animal, counter, animal-counter interaction, or duplicate count. The standard error of a rate was further developed and consideration was given to the transformation of data to the square root in order to achieve equal residual components of variance (CRAMÉR, 1946, p. 367).

The construction of MPRE tables was performed in a hypothetical versus test case. The original counting data from normal animals and from animals subjected to a liver or pancreas operation (see Section 3) was used for construction of MPRE tables. An analysis of variance was performed separately on the square roots of numerators and denominators of the labeling indices of the data classified by animal, intercounter, and intracounter. The data classified by animal and intercounter was also used. Variance components caused by these factors were derived (SCHEFFÉ, 1959). Similarly, an analysis of components was performed on cross products of deviations from means, analogous to the analysis of variance. Corresponding covariance components were derived.

After mean squares and cross products caused by various factors were derived by dividing appropriate sums of squares and cross products by degrees of freedom, variance and covariance components were obtained for the chosen factors of classification. These results were used to derive the standard error of a ratio taking into consideration the transformation back from square roots of numerators and denominators to their original values. These standard errors incorporated the numbers of counters, duplicate counts, animals, and the number of nuclei counted per single count. The last unit affected residual error.

Our approximate tables were based on varying the number of the units of variance components and the number of nuclei counted per count. The tables assumed for each combination of components an equal number of nuclei counted per count, such as 1,000, 2,000, 3,000, etc. The procedure generalizes to other similar problems.

One can multiply the standard error by a suitable factor and add and subtract from the overall sample average of a labeling index (or mean of the indices) to derive a confidence bound. We used 1.96 for 95 % confidence as the factor from the normal table as a large sample approximation, assuming a Gaussian curve. Dividing half the length of the 2-tailed 95 % confidence interval by the SA of the problem gave a rough estimate of MPRE with respect to the sample average with 95 % confidence.

By systematically varying the number of animals, counters, duplicate counts and number of nuclei counted in a single denominator tables of MPRE were produced by a computer. Tables for all combinations of up to 6 animals 6 counters, 6 counts and 6,000 nuclei per count were printed. Additional, tables were obtained for all combinations of up to 10 animals, up to 3 counters, 1 count and 1,000, 2,000 and 3,000 nuclei counted per count. Such a MPRE table could be used where a hypothetical value, determined by many previous experiments, was known and could be used as a control value (Carol and Fitzgerald, 1968).

A. Method of Calculating Maximum per Cent Possible Error (MPRE) Due to Indices with Random Denominators

Using varying numbers of animals, counters, duplicate counts and auto-radiograms, the labeling indices were obtained by adding counts of labeled nuclei and dividing by the sum of total nuclei counted. Both sums were random because all terms were the result of a random field selection method (Fitz-gerald et al., 1968b).

The ratio of the labeling index is

$$\frac{\text{Sum of squares of square roots of terms making up the numerator}}{\text{Sum of squares of square roots of terms making up the denominator}}. \tag{1}$$

It was cast in this form because square roots of counts tend to obey the requirement of equal residual error variability in Model II covariance analysis. Covariance components as well as variance components were derived analogous to a previous paper (Carol and Fitzgerald, 1968) (Fitzgerald et al., 1968b) for both square roots of numerators and denominators. These latter components had been derived by solving equations for components in terms of mean squares (Scheffé, Chap. 7, 1959).

For example, in Problem III (1) classified by animal and counter the equations were, using square roots of numerators and denominators:

$$\text{Mean square}_{\text{animal}} = \text{var comp}_{\text{random error}} + \text{var comp}_{\text{int}}$$
$$+ (\text{ctr}) \text{ var comp}_{\text{animal}}$$
$$\text{Mean square}_{\text{counter}} = \text{var comp}_{\text{random error}} + \text{var comp}_{\text{int}}$$
$$+ (\text{an}) \text{ var comp}_{\text{counter}}$$
$$\text{Mean square}_{\text{int}} \quad = \text{var comp}_{\text{random error}} + \text{var comp}_{\text{int}}$$

where

$$\text{var comp}_Z = \text{variance component due to factor } Z$$
$$\text{int} = \text{interaction}$$
$$\text{ctr} = \text{number of counters}$$
$$\text{an} = \text{number of animals}$$

Covariance analysis of square roots of numerators with square roots of de-nominators as covariates gave us the variance and covariance (cross product) components for square roots of numerators and denominators. Using the delta method (CRAMÉR, 1946, p. 353) and the fact that we transformed back to the numerators and denominators themselves, we derived the variance of an index such as (1) taking into consideration that the components of variance were based on square roots of numerators and denominators as follows:

The large sample variance of a function H of $2n$ variables $X_1, \ldots, X_n$, $Y_1, \ldots, Y_n$, generalizing as to the number of variables from (CRAMÉR, 1946 p. 354) is

$$\operatorname{var} H = \sum_{i=1}^{n} \sum_{j=1}^{n} \operatorname{cov}\left(x_i, x_j\right)\left(\frac{\partial H}{\partial x_i}\Big|_{x_i=E\,x_i}\right)\left(\frac{\partial H}{\partial x_j}\Big|_{x_j=E\,x_j}\right)$$
$$+ \sum_{i=1}^{n} \sum_{j=1}^{n} \operatorname{cov}\left(y_i, y_j\right)\left(\frac{\partial H}{\partial y_i}\Big|_{y_i=E\,y_i}\right)\left(\frac{\partial H}{\partial y_j}\Big|_{y_j=E\,y_j}\right)$$
$$+ 2\sum_{i=1}^{n} \sum_{j=1}^{n} \operatorname{cov}\left(x_i, y_j\right)\left(\frac{\partial H}{\partial x_i}\Big|_{x_i=E\,x_i}\right)\left(\frac{\partial H}{\partial y_j}\Big|_{y_j=E\,y_j}\right)$$

where $\frac{\partial Z}{\partial t}\Big|_{t=t_0}$ means partial derivative with respect to t at $t=t_0$, $Et=$ expected value of t, $\operatorname{cov}(t, u) =$ covariance of t and u.

The resulting variance of the ratio $H = \dfrac{\sum\limits_{i=1}^{n} X_i^2}{\sum\limits_{i=1}^{n} Y_i^2}$ where $X_i =$ square root of the numerator of the ith index and $Y_i =$ square root of the denominator of the ith index is, considering the transformation count_i of labeled nuclei $= X_i^2$ and count_i of total nuclei $= Y_i^2$,

$$4\left[\frac{EX_i}{EY_i}\right]^4 \left\{\frac{\operatorname{var}(\text{sample mean } X_i)}{(EX_i)^2} + \frac{\operatorname{var}(\text{sample mean } Y_i)}{(EY_i)^2}\right.$$
$$\left. - 2\,\frac{\operatorname{cov}(\text{sample mean } X_i, \text{ sample mean } Y_i)}{EX_i\,EY_i}\right\}.$$

Note that $\operatorname{var}(Z)$ indicates variance of Z, $\operatorname{cov}(m, q)$ indicates covariance of m and q, $n =$ no. of terms making up a numerator as well as a denominator of an index and var (sample mean) of Problem II was expressed in variance components as:

$$\frac{\text{var component}_{\text{animal}}}{\text{no. of animals}} + \frac{\text{variance component}_{\text{counter}}}{\text{no. of counters}}$$

$$+ \frac{\text{variance component}_{\text{duplicate counts}}}{(\text{no. of duplicate counts}) \,(\text{no. of animals}) \,(\text{no. of counters})}$$

$$+ \frac{\text{variance component}_{\text{interaction between counter and animal}}}{(\text{no. of animals}) \,(\text{no. of counters})}$$

$$+ \frac{\text{residual variance}}{(\text{no. of animals}) \,(\text{no. of counters}) \,(\text{no. of duplicate counts})}$$

since our model was $\sqrt{\text{numerator}} = \begin{cases} \text{constant} + \text{animal effect} \\ + \text{ intercounter effect} \\ + \text{ counter-animal interaction} \\ + \text{ intracounter effect nested} \\ \text{within animal and intercounter} \\ + \text{ random error (all independent)} \end{cases}$

and similarly for $\sqrt{\text{denominator}}$. Covariance was analogously treated. Sample means were used for expected values.

Problem III was the same without the duplicate count component. Actually residual variance cannot be separated out from the highest order interaction or, in the case of II, from the nested duplicate count component.

B. 1. Method of Calculating Standard Error Assuming Labeling Index to be a Rate with Constant Denominator

Although our field selection method involved a random denominator, we nevertheless developed a procedure for a fixed denominator and mention it for use where it might apply.

We presume the model of Problem III:

$$Y = \frac{\text{rate}}{\sqrt{\dfrac{\text{rate}\,(1-\text{rate})}{\text{denominator}}}} = \mu + \alpha_a + \alpha_c + \alpha_{ac} + e_{ac} \qquad (2)$$

where rate was any index, μ was a constant, α_a was random animal effect, α_c was random counter effect, α_{ac} was random animal-counter interaction, and e_{ac} was random residual effect. All random effects have a mean of zero. We had performed a component analysis of variance on Eq. (2). This expression could be written as

$$Y = \frac{\sqrt{(\text{rate})\,(\text{den})}}{\sqrt{1-\text{rate}}} = \frac{\sqrt{\text{den}}}{\sqrt{\dfrac{1}{\text{rate}} - 1}}$$

$$\sqrt{\frac{1}{\text{rate}} - 1} = \frac{\sqrt{\text{den}}}{Y}$$

$$\frac{1}{\text{rate}} = \frac{\text{den}}{Y^2} + 1$$

$$\text{rate} = \frac{1}{\dfrac{\text{den}}{Y^2} + 1}$$

where den means denominator of a single counting.

Then the variance of the average of several rates over animals and counters equals

$$\text{var}\left(\sum_{a=1}^{A}\sum_{c=1}^{C} \frac{1}{\dfrac{\dfrac{\text{den}}{Y_{ac}^{2}} + 1}{AC}}\right) = \frac{\sum\limits_{a}^{A}\sum\limits_{c}^{C}\sum\limits_{a'}^{A}\sum\limits_{c'}^{C} \text{cov}\,(Y_{ac},\, Y_{a'c'})}{A^2 C^2} \left(\frac{\partial \dfrac{1}{\dfrac{\text{den}}{Y_{ac}^{2}} + 1}}{\partial Y_{ac}}\Bigg|_{Y_{ac}=EY_{ac}}\right)$$

$$\times \left(\frac{\partial \dfrac{1}{\dfrac{\text{den}}{Y_{a'c'}^{2}} + 1}}{\partial Y_{a'c'}}\Bigg|_{Y_{a'c'}=EY_{a'c'}}\right)$$

where

    var t means variance of t

    A = total number of animals

    C = total number of counters

    a refers to a^{th} animal

    c refers to c^{th} counter

$\dfrac{\partial Z}{\partial t}\Big|_{t=Et}$ means partial derivative of Z with respect to

$$t \text{ at } t = E\,t$$

$E\,Y_{ac} = \mu = $ expected value of Y_{ac}

$\mathrm{cov}\,(Y_{ac}, Y_{a'c'}) = $ covariance of Y_{ac} and $Y_{a'c'}$.

Then for large denominators the variance of the average rate is

$$\left[\frac{\mathrm{var}\,\alpha_a}{A} + \frac{\mathrm{var}\,\alpha_c}{C} + \frac{\mathrm{var}\,\alpha_{ac}}{AC} + \frac{\mathrm{var}\,e_{ac}}{AC}\right] \left. \frac{4\,(-1)^2\,\dfrac{\mathrm{den}^2}{Y_{ac}{}^6}}{\left(\dfrac{\mathrm{den}}{Y_{ac}{}^2}+1\right)^4} \right|_{Y_{ac}=\mu}.$$

Since μ^2 was equivalent to $\dfrac{p^2\,\mathrm{den}}{p\,(1-p)} = \dfrac{p\,\mathrm{den}}{1-p}$, then for large den, where p is the true proportion, the variance of the average rate is

$$\left[\frac{\mathrm{var}\,\alpha_a}{A} + \frac{\mathrm{var}\,\alpha_c}{C} + \frac{\mathrm{var}\,\alpha_{ac}}{AC} + \frac{\mathrm{var}\,e_{ac}}{AC}\right] \frac{\dfrac{4p\,\mathrm{den}^3}{1-p}}{\left(\mathrm{den}+\dfrac{p\,\mathrm{den}}{1-p}\right)^4}$$

$$= \left(\frac{\mathrm{var}\,\alpha_a}{A} + \frac{\mathrm{var}\,\alpha_c}{C} + \frac{\mathrm{var}\,\alpha_{ac}}{AC} + \frac{\mathrm{var}\,e_{ac}}{AC}\right) \frac{4p\,(1-p)^3}{\mathrm{den}}.$$

As in the random denominator case, we used the interaction component for both interaction and random residual error, multiplying it by the ratio of the average denominator of a single experimental count to the actual one in the table. The square root of the variance or standard error was used to get the MPRE and sensitivity as in the first method.

B. 2. Method of Calculating Standard Error Assuming Labeling Index to be the Sum of Squares of Square Roots of Random Numerators Divided by a Fixed Overall Denominator

Having done a component analysis on square roots of counts of labeled nuclei using a two-way design as an example (Problem III), we obtained variance of an average rate

$$= \mathrm{var}\sum_{a=1}^{A}\sum_{c=1}^{C}\left(\frac{(\sqrt{\mathrm{counts}_{ac}}\text{ of labeled nuclei})^2}{(\text{no. of countings})\,(\text{total nuclei in a single counting})}\right)$$

$$= \sum_{a}^{A}\sum_{c}^{C}\sum_{a'}^{A}\sum_{c'}^{C}\mathrm{cov}\,(\sqrt{\mathrm{count}_{ac}},\,\sqrt{\mathrm{count}_{a'c'}})\,2\,\sqrt{\mathrm{single\ count}_{ac}}\Big|_{\substack{\sqrt{\mathrm{single\ count}_{ac}}\\=E\sqrt{\mathrm{single\ count}_{ac}}}}$$

$$\frac{\text{times }2\sqrt{\mathrm{single\ count}_{a'c'}}\Big|_{\sqrt{\mathrm{single\ count}_{a'c'}}=E\sqrt{\mathrm{single\ count}_{a'c'}}}}{(\text{no. of countings})^2\,(\text{total nuclei in a single counting})^2}$$

$$= \frac{\left(\dfrac{\mathrm{var}_a\,\alpha}{A} + \dfrac{\mathrm{var}\,\alpha_c}{C} + \dfrac{\mathrm{var}\,\alpha_{ac}}{AC} + \dfrac{\mathrm{var}\,e_{ac}}{AC}\right)4\,(E\,\sqrt{\mathrm{single\ count}})^2}{(\text{total nuclei in a single counting})^2}.$$

Count_{ac} is the count of the ath animal and the cth counter. We proceeded as in previous methods. The number of nuclei in a single count was set at the average of the pilot experiment when we evolved MPRE and sensitivity tables, as before. A, C and denominators of single countings were varied to make up tables as in previous sections.

B. 3. Method of Calculating Standard Error where Variance Components were Based on a Covariance Analysis of $\sqrt{Numerator}$ with $\sqrt{Denominator}$ as a Covariate

Using square root of numerator with square root of denominator as a covariate, if

$$\sqrt{n_{ac}} = \mu + \alpha_a + \alpha_c + \alpha_{ac} + e_{ac} + \pi \sqrt{d_{ac}}$$

where n_{ac} is numerator in ac cell, d_{ac} is denominator in ac cell, π is a weight multiplying the covariate, then

$$\text{var} \left[\sum_a^A \sum_c^C \frac{(\sqrt{n_{ac}} - \Pi \sqrt{d_{ac}})^2}{\text{no. of countings}} \right]$$

$$= \sum_a^A \sum_c^C \sum_{a'}^{A'} \sum_{c'}^{C'} \text{cov}\,(\sqrt{n_{ac}} - \Pi \sqrt{d_{ac}},\, \sqrt{n_{a'c'}} - \Pi \sqrt{d_{a'c'}})$$

$$\times 2\,(\sqrt{n_{ac}} - \Pi \sqrt{d_{ac}}) \bigg|_{\sqrt{n_{ac}} - \Pi \sqrt{d_{ac}} = E\,(\sqrt{n_{ac}} - \Pi \sqrt{d_{ac}})}$$

$$\frac{\times 2\,(\sqrt{n_{a'c'}} - \Pi \sqrt{d_{a'c'}}) \bigg|_{\sqrt{n_{a'c'}} - \Pi \sqrt{d_{a'c'}} = E\,(\sqrt{n_{a'c'}} - \Pi \sqrt{d_{a'c'}})}}{\text{no. of countings}^2}$$

$$= 4\,[E\,(\sqrt{n_{ac}} - \Pi \sqrt{d_{ac}})]^2 \left[\frac{\text{var } \alpha_A}{A} + \frac{\text{var } \alpha_c}{C} + \frac{\text{var } \alpha_{ac}}{AC} + \frac{\text{var } e_{ac}}{AC} \right].$$

Residual random error was multiplied by the ratio of the average denominator of the experiment to the actual denominator in the table as in B_1 and B_2. Also, we actually used the interaction term as an estimage of the random residual term, particularly since interactions were usually non-significant.

B. 4. Methods of Squaring Back from Confidence Intervals for Square Roots of Numerators and Denominators

We performed analyses on square roots of data without using the square of the derivative of the transformation as a factor multiplying the variance. We squared back to get confidence intervals and therefore MPRE. Tests were performed on square roots of rates to get sensitivities.

Footnote to Table 3:

MPRED values for combinations of components in Problem III, liver-operated animals versus control animals.

[a] The MPRED, a case of test versus control, has a different meaning from the MPRE, a concept used for hypothetical-versus-test values (Fig. 5). The MPRED measures the ratio (percent) of the half length of a 95% confidence interval for an average difference in labeling indexes to the difference in sample means (SD) — not to the sample average (SA), as previously described and illustrated (Fig. 5). The MPRED is larger than the MPRE because the latter reflects the variability of a single sample average (SA), whereas, the former represents the difference between two sample averages, the variances of which are additive (Carol and Fitzgerald, 1968).

Table 3. *MPRED*[a] *with combinations of components, test vs. controls. (Problem III —
liver operation vs. control)*

Animal	Counter	Nuclei per count	Total nuclei counted	MPRED (%)
1	1	1,000	1,000	328
1	1	2,000	2,000	288
1	2	1,000	2,000	277
2	1	1,000	2,000	245
1	1	3,000	3,000	273
1	3	1,000	3,000	258
3	1	1,000	3,000	210
1	2	2,000	4,000	254
2	1	2,000	4,000	218
2	2	1,000	4,000	204
1	1	4,000	4,000	266
1	4	1,000	4,000	248
4	1	1,000	4,000	190
1	2	3,000	6,000	246
1	3	2,000	6,000	241
2	1	3,000	6,000	208
2	3	1,000	6,000	188
3	1	2,000	6,000	189
3	2	1,000	6,000	172
1	1	6,000	6,000	258
1	6	1,000	6,000	237
6	1	1,000	6,000	167
3	4	1,000	12,000	150
4	3	1,000	12,000	140
1	6	2,000	12,000	228
2	6	1,000	12,000	171
6	1	2,000	12,000	155
6	2	1,000	12,000	134
6	3	1,000	18,000	120
6	2	2,000	24,000	126
6	3	2,000	36,000	114
6	3	3,000	54,000	112
8	1	1,000	8,000	155
8	1	2,000	16,000	145
8	2	1,000	16,000	122
8	2	2,000	32,000	116
8	2	3,000	48,000	113
10	1	1,000	10,000	147
10	1	2,000	20,000	139
10	2	1,000	20,000	115
10	2	2,000	40,000	109
10	3	1,000	30,000	101
10	3	2,000	60,000	97
10	3	3,000	90,000	96

C. Method for Calculating MPRED Tables for Two Sample Tests (Test Versus Control)

The analogous extension of (3.B) for 2 samples can be made for a different derivation of the MPRE concept—called the MPRED. The half length of a 95 % confidence interval for a mean difference is divided by the difference (SD) between sample means of the pilot experiment. The SD functions as a measure of the order of magnitude. It divides into the sample difference minus the most conservative true difference (95 % confidence).

The formula is:

$$\frac{\text{Sample difference between test and control} - 95\,\% \text{ most conservative true difference between test and control}}{\text{Sample average difference}}$$

or

$$\frac{\text{SD} - \text{TD}}{\text{SD}}.$$

The MPRE concept was extended to a test-versus-control design and the latter was called the MPRED index (Table 3), (Carol and Fitzgerald, 1968). The MPRED technique evaluates the comparison of results from experimental test animals with those of control animals simultaneously examined (MPRED), rather than the comparison with hypothetical averages (MPRE) obtained earlier from large samples. Experimental pathologists generally prefer to use the test-versus-control design because of the known susceptibility of control animals to the influence of environmental factors.

2. Estimation of the Sensitivity of the Labeling Index Determination

Sensitivity (S) tables detecting a two-tailed alternate hypothesis to a null hypothesis regarding average labeling indices were also constructed (Carol and Fitzgerald, 1968; Cramér, 1946). For convenience we used the SA itself as the null hypothesis. The difference between two hypotheses was scaled by the standard error and the sensitivity was determined by the number of counters, animals, duplicate counts (Problem II only) and the total number of nuclei counted along with the above deviation between contrasting hypotheses. These were varied to form a table. A test of hypothesis was set at a 95 % probability of detecting the null hypothesis.

We also developed S tables for determining the average difference in labeling indices between test-versus-control groups (Table 4) (Carol and Fitzgerald, 1968). The null hypothesis was zero in these tables. As with the MPRED tables, test versus control tables are necessary for most experimental pathology studies.

Programs were written and used with a subroutine deriving the probability under the normal curve called ARNORM. The programs were written in Fortran II-D and are available from one of the authors (B.C.). They were used with an International Business Machine Company Computer No. 1620, Model II.

Methods

By varying numbers of levels of factors, using a large sample approach, the standard error of a mean can be made to vary systematically to produce a table of 2-tailed confidence intervals. We chose a confidence coefficient of 95 %, thus using 1.96 as a factor. We also varied the total nuclei counted in a single counting and accounted for it approximately by multiplying the highest order interaction variance component which contains the residual variance in a single observation per cell design by the ratio of the average single count of nuclei in denominators of the underlying experiment to the single count denominator of the table mentioned above. Usually these highest order interactions do not test significant.

A. Method of Calculating Table of Sensitivity with a Random Denominator

The standard error was similarly used to derive two-tailed sensitivity tables (power functions) for various separations between the null hypothesis (we used the sample average of the experiment) and the alternative hypothesis assuming a 5 % level of significance. The tables were varied also by number of counters, animals, duplicate counts and sizes of a single denominator.

A typical sensitivity was determined by the probability (using the normal distribution) greater than

$$\left[1.96 - \frac{\text{index under null hypothesis-index under alternate hypothesis}}{\substack{\text{standard error of an index for a certain number of counters, animals,}\\ \text{duplicate counts and nuclei counted in a single counting}}} \right]$$

— prob. to right of

$$\left[-1.96 - \frac{\text{index under null hypothesis-index under alternate hypothesis}}{\substack{\text{standard error of an index for a certain number of counters, animals,}\\ \text{duplicate counts and nuclei counted in a single counting}}} \right]$$

$$+ 1.$$

B. Method for Calculating Sensitivity (S) Tables for 2 Sample Test, Test Versus Control

For two-sample tests, asymptotically, use as standard error the square root of the sum of squares of standard errors for each sample as calculated in the one sample case.

Results
MPRE Tables

In Problem II (A) increases in the number of animals, counters, duplicate counts and the number of nuclei counted per count all reduced MPRE. When one component was increased by a factor and the other components were kept constant at 1 the largest reduction of MPRE occurred with the increase in the number of animals. Comparable increase in the number of other component had much less effect (Fig. 6). The three groups of Problem III demonstrated the same general decrease of MPRE with increase in component number as noted in Problem II but differed somewhat between groups and had a lower MPRE (Table 3, CAROL and FITZGERALD, 1968).

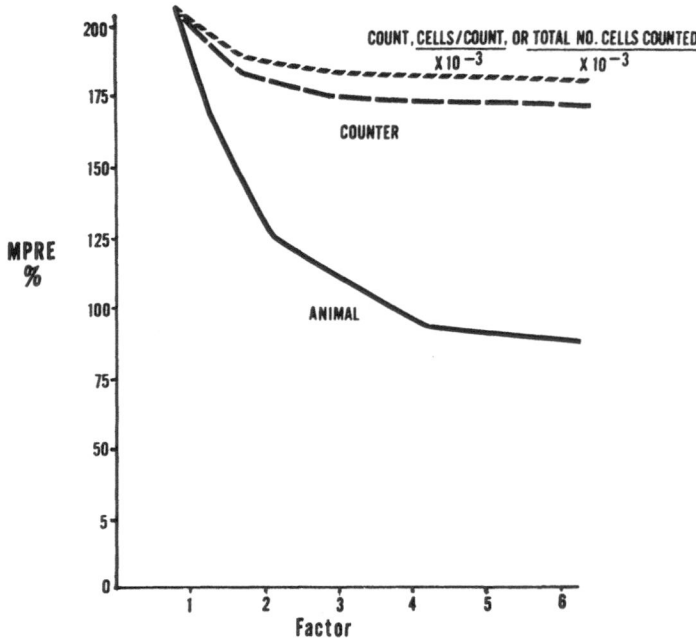

Fig. 6. Change in maximum possible relative error (MPRE) of the labeling index, when each component was separately increased by a unit and the other components remained fixed at one. Relatively little change in MPRE with increase of counters from 1 to 6 or when nuclei per count increased from 1000 to 6000. However, when the number of animals was increased from 1 to 6 the MPRE was decreased by over 100% (Problem II)

MPRED tables showed results similar to the MPRE tables except that the error was much higher.

S Tables

The S tables showed an increase of sensitivity with the increase of component numbers. The probability of detecting comparable differences was less in the test-versus-control tables than in the hypothetical-versus-test case (Table 4). Again, the most significant factor in increasing sensitivity was an increase of animal number. Increasing the number of counters was the next most efficient means of increasing sensitivity whereas increasing the number of nuclei counted per count (in thousands of nuclei counted) had the least effect.

Discussion

Reductions in MPRE with an increase in the number of each component would be expected from statistical principles. The decrease of MPRE to different degrees by different components was shown in a previous study (CAROL and FITZGERALD, 1968) where the variance components made up different percents of the total variance (Section 3) (FITZGERALD et al., 1968b).

The greatest comparable reduction of MPRE occurring with an increase of animal number is consistent with the analysis of variance in Section 3 A

Table 4. *Sensitivity with combinations of components test vs. control (problem III — liver operation vs. control)*

Animal	Counter	Nuclei per count	Total nuclei counted	Interval[a] (%)	Sensitivity[b] (%)
1	1	1,000	1,000	0.3	6
1	1	1,000	1,000	0.6	10
1	1	1,000	1,000	0.9	16
1	1	1,000	1,000	1.2	25
1	1	1,000	1,000	1.5	36
1	1	6,000	6,000	0.3	7
1	1	6,000	6,000	0.6	12
1	1	6,000	6,000	0.9	21
1	1	6,000	6,000	1.2	34
1	1	6,000	6,000	1.5	48
3	2	1,000	6,000	0.3	9
3	2	1,000	6,000	0.6	22
3	2	1,000	6,000	0.9	43
3	2	1,000	6,000	1.2	66
3	2	1,000	6,000	1.5	84
3	2	2,000	12,000	0.3	10
3	2	2,000	12,000	0.6	24
3	2	2,000	12,000	0.9	47
3	2	2,000	12,000	1.2	71
3	2	2,000	12,000	1.5	88
6	1	1,000	6,000	0.3	9
6	1	1,000	6,000	0.6	23
6	1	1,000	6,000	0.9	45
6	1	1,000	6,000	1.2	69
6	1	1,000	6,000	1.5	86
6	2	1,000	12,000	0.3	12
6	2	1,000	12,000	0.6	33
6	2	1,000	12,000	0.9	63
6	2	1,000	12,000	1.2	86
6	2	1,000	12,000	1.5	97
8	1	1,000	8,000	0.3	10
8	1	1,000	8,000	0.6	26
8	1	1,000	8,000	0.9	51
8	1	1,000	8,000	1.2	75
8	1	1,000	8,000	1.5	91
8	2	1,000	16,000	0.3	13
8	2	1,000	16,000	0.6	38
8	2	1,000	16,000	0.9	70
8	2	1,000	16,000	1.2	91
8	2	1,000	16,000	1.5	99
10	1	1,000	10,000	0.3	11
10	1	1,000	10,000	0.6	28
10	1	1,000	10,000	0.9	54
10	1	1,000	10,000	1.2	79
10	1	1,000	10,000	1.5	93

Table 4 (continued)

Animal	Counter	Nuclei per count	Total nuclei counted	Interval[a] (%)	Sensitivity[b] (%)
10	2	1,000	20,000	0.3	14
10	2	1,000	20,000	0.6	42
10	2	1,000	20,000	0.9	75
10	2	1,000	20,000	1.2	94
10	2	1,000	20,000	1.5	99
10	3	2,000	60,000	0.3	18
10	3	2,000	60,000	0.6	54
10	3	2,000	60,000	0.9	87
10	3	2,000	60,000	1.2	98
10	3	2,000	60,000	1.5	100

S values for combinations of components in Problem III, liver-operated animals versus control animals.

Problem III_3 represents a sample of autoradiograms from a group of animals with liver operations and Problem III_1 a sample of autoradiograms from the control group of the same experiment. In a test-versus-control set of circumstances, the variation will be greater than with a hypothetical-versus-test case because in the former, the variances will be additive, whereas in the hypothetical-versus-test situation, a single sample is used.

[a] Interval is the specified difference in percent in labeling index between the null hypothesis of zero average difference and the competing hypothesis.

[b] Sensitivity is the probability (in percent), in testing for average differences between labeling indexes, of detecting a competing hypothesis differing from the null hypothesis by a specified amount (Carol and Fitzgerald, 1968).

which showed that animal variance made up the highest percent of total variance. Variation in response from animal to animal is axiomatic in biology but the relative importance of this component in relation to other components is usually not assessed (Fig. 7).

The lesser effect on MPRE of increasing the number of counters is also consistent with a similar analysis of variance of the previous section where intercounter percent of total variance was small. As in the counting of spermatozoa (Freund and Carol, 1964), however, differences between counters were noted.

The lack of significant effect of duplicate counts of the same autoradiogram would suggest that a duplicate count of the same autoradiogram would not greatly decrease the MPRE and an analysis of variance in a prior study (Fitzgerald et al., 1968b) also indicated that the number of autoradiograms was not a significant component contributing to total variance (Freund and Carol, 1964).

The number of nuclei counted per count was not analyzed as a component of variance but it was varied and made part of our tables (Freund and Carol, 1964). It affected the residual error and therefore an increase in the number of nuclei counter per count decreased MPRE. It is somewhat surprising that the increased number of nuclei counted did not have more effect. It would

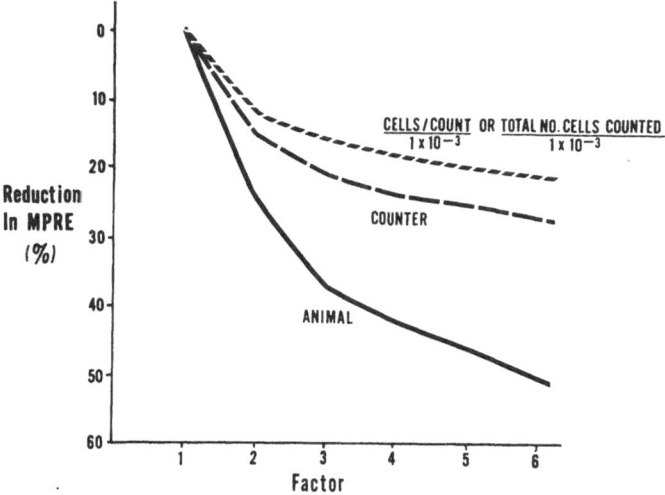

Fig. 7. Relative reduction of MPRE in an experiment where the effect of liver operations on the pancreas acinar cell labeling index was studied (Problem III_2). As in Fig. 6, each component was increased by a unit while other components remained fixed at 1. However, in this figure the cumulative reduction in MPRE, as a percent of the MPRE, when all other components were 1 is indicated. In this experiment the increase of animal number from 1 to 6 gives a greater reduction of MPRE than does increasing the number of cells counted per count, or increasing the number of counters, as in Problem II (Fig. 6). However, the reduction of MPRE by increasing animal number from 1 to 6 does not give as great a reduction of MPRE as occurs in Problem II (Fig. 6)

suggest that in our studies 1,000 to 2,000 nuclei gives a fairly representative sample.

If one had a known control value derived from thousands of samples one might dispense with parallel controls and use the hypothetical-versus-test tables for the derivation of S tables. Simultaneous controls are necessary in most experimental pathology studies so for that reason test-versus-control tables were also developed. It should be noted that in contrast to the MPRE which is related to a sample average (SA), the MPRED table (Table 3) is related to the differences between means (CAROL and FITZGERALD, 1968). A preliminary experiment must be done to obtain the magnitude of variance components of the two samples in order to develop the MPRED tables.

When a total of 6,000 nuclei is counted by the combination of one counter, counting 6,000 nuclei in one animal the MPRE would be 258%. Where one counter counts 1,000 nuclei in an autoradiogram from each of 6 animals for the same total of 6,000 nuclei counted the MPRE would be 167%. If 10 animals, 1 counter and 1,000 nuclei per count for a total of 10,000 nuclei counted were employed the MPRE would be 147% (CAROL and FITZGERALD, 1968). The increase of animal number gives a significant decrease of MPRE.

The S tables showed a roughly inverse relationship to the MPRED tables, i.e., for the same combinations of components a decrease of MPRED was accompanied by an increase of sensitivity and vice versa. A high sensitivity may not necessarily indicate a low MPRED, or the reverse, because in the MPRED the variation of the sample average and the sample average itself are involved but in the sensitivity derivation the sample average is not involved.

There was a change of sensitivity (S), as with the MPRED, when the animal component was increased, so that sensitivity was greater with increase of animal number than when any other component was changed by the same factor. Other components affected the sensitivity (Table 4) in the same order as they did the MPRED. However, the degree of change differed in the groups. The sensitivity was higher in the liver operations than in the pancreas-operations (Table 4) and (Table 5, CAROL and FITZGERALD, 1968). If 6,000 nuclei were counted in the autoradiogram of 1 animal by 1 counter in the animals with a liver operation the probability in detecting a difference of labeling indices of 1.5 % would be 48 %. In the same experimental group if 6,000 nuclei were counted by the combination of 6 animals, 1 counter and 1,000 nuclei per count the probability of detecting 1.5 % difference would be 86 % (Table 4). The respective comparable probabilities (S) for the pancreas-operations were 27 % and 72 % (Table 5, CAROL and FITZGERALD, 1968).

Our results showed many differences of MPRE and S in different subgroups of the same experiment (Tables 3 and 5, CAROL and FITZGERALD, 1968). The analysis of variance in section 3 A indicated differences in percents of total variance within the same experiment. MPRE and S tables should, therefore, be made up for major groups of an experiment.

From our studies we have formulated general procedures for our own experiments using the acinar cell nuclear labeling index of the rat pancreas. Two counters are employed for counting the 2 autoradiograms of each animal —one for each of the 2 samples of pancreas tissue taken for study from each animal. A minimum of 3 animals in each of the test and control groups is taken at each sacrifice. An experiment is repeated at least once. In each autoradiogram 1,000—2,000 nuclei are counted. The minimum figures, therefore, are: 2 experiments; 6 animals; 2 counters; and 1,000 nuclei per count to give a total of 12,000 nuclei counted per test or control group. Usually higher numbers are obtained at the important time points (FITZGERALD et al., 1968a).

The principles utilized and allied techniques developed herein may be applied to other types of experiments, particularly where ratios are involved. The methods could be further extended into assigning costs for different kinds of error in decision-making based on specific experimental designs (WALD, 1950).

Summary

An attempt has been made to analyze the autoradiographic method as employed for the DNA labeling index determination of the percent of labeled rat pancreas acinar cell nuclei after the administration of thymidine-H^3. A technique to insure a wide random sampling of the autoradiogram was described. An analysis of variance was performed on the data from an experiment involving the labeling index of pancreas acinar cells of control animals and those subjected to pancreas degeneration and regeneration. The largest source of variance was the animal component. Other components were much less significant. The autoradiographic technique per se was relatively unimportant as a source of variation. Tables of maximum possible error (MPRE) relative to the sample average and tables of sensitivity (S) for the labeling index were developed by a computer. These tables indicated the relative importance of components such as the number of animals, the number of counters, and the number of nuclei counted per count in reducing error and increasing the sensitivity of the labeling index determination. Comparable tables would give an investigator flexibility in the design of his experiments because they would give a practical estimate of the number of individual components needed to reduce error and indicate the probability of detecting specified differences in labeling indices.

Bibliography

BASERGA, R.: Biochemistry of the cell cycle: a review. Cell Tiss. Kinet. 1, 167—191 (1968).

CAROL, B., FITZGERALD, P. J.: Pancreatic acinar cell regeneration. VI. Estimation of error of the autoradiographic labeling index (thymidine-H³)—maximum possible error (MPRE) and sensitivity (S). Amer. J. Path. 53, 971—987 (1968).

CHALKLEY, H. W.: Method for quantitative morphologic analysis of tissue. J. Nat. Cancer Inst. 4, 47—53 (1943).

— CORNFIELD, J., PARK, H.: A method for estimating volume-surface ratios. Science 110, 295—297 (1949).

CRAMÉR, H.: Mathematical methods of statistics. Princeton, N. J.: Princeton Univ. Press 1946.

ERÄNKÖ, O.: Quantitative methods in histology and microscopic histochemistry. Boston: Little Brown 1955.

FISHER, R. A.: Statistical methods for research workers (ed. 12). New York: Hafner 1954.

FITZGERALD, P. J.: The problem of the precursor cell of regenerating pancreatic acinar epithelium. Lab. Invest. 9, 67—85 (1960).

— Autoradiographic labeling of pancreatic acinar cells with thymidine-H³ during degeneration and regeneration. Canad. Med. Ass. J. 88, 480—482 (1963).

— CAROL, B., LIPKIN, L., ROSENSTOCK, L.: Pancreactic acinar cell regeneration. V. Analysis of variance of the autoradiographic labeling index (thymidine-H³). Amer. J. Path. 53, 953—970 (1968b).

— EIDINOFF, M. L., KNOLL, J. E., SIMMEL, E. B.: Tritium in radioautograhpy. Science 114, 494—498 (1951).

— RICHARDS, C., LIPKIN, L., ROSENSTOCK, L.: Increased autoradiographic labeling (thymidine-H³) of pancreatic acinar cell nuclei during degeneration. (Abst.) Fed. Proc. 22, 603 (1963).

— VINIJCHAIKUL, K.: Nucleic acid metabolism of pancreatic cells as revealed by cytidine-H³ and thymidine-H³. Lab. Invest. 8, 319—329 (1959).

— — CAROL, B., ROSENSTOCK, L.: Pancreatic acinar cell regeneration. III. DNA synthesis of pancreas nuclei as indicated by thymidine-H³ autoradiography. Amer. J. Path. 52, 1039—1066 (1968a).

FREUND, M., CAROL, B.: Factors affecting haemocytometer counts of sperm concentrations in human semen. J. Reprod. Fertil. 8, 149—155 (1964).

Hennig, A.: Bestimmung der Oberfläche beliebig geformter Körper mit besonderer Anwendung auf Körperhaufen im mikroskopischen Bereich. Mikroskopie **11**, 1—20 (1956).
— Meyer-Arendt, J. R.: Microscopic volume determination and probability. Lab. Invest. **12**, 460—464 (1963).
Howard, A., Pelc, S. R.: Synthesis of desoxyribonucleic acid in normal and irradiated cells and its relation to chromosome breakage. Heredity, Suppl. **6**, 261—273 (1953).
Leblond, C. P., Walker, B. E.: Renewal of cell populations. Physiol. Rev. **36**, 255—276 (1956).
Mauer, M.: Quoted by Belanger, L., The use of radioautography in investigating protein synthesis, ed. C. P. Leblond and K. B. Warren. Symposium, Internat. Soc. For Cell Biology, p. 3—4, New York: Academic Press 1954.
Richards, C., Fitzgerald, P. J., Carol, B., Rosenstock, L., Lipkin, L.: Segmental division of the rat pancreas for experimental procedures. Lab. Invest. **13**, 1303—1321 (1964).
Scheffé, H.: The analysis of variance. New York: Wiley 1959.
Schultze, B., Citoler, P., Hempel, K., Citoler, K., Mauer, W.: Cytoplasmic protein synthesis in cells of various types and its relation to nuclear protein synthesis. In: The use of radioautography in investigating protein synthesis, ed. C. P. Leblond and K. B. Warren. Symposium, Internat. Soc. For Cell Biology, vol. 4, p. 107—139. New York: Academic Press 1965.
Taylor, J. B., Woods, P. S., Hughes, W. L.: The organization and duplication of chromosomes as revealed by autoradiographic studies using tritium-labeled thymidine. Proc. Nat. Acad. Sci. **43**, 122—128 (1957).
Verley, W. G., Hunebelle, G.: Preparation de thymidine. Marquée avec du tritium. Bull. Soc. Chim. Belges **66**, 640—649 (1957).
Wald, A.: Statistical decision functions. New York: Wiley 1950.
Weibel, E. R.: Morphometry of the human lung, p. 47. New York: Acad. Press 1963 a.
— Principles and methods for the morphometric study of the lung and other organs. Lab. Invest. **12**, 131—155 (1963 b).

Department of Pathology, University of Kiel, Head: Prof. Dr. K. LENNERT

Renal Siderosis
Morphology, Etiology, Pathogenesis and Differential Diagnosis
With Special Reference to Traumatic Hemolytic Anemia

WOLFGANG REMMELE and ANNE HINRICHS

With 11 Figures

Table of Contents

A. Introduction

Only few pathological conditions are known which are accompanied by deposition of hemosiderin in the kidney. In the past it was considered a rule that only in patients with primary hemochromatosis and paroxysmal nocturnal hemoglobinuria could considerable amounts of hemosiderin be found in the tubular epithelium of the kidney. This view is no longer true. Meanwhile some more conditions associated with renal hemosiderosis have been described. Among them are traumatic hemolytic anemias related to cardiac valvular disease, implantation of prosthetic heart valves, and microangiopathy of different origin as well as special types of sideroachrestic anemia. Cardiac surgery may be followed by such extensive siderosis of the kidney that the term "blue kidney" has been introduced (Roberts, 1966) to describe the aspect of the kidney after staining with Prussian blue.

This article contains our present knowledge of renal siderosis and deals with the problems of morphology, etiology, pathogenesis, and differential diagnosis. It presents a review of the literature to date and the results of personal investigations.

B. Kidney and Iron Metabolism

The adult looses 0.5—1.0 mg of iron per day. This is the same amount as excreted by the rabbit (Muir and Dunn, 1914/15). 90—95 % is contained in leukocytes, epithelial cells, and body secretes. Desquamation of epithelial cells of the skin, the mucous membranes, the gastrointestinal tract and the sweat glands mainly attribute to the loss of iron (Moore and Dubach, 1959; Finch, 1964).

Only 0.05 mg, i.e. 5—10% of the daily loss of iron, is excreted with the urine (Cartwright et al., 1954; Plötner and Petzel, 1954; Gisinger and Puxkandl, 1955). The question as to whether the iron contained in urine is free iron or iron bound to transferrin (Najean, 1964) has not yet been definitely settled. According to Finch (1964) most of it is free iron. However, the urine contains transferrin even under normal conditions (Schultze and Heremans, 1966).

The transferrin content of blood plasma amounts to 250—300 mg-% which can bind 280—371 (Dreyfus and Schapira, 1964) and 250—400 µg of iron (Laurell, 1959), respectively. Transferrin is not saturated by the usual amount of iron in blood (140 µg-%). The level of free iron in blood is far below 1 µg-%, and an active reabsorption by the tubular epithelium has not yet been established (Laurell, 1959). If the iron in urine is predominantly free iron, as mentioned above, urinary iron excretion is due to either ultrafiltration of free iron or uncoupling of the iron-protein complex during its passage through the tubular apparatus. The site where the complex is split in the tubular apparatus is unknown.

Furthermore, some of the iron enters the urine bound to hemopexin (Schultze and Heremans, 1966).

In some diseases the amount of iron excreted in urine may increase considerably. Values of 1.2 mg/die were estimated in hemochromatosis (SCHWARZMANN, 1962). This may partly be explained by the fact that subsequent complete saturation of transferrin free iron appears in the serum which is subject to ultrafiltration. As mentioned above, reabsorption of free iron has not yet been proved.

Modern therapy of primary hemochromatosis with chelating agents (EDTA, DTPA, desferrioxamine) may increase urinary iron excretion to values of about 15 mg per day (DREYFUS and SCHAPIRA, 1964).

Corresponding to the insignificant rôle of the kidney in iron metabolism and to the undoubtedly high turnover rate of reabsorbed iron within the tubular epithelial cells the iron content of renal tissue is very low. It amounts to 0.0038—0.0187 (average 0.0104) g per kidney or 0.0101—0.0498 (average 0.0277) g per 100 g dry weight (MACDONALD, 1964). In the rabbit the iron content appears to be higher (0.42 mg in the kidneys according to MUIR and DUNN, 1914/15). The same is true for the dog (about 6 mg per 100 g tissue, NEWMAN and WHIPPLE, 1932). No iron is visible in the normal kidney when stained with Prussian blue.

C. General Pathogenesis of Renal Siderosis

As a rule, the development of renal siderosis depends on either erythrocyturia or hemoglobinuria. Exceptions are primary and secondary hemochromatosis (see below). Another exception is the entry of erythrocytes from hemorrhages in the interstitium into the lumina of the renal tubules which is said to play an important rôle in sickle cell anemia (MOSTOFI et al., 1957; RANDERATH and BOHLE, 1959).

1. Erythrocyturia

Even under normal conditions, urine contains small numbers of erythrocytes up to 500,000 per day (BELL, 1947; ADDIS, 1948; ALLEN, 1951) corresponding to the number of erythrocytes in 0.1 mm³ blood.

Undoubtedly, the erythrocytes may be disrupted within the renal tubules. The liberated hemoglobin is partially excreted in the urine, partially reabsorbed by the epithelial cells and transformed into hemosiderin. It can be expected from this that recurring erythrocyturia, e.g. in sickle cell anemia, may lead to renal hemosiderosis.

2. Hemoglobinuria

In most cases, Hb-uria is the result of hemoglobinemia.

The normal *Hb content of blood plasma* varies between 0 and 0.5 mg-% (SHINOWARA, 1954; HAM, 1955; Geigy-tables, 1960). The Hb levels estimated by CROSBY and DAMESHEK (1951) never exceeded 4 mg-% and most frequently amounted to 2—3 mg-%. CROSBY (1955) found normal values up to 5 mg-%. There is no doubt that the level of Hb in blood largely depends on how carefully blood is taken from the veins. Traumatic hemolysis may simulate higher "normal" values.

If *intravascular hemolysis* has taken place the Hb content of blood plasma may rise to values of about 1 g-% (Ham, 1955). Hb is eliminated from the blood in 3 ways (Ham, 1955): 1. by urinary excretion (10—33 %), 2. by intracellular transformation of Hb into bilirubin (increase of bilirubin in blood serum), and 3. by formation and possibly urinary excretion of methemalbumin (heme from Hb, bound to albumin). Renal siderosis may follow urinary excretion of Hb and perhaps of methemalbumin. However, methemalbumin does not appear in the final urine. The question, therefore, as to whether it is not subject to ultrafiltration or reabsorbed quantitatively, has not yet been settled (Lathem, 1959).

The *renal threshold for Hb* lies between 100 (Ham, 1955) and 150 (Geigy-tables 1960) mg-%. Hb is excreted via the glomeruli and not via the tubuli (Randerath and Krückemeyer, 1949).

Careful studies concerning the renal threshold for Hb have been carried out by Gilligan, Altschule and Katersky (1941). They injected hemolysates of different volumes and concentrations into 10 healthy individuals, 4 patients with cardiac insufficiency, and 1 patient with metastatic cancer of the colon. The amount of Hb given varied between 1.3 and 16.4 g. The Hb content of plasma rose to 40—380 mg-%. The clearance of Hb was enhanced when high values of Hb were measured in the plasma. Hb-uria appeared in normal individuals at Hb levels above 135 mg-% and continued until Hb had fallen to 30—50 mg-%. Patients with preexisting proteinuria developed Hb-uria at Hb serum levels of only 40—50 mg-%. Renal function appeared to be unchanged by Hb-uria. In one case the clearance of urea amounted to 83 % in the 3 hours prior to injection of Hb and to 76% in the 3 hours after.

The renal threshold for Hb may decrease in chronic Hb-uria (Ham, 1955). This finding is consistent with experiments in animals (Lichty et al., 1932; Newman and Whipple, 1932). The renal threshold is also decreased in pre-existent proteinuria (Gilligan et al., 1941), probably as a result of disturbed glomerular permeability. In animal experiments, spasms of the renal arterioles could be produced by injections of Hb (Reid, 1929; Mason and Mann, 1931; Hesse and Filatov, 1933). The lowering of the renal threshold for Hb may further be the consequence of 1. a decrease of tubular reabsorptive capacity after repeated Hb-uria or other types of proteinuria (e.g. injections of bovine albumin in animals, for ref. see Randerath and Bohle, 1959) and 2. loss of haptoglobin in the course of proteinuria. This may be discussed at least for haptoglobin Hp 1-1, the low molecular form of haptoglobin (molecular weight = 85,000) while the higher molecular haptoglobins (Hp 1-2 and Hp 2-2, molecular weight = 160,000) are not excreted in the urine (Schumacher and Schlumberger, 1962; Schultze and Heremans, 1966).

The renal threshold is essentially determined by the level and saturation of haptoglobin. Hb is transported in blood plasma partially bound to haptoglobin and partially as free Hb. The haptoglobin level amounts to 113 ±

43 mg-% in normal men and 90 ± 30 mg-% in normal women (NYMAN, 1959). The binding capacity is restricted to 90—140 mg-% of iron (LAURELL and NYMAN, 1957; ALLISON, 1959; LATHEM and WORLEY, 1959). Free Hb appears in the blood only after this value has been exceeded. Then methemalbumin is also observed in blood (LATHEM and WORLEY, 1959).

Free Hb is excreted in the urine at a rate of 8—10 mg/min. The concentration in the glomerular filtrate is 5 % of that in the blood plasma. Tubular reabsorption is low (0—2.6, mean 1.3 ± 0.9 mg/min), yet sufficient in order to prevent Hb-uria up to Hb levels in blood plasma of 60 mg-% (mean 27 mg-%; LATHEM, 1959).

The Hp-Hb complex and methemalbumin do not appear in the final urine, probably because their molecular weight (155,000 for the Hp 1-1-Hb complex; GUINAND et al., 1956) is too high. This has been confirmed for the Hp-Hb complex by LAURELL and NYMAN (1957). It disappears from the serum at a rate of about 13 mg Hb/100 ml/hr and is probably removed by the RES (LAURELL and NYMAN, 1957). If nephrectomized animals are used Hb is also eliminated from the plasma. Apparently, this process does not depend on the presence of the kidneys (FURTH, 1955).

The *renal function* is influenced by hemoglobinemia if it is high enough. BRANDT et al. (1951) observed an increase of the glomerular filtration rate in one third and a decrease in two thirds of their cases following infusion of a 6 % Hb solution. In all cases a significant decrease of renal plasma flow rate, urinary excretion and sodium excretion took place while the PAH clearance, hematocrit, pulse frequency and blood pressure remained unchanged.

Hemosiderin develops from excreted hemoglobin as follows: First globin is split off the hemoglobin molecule within the tubular epithelial cell, and the protein component is broken down by the mitochondrial enzymes (ZINGG and ZOLLINGER, 1951). According to STURGEON and SHODEN (1964) the intracellularly dispersed ferritin becomes concentrated in vacuoles as the iron level increases. Denaturation of the apoferritin matrix is associated with loss of water solubility, which in biochemical terms marks the change from ferritin to hemosiderin. Then the iron micelles are aggregated into what STURGEON and SHODEN call true or mature hemosiderin.

There are many causes of Hb-uria. Among them the following are the most important (ROSS, 1945; HAM, 1955; RANDERATH and BOHLE, 1959): Intravascular hemolysis following strenuous physical exertion (so-called athletic and march Hb-uria), intravascular hemolysis due to hypotonicity of blood plasma (intravenous injection of distilled water), paroxysmal nocturnal hemoglobinuria Strübing-Marchiafava-Micheli, paroxysmal cold hemoglobinuria, incompatible blood transfusions, acquired hemolytic anemias, thermic lesions of erythrocytes (in burns), hemolysis caused by chemical agents (As, sulfonamides, phenylhydrazine, naphthaline, quinine, mushroom intoxications, potassium chlorate, KMnO4, phenol, lysol, carbon tetrachloride), hemolysis by blood parasites (malaria = black water fever, Oroya fever), enzymopenic hemolytic anemias (favism) and toxemia of pregnancy. The following causes have to be added: traumatic hemolytic anemias in cardiac valvular disease and after implantation of heart valve prostheses, and the traumatic hemolytic anemias in microangiopathy.

D. Etiology and Morphology of Renal Siderosis
I. Primary Hemochromatosis

According to MACDONALD (1964) hemochromatosis is defined by the association of portal cirrhosis with an elevated iron content in the liver, pancreas, gastrointestinal tract, kidney and other organs, while enlarged liver, diabetes mellitus, skin pigmentation, elevated serum iron, hemofuscin pigment, and iron in certain locations such as in bile duct epithelium may be present but are not necessary for the diagnosis. MACDONALD's classification of hemochromatosis has to be modified in so far as group I A ("Idiopathic" hemochromatosis associated with anemia, particularly megaloblastic, pyridoxine responsive) is characterized by secondary hemochromatosis in the course of symptomatic sideroachrestic anemias (see below).

In hemochromatosis the kidney contains 0.005—0.42 (average 0.182) g iron corresponding to 0.02—0.21 (average 0.11) g per 100 g of wet tissue and 0.01—0.48 (average 0.2) g per 100 g dry weight (MACDONALD, 1964). CLETON and BLOK (1963) found an iron content of 0.038 g in their case.

Microscopically, 83 % of 57 cases had renal siderosis (MACDONALD and MALLORY, 1960). HEDINGER (1953) gives a somewhat lower figure (15 out of 22 cases = 68.2 %).

The hemosiderin is predominantly localized in the epithelial cells of the distal convoluted tubules and in the ascending part of Henle's loops (WALTHARD, 1946; HEDINGER, 1953; RANDERATH and BOHLE, 1959; MACDONALD, 1964). The proximal convoluted tubules are the site of hemosiderosis less often (Fig. 1 and 6). If present there, hemosiderosis is not the result of transfusion therapy because in 5 cases with siderosis of the proximal convoluted tubules no transfusions has been given before (HEDINGER, 1953). The cells of the glomerular tuft may also show hemosiderin granules (HEDINGER, 1953).

These results of former authors correspond to our personal investigations in 4 cases of primary hemochromatosis.

Case No. 1

D. K., 64 y. old woman.

Clinical diagnosis: Diabetes mellitus. Coma of unknown origin (cancer with metastatic lesions in the brain?).

Autopsy (S 587/65): Hemochromatosis with massive siderosis of the liver. Slight fibrosis of the pancreas without siderosis. Perivenous lymphocytic meningoencephalomyelitis.

Kidneys: Normal size (280 g). Very slight siderosis of some epithelial cells of the proximal and distal convoluted tubules. Considerable siderosis of the endothelial cells of the renal vessels, especially of the medullary vasa recta.

Case No. 2

G. B., 44 y. old man.

Clinical diagnosis: Decompensated liver cirrhosis (primary cancer of the liver?).

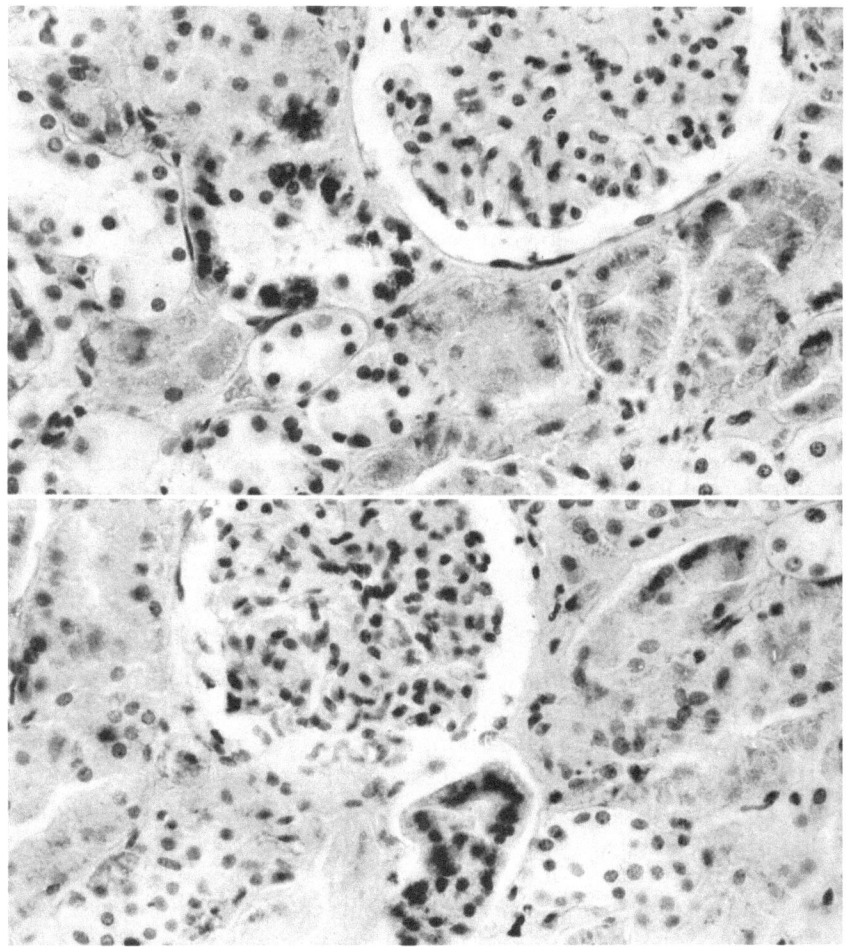

Fig. 1. Renal siderosis in primary hemochromatosis. Hemosiderin deposits are restricted to the epithelial cells of the distal convoluted tubules. The proximal convoluted tubules are free of iron pigment. Case No. 3. Prussian blue reaction. 340 ×

Autopsy (S 784/65): Nodular cirrhosis of the liver (1270 g) with moderate hemochromatosis. Fibrosis and hemochromatosis of the pancreas. Moderate siderosis of myocardium, adrenal glands, pituitary gland and parotid gland.

Kidneys: Normal size (310 g). Slight siderosis of few distal convoluted tubules and Henle's loops. Pigmented casts in several tubuli.

Case No. 3

J. v. H., 67 y. old woman.

Clinical diagnosis: Liver cirrhosis. Coma hepaticum. Macrocytic hemolytic anemia with free serum Hb (beginning some months prior to death following porto-caval anastomosis, no erythrocyte antibodies observed).

Autopsy (S 62/56): Nodular portal cirrhosis with fatty degeneration of the liver. Considerable hemochromatosis of the liver, pancreas, myocardium, adrenal glands, thyroid gland and pituitary gland.

Kidneys: Normal size (285 g). Considerable hemochromatosis of the proximal and distal convoluted tubules and Henle's loops. The degree of siderosis of the proximal and distal convoluted tubules changes from one part of the microscopic slide to the other (Fig. 1). Henle's loops are extremely siderotic. Some of the epithelial cells of Bowman's capsule contain hemosiderin. Iron positive amorphous material in some Bowman's spaces and tubules.

Case No. 4

J. R., 24 y. old man.

Clinical diagnosis: Panmyelophthisis (Hb 42%, 1600 leukocytes, 10,000 platelets). Hemorrhagic diathesis.

Autopsy (S 430/66): Panmyelophthisis with increase of fatty marrow in vertebrae, sternum and femur. Severe hemorrhagic diathesis and pulmonary edema. Subchronic liver dystrophy with moderate siderosis. Fibrosis and hemochromatosis of the pancreas. Hemochromatosis of the adrenal glands, myocardium and testes. Insignificant siderosis of spleen and bone marrow in the femur (following blood transfusions).

Kidneys: Slightly enlarged (350 g). Moderate siderosis of the distal convoluted tubules and Henle's loops. Diffuse slight siderosis of the proximal convoluted tubules. Focal siderosis of the epithelial cells of Bowman's capsule and of few glomerular podocytes. Iron positive amorphous material in numerous tubules, especially proximal convoluted tubules and Henle's loops.

II. Sideroachrestic Anemia with Secondary Hemochromatosis

According to HEILMEYER (1961) and VERLOOP (1965) sideroachrestic anemias are divided into connatal and acquired idiopathic anemias and symptomatic anemias. Only the idiopathic anemias show general secondary hemochromatosis while the symptomatic forms merely have a more or less significant siderosis (LENNERT and OERKERMANN, 1967). Differential diagnosis between secondary and primary hemochromatosis is based mainly upon the following features present only in sideroachrestic anemia: Anemia, hyperplasia of bone marrow, and occurrence of numerous sideroblasts in the bone marrow (VERLOOP et al., 1962, LENNERT and OERKERMANN, 1967).

In several cases siderosis of the kidney has been described (GOLDISH and AUFDERHEIDE, 1953; FEIT and BELUSA, 1961; VERLOOP et al., 1962; LENNERT and OERKERMANN, 1967). In one case chromoprotein casts were observed within the renal tubules (MÄHR and WUKETICH, 1961). Often, however, no data are given concerning the hemosiderin content of the kidney (COOLEY, 1945; MILLS and LUCIA, 1949; CROSBY and SHEEHY, 1956; GELPI and ENDE, 1958; DACIE et al., 1959; GERHARTZ, 1963).

The localization of hemosiderin within the tubular apparatus differs. GOLDISH and AUFDERHEIDE (1953) and LENNERT and OERKERMANN (1967) observed hemosiderin in the distal convoluted tubules, FEIT and BELUSA (1961) also in the proximal convoluted tubules which contained no iron in the case of LENNERT and OERKERMANN. GOLDISH and AUFDERHEIDE described hemosiderin also in the collecting tubules, LENNERT and OERKERMANN in Henle's loops. VERLOOP et al. (1962) give no precise localization. Our own material comprises the cases published by LENNERT and OERKERMANN and one more patient observed in the last year.

Case No. 5

E. T., 76 y. old woman.

Clinical diagnosis: Diabetes mellitus, parotitis, hemolytic anemia, broncho-pneumonia. Hb 3.9 g-%.

Autopsy (S 762/67): Acquired idiopathic sideroachrestic anemia: Deeply reddish-brown marrow in the spine and femur. Liver dark brown (1400 g), moderately consistent. Spleen moderately enlarged (180 g), dark red color. Severe secondary hemochromatosis of the liver, thyroid gland, adrenal cortex and pancreas. Moderate siderosis of the myocardium (predominantly of the left chamber). Siderosis of the arterial walls in the spleen. Severe siderosis of the lymph nodes.

Kidneys: Size moderately diminished (200 g). Moderate to slight siderosis of the distal convoluted tubules and the Henle's loops. Proximal convoluted tubules and collecting tubules free of hemosiderin.

It appears from the above that in secondary hemochromatosis associated with sideroachrestic anemia the same parts of the nephron are affected by siderosis as in primary hemochromatosis. Although few cases with renal siderosis have been published to date, the siderosis apparently prefers the distal convoluted tubules.

Iron deposition seems to be less severe in cases of symptomatic sideroachrestic anemia (LENNERT and OERKERMANN, 1967). This is in accordance with the fact that general hemochromatosis is missing in this type of sideroachrestic anemia.

In some cases of symptomatic sideroachrestic anemia due to pyridoxin deficiency (MAIER, 1957; VEYRAT and MAURICE, 1960) no renal siderosis was described. The same is true for several cases of sideroachrestic anemia due to folic acid deficiency (FRICK and BRUNNER, 1963: no detailed description; MUGGIA and OLIVETTI, 1967: Kidney free of hemosiderin) and to lack of vitamin B 12 (KOSZEWSKI, 1952).

In one case of pernicious anemia an extensive deposition of hemosiderin was found (YATES and THALHIMER, 1926), but the patient had received 113 blood transfusions (corresponding to 52 l of native blood) within a space of 3 years. Apparently blood transfusions do not produce renal siderosis (ROBERTS and MORROW, 1966; HEDINGER, 1953; personal observations); it is, however, doubtful whether this may be considered true for cases with blood transfusions in such high numbers as in the case of YATES and THALHIMER.

III. Hemolytic Anemias

a) Paroxysmal Nocturnal Hemoglobinuria Strübing-Marchiafava-Micheli (PNH)

In contrast to the majority of hemolytic anemias erythrocytes are destroyed in PNH not by the cells of the RES but within the blood. Anomalies of erythrocyte membrane and disturbances of erythrocyte lipid metabolism are considered to be important factors in the pathogenesis of this disease (for ref. see MENGEL *et al.*, 1967). Plasma Hb level is elevated to values above 100 mg-% (Case 2 of HUTT *et al.*, 1961: 105 mg-%; CROSBY, 1953: 180 mg-%).

The renal threshold which normally lies at 135 mg-% may be lowered to 50—100 mg-% (CROSBY, 1953).

In PNH the kidney contains considerable amounts of hemosiderin. In one case (HEITZMAN et al., 1953) the total amount of iron within the kidney was estimated as 3.22 g/100 g dry weight.

Macroscopically the kidneys are dark brown and often enlarged. Microscopically a marked hemosiderosis of the tubular epithelial cells exists in all cases. This was confirmed by HEITZMAN et al. (1953) in a review of 19 autopsied cases since MARCHIAFAVA's first description of the disease.

Basically, all parts of the tubular apparatus may take part in hemosiderosis, from the proximal convoluted tubules to the collecting tubules (HEITZMAN et al., 1953). Apparently the most profound changes, however, concern the proximal convoluted tubules and Henle's loops (WITTS, 1936; RANDERATH and BOHLE, 1959; HUTT et al., 1961; ALTHOFF, 1966, 1967; see Fig. 6). Renal hemosiderosis may be accompanied by intense hemosiderinuria (CROIZAT et al., 1948; JACQUET et al., 1949; HEITZMAN et al., 1953; GAITHER, 1961).

Electronmicroscopic studies have demonstrated that the hemoglobin entering the lumen of the tubuli is reabsorbed by the epithelial cells and transformed into hemosiderin and ferritin (HUTT et al., 1961). The possibility that hemoglobin or ferritin might enter the epithelial cells from the capillaries surrounding the epithelial cells could not be denied but was considered to be less probable. Ferritin could be observed within the glomerular podocytes, in the free space of Bowman's capsule, in the parietal cells of Bowman's capsule, in the lumina of the tubuli and in higher concentration inside the tubular epithelial cells. The high ferritin content of the epithelial cells indicates that the rate of accumulation by far exceeds the delivery of ferritin from the cells. The ferritin may leave the cells in four different ways: 1. by secretion into the tubular lumen, 2. by desquamation of cells loaded with ferritin and hemosiderin, 3. by entering the peritubular capillaries via the epithelial basal membrane, and 4. by transformation into a non-ferritin form which might leave the cell in one of the first three ways mentioned. Since the peritubular capillaries contained more ferritin than the capillaries of the glomerular tuft, the third way appeared to be possible. The second way has been established by light and electron microscopy.

The question as to whether hemosiderosis might disturb renal function can be denied for all but two cases (CROSBY, 1953) and is discussed only by few authors (MARCHIAFAVA, 1911; SUSSMAN and KAYDEN, 1948; JACQUET et al., 1949; HEITZMAN et al., 1953).

In the case of HEITZMAN et al. (1953) each kidney weighed 40 g. The capsule stripped with great difficulty, and the subcapsular surfaces were nodular, rough, moist and brown. The cut surfaces showed indistinctly demarcated cortices and medullary pyramids; there was striking, dark brown, granular pigmentation of the cortices. Microscopically, many of the convoluted tubules and Henle's loops showed marked atrophy, with areas of interstitial fibrosis. Many of the remaining tubules, especially the proximal convoluted tubules, were markedly enlarged.

Hemosiderin was found inside the tubular epithelial cells, in the lumina of the tubules, and predominantly in the interstitial connective tissue. Glomeruli, arterioles and arteries were free of hemosiderin. About half of the glomeruli were completely hyalinized and many others showed thickened and scarred Bowman's capsules, together with focal fibrosis of individual tufts.

HEITZMAN et al. interpreted the picture as "hemosiderin nephrosis with renal failure".

Obviously, it appears more probable that the morphologic changes in the kidneys corresponded to hemosiderin nephrosis in connection with PNH on one hand and to chronic pyelonephritis on the other hand. This is also CROSBY's (1953) opinion who thinks that renal failure in PNH is not the results of massive hemosiderin deposits but of recurring pyelonephritis. In two cases renal failure was caused by nephrosclerosis (GLASER, 1948) and "lower nephron nephrosis" (CROSBY, 1953).

Theoretical arguments also exist against the production of contracted kidneys by intense hemosiderosis. So far no substantial evidence has been obtained in favor of a "cirrhogenous" action of hemosiderin (MACDONALD, 1964). According to MACDONALD liver cirrhosis in hemochromatosis is nothing but an ordinary cirrhosis caused by additional factors independent of hemochromatosis such as alcoholism, dietary deficiency or virus hepatitis. In primary hemochromatosis the weight of the kidneys is in the normal range (SHELDON, 1935; MACDONALD, 1964).

The differential diagnosis between PNH and other types of general siderosis is facilitated by the fact that liver and spleen are usually free of hemosiderin (MERLISS, 1952; for ref. see Table 2 of HEITZMAN et al., 1953). There are, however, exceptions to this rule. In most cases the bone marrow appears to be normal or hyperplastic (HEITZMAN et al., 1953).

b) Traumatic Hemolytic Anemias

To date about 5 hemolytic conditions are known which are characterized by mechanical, traumatic origin of hemolysis. In two of them (so-called athletic and march hemoglobinuria) alterations of renal morphology are unknown. Morphologic changes of the kidney in the other types of traumatic hemolytic anemias and hemoglobinuria have become known only in the last years. This group comprises the following conditions: Hemoglobinuria and renal siderosis in chronic cardiac valvular disease, following implantation of valvular prostheses, and in microangiopathy.

1. Athletic Hemoglobinuria

Normal individuals performing long strenuous runs often develop severe hemoglobinemia and hemoglobinuria. JUNDELL and FRIES (1911) found 4 cases with intense hemoglobinuria among 39 subjects who ran distances of 10,000 to 42,194 meters. GILLIGAN et al. (1943) described moderate hemoglobinemia in 10 out of 22 men who had run races of 2.6—2.8 and 4.5—5.1 miles. 18 out of 22 men who had run 26.2 miles in the marathon race developed severe hemoglobinemia up to 44 mg-% at the end of the race. After the marathon race hemoglobinuria was observed in 4 of 5 subjects who had plasma hemoglobin levels of between 20 and 44 mg-%. Most of the marathon runners showed formed elements in the urine. Anomalies of erythrocyte morphology were not, however, to be seen. Hemolysis was never followed by hemolytic anemia. Proteinuria was observed in all the marathon runners including those who did not develop hemoglobinuria. This is remarkable since the renal threshold for hemoglobin may be lowered by preexisting proteinuria to values of about 30—50 mg-% (see p. 100). This may explain hemoglobinuria in those subjects whose serum level of hemoglobin amounted to less than 50 mg-%. The proteinuria may last longer than the hemoglobinuria (FINNY, 1926). Hemoglobinuria has also been described in football players (according to BOONE et al., 1955, in 16.2%).

Though renal siderosis has not yet been described in athletic hemoglobinuria it can be anticipated that transitory renal siderosis might develop in this condition.

2. March Hemoglobinuria

March hemoglobinuria is observed exclusively in healthy young men and may presumably also lead to transitory renal siderosis. It is independent of fever, hyperventilation, other physical disturbances, familial or racial factors (GILLIGAN and BLUMGART, 1941). Usually hemoglobinuria disappears within hours. In rare cases it may last some days. Spleen and liver are transiently enlarged (for ref. see ROSS, 1945). Usually the attacks of hemoglobinuria disappear without any therapy within several months to years. Only in exceptional cases can they be observed over many years (FÖRSTER, 1919: more than 20 years). They are not followed by hemolytic anemia since the amount of blood destroyed does not exceed 40 ml. There are no anomalies of the blood cells incl. leukocytes and thrombocytes. Osmotic fragility of erythrocytes is normal. The serum does not contain agglutinins or hemolysins (GILLIGAN and BLUMGART, 1941).

Plasma-Hb may reach values of up to 200 mg-%, the urine may contain 1.5 g Hb/100 ml. Regularly, hemoglobinuria is accompanied by proteinuria.

March hemoglobinuria is produced by short brisk walks or fast runs in the lordotic (upright) posture. Hemoglobinuria does not appear in the same persons if they undergo physical exercise in kyphotic (bent over) position (WITTS, 1936; PORGES and STRISOWER, 1914; GILLIGAN and BLUMGART, 1941). In march hemoglobinuria the renal threshold for hemoglobin is markedly lowered (GILLIGAN and BLUMGART, 1941).

According to ROBERTS and MORROW (1966) march hemoglobinuria may be associated with renal siderosis in biopsy specimens. The publication cited by ROBERTS and MORROW (LEONARDI and RUOL, 1960) does not, however, contain evidence in favor of this statement.

Finally, it must be pointed out that the pigment appearing in blood and urine is hemoglobin and not myoglobin. This is true for march hemoglobinuria as well as for athletic hemoglobinuria.

3. Traumatic Hemolytic Anemia in Chronic Cardiac Valvular Disease

Only during the last few years have we learnt that chronic cardiac valvular disease may be the cause of traumatic hemolytic anemias. The first case was published by DAMESHEK in 1964. A 64-year old woman showed a hemolytic anemia with reticulocyte counts up to 18%. Clinical diagnosis was "hemolytic anemia of unknown type and rheumatic heart disease, with aortic and mitral stenosis and regurgitation". Autopsy revealed "hemolytic anemia, with renal tubular hemosiderosis, due to paroxysmal nocturnal hemoglobinuria or erythrocyte trauma caused by calcified heart valves" and "rheumatic heart disease, severe, with aortic stenosis and insufficiency, mitral stenosis and insufficiency and tricuspid stenosis". The blood smear of the patient contained numerous "helmet cells" (see p. 124). DAMESHEK pointed out that the same type of disrupted erythrocytes is to be observed in thrombotic thrombocytopenic purpura, and he considered it probable that the fragmentation of the erythrocytes might be caused by passage of the blood through the narrowed small vessels. He felt that the same mechanism of traumatic hemolysis might be responsible for the appearance of helmet cells in cardiac valvular disease and might be the cause of hemosiderosis of the kidneys. Hemosiderin was found in the epithelial cells of the convoluted tubules and Henle's loops. Little pigment was contained in the proximal collecting tubules and in Bowman's spaces but none in the distal collecting tubules. Spleen, liver and bone marrow were free of hemosiderin. Bone marrow erythropoiesis was somewhat hyperplastic.

First investigations using ferrokinetic methods were carried out by BRODEUR et al. (1965a and b). Erythrocyte life span proved to be shortened in 15 out of 21 patients with aortic valvular disease. This observation was thought to be due to traumatic mechanical hemolysis. Only one patient showed a compensated hemolytic anemia (hematocrit 35%, reticulocyte count 4%). A shortening of erythrocyte life span was also found in 14 patients with chronic mitral valvular disease in spite of normal reticulocyte numbers and hematocrit values (BRODEUR et al., 1966).

GEHRMANN and LOOGEN (1966) described compensated hemolysis in 17 out of 47 patients with different types of valvular disease. Erythrocyte life span was most frequently shortened in the group with valvular stenosis (6 out of 9 cases with aortic stenosis, all 3 cases of mitral stenosis). On the other hand, erythrocyte life span was normal in 7 out of 11 cases with aortic insufficiency and all cases of mitral insufficiency. The observations of DAMESHEK, BRODEUR et al. and GEHRMANN and LOOGEN could be confirmed by several authors, in some cases by establishing renal siderosis at autopsy.

MILLER et al. (1966) described a 27 year old man with moderate aortic and mitral stenosis and insufficiency. Hb amounted to 11.4—11.7 g-%, the reticulocyte count to 30—63 % and hematocrit to 39%. Mechanic fragility of erythrocytes in vitro was normal, the Coombs test negative, complete or incomplete warm and cold hemolysins and agglutinins could not be established. The erythrocytes were normochromic, the blood smear contained several fragmented erythrocytes. Bone marrow erythropoiesis was hyperplastic. In a first set of investigations during which the patient was bedridden, erythrocyte life span was normal. In a second set the patient was exhausted twice daily until dyspnea and tachycardia (100—125/min) developed. During this period erythrocyte life span decreased markedly. Surgical biopsy of the kidney was not performed but the cells of the urinary sediment gave a strongly positive Prussian blue reaction.

Another case was reported by Westring (1966). The 20 year old woman was suffering from aortic insufficiency and showed a hemolytic anemia with hemoglobin values of 9.5 g-%, a hematocrit of 27% and reticulocyte counts of 27 to 43 $^o/_{oo}$. The Coombs test was negative. The erythrocytes were morphologically intact. Six months after the implantation of an aortic prosthesis (Starr-Edwards) Hb had fallen to 6.8 g-% and the hematocrit to 21% while the reticulocyte count had increased to 68$^o/_{oo}$. The mechanic fragility of the erythrocytes was normal, the urinary sediment did not contain hemosiderin. Later on the blood smear showed numerous fragmentocytes. At autopsy 18 months after the operation the tubular epithelial cells showed a marked hemosiderosis. Since symptoms of a hemolytic anemia had been found preoperatively, it may be concluded that the siderosis of the kidney had also developed before the times of operation, but that it was enhanced by the implantation of the prosthesis and tearing of the prosthesis which had demanded a second operation 8 months prior to death.

Westring investigated 12 more cases with aortic valvular disease and among them found one woman with hemolytic anemia and shortened erythrocyte life span, high reticulocyte count and fragmentocytes (schistocytes) in peripheral blood. At the same time the patient was suffering from Lues III. The Donath-Landsteiner test and the Coombs test were negative. Two more patients had a shortened erythrocyte life span, three a reticulocytosis above 20$^o/_{oo}$. The number of schistocytes in blood did not differ significantly between the group of patients with valvular disease and a control group consisting of 35 healthy individuals. The control group showed 2.8$^o/_{oo}$ schistocytes (mean value), the cardiac disease group 2.1$^o/_{oo}$. The range, 0—6$^o/_{oo}$ schistocytes, was the same for both groups.

Ziperovich and Paley (1966) mentioned a 23 year old woman with mitral stenosis and insufficiency who developed a hemolytic anemia following suture of a cleft in the anterior mitral valve. It was accompanied by reticulocytosis, poikilocytosis and anisocytosis in peripheral blood and by Hb-uria. The hemolytic anemia disappeared within 15 days after implantation of a Starr-Edwards ball prosthesis.

19 patients (= 3%) out of about 600 with different cardiac valvular diseases showed anomalies of erythrocyte morphology, 17 without any symptoms of anemia (Forshaw and Harwood, 1967). The authors think that the negative results of Miller et al. (1966) and Westring (1966) are due to the small number of cases investigated by these authors.

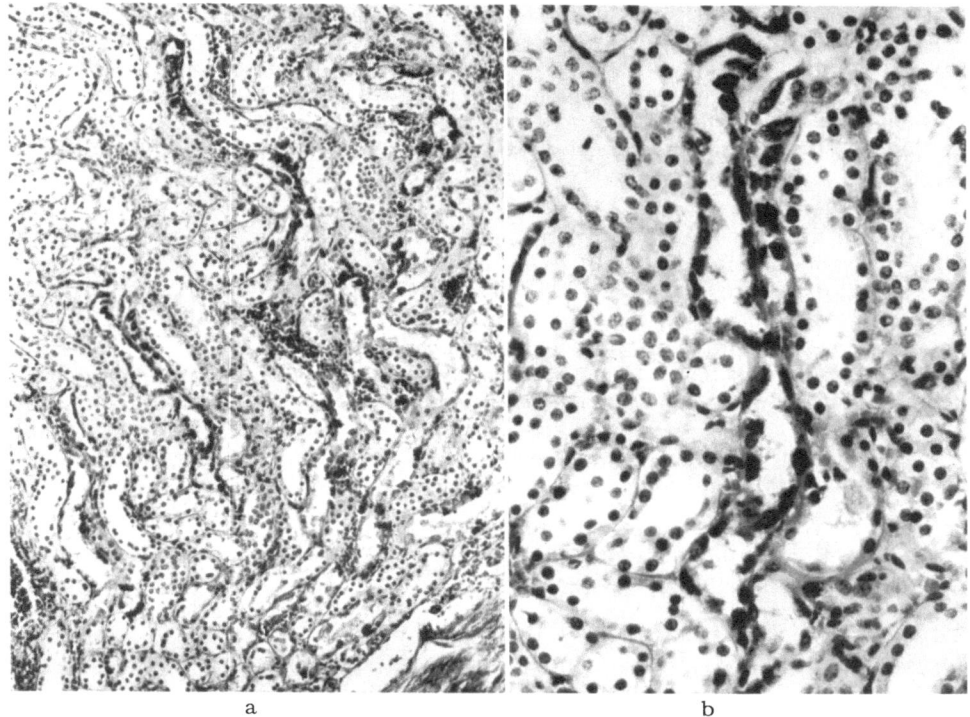

a   b

Fig. 2a and b. Renal siderosis in chronic ulcerative aortic endocarditis with destruction
of the aortic valves and calcification. Deposition of hemosiderin inside the epithelial cells
of the loops of Henle. Case No. 7. Prussian blue reaction. a 110×. b 280×

A study of the pathology of renal siderosis in chronic cardiac valvular
disease was published by ROBERTS in 1966. Four cases out of a group of
135 patients with severe stenosis and/or insufficiency of the heart valves
(functional classes III to IV according to the classification of the New York
Heart Association) had intense hemosiderosis of the kidneys, predominantly
of the proximal convoluted tubules. On no occasion was a hemosiderosis of
the liver and spleen observed. In 3 cases hemosiderin was diminished in the
bone marrow, in one case it was elevated. The erythropoiesis was hyperplastic
in all cases. The hematocrit values prior to death had amounted to 33—42%,
in one case the reticulocyte count had been slightly elevated (23°/$_{00}$). These
4 patients had aortic stenosis and insufficiency, and their aortic valves were
severely calcified.

Our material of mitral and aortic insufficiency and stenosis contains
2 cases with renal siderosis among a total number of 107.

Case No. 6

A. H., 62 y. old woman.

Clinical diagnosis: Aortic stenosis and insufficiency, severe congestive heart
failure.

Autopsy (S 275/64): Severe aortic stenosis with calcification. Recurrent verrucous endocarditis of the mitral valve. Scar in the apex of the left chamber following myocardial infarction. Both ventricles hypertrophied and dilated (heart 585 g).

Kidneys: Chronic congestion of the kidneys (275 g). Occasional siderosis of the epithelial cells of the proximal convoluted tubules. Few Henle's loops contain casts giving a positive granular Prussian blue reaction.

Case No. 7

W. B., 43 y. old woman.

Clinical diagnosis: Aortic vitium known for several years. Recurrent subacute bacterial endocarditis (SR 40/80, 10,000 leukocytes)?

Autopsy (S 467/67): Chronic ulcerative aortic endocarditis with destruction of the aortic valves and calcification. Severe hypertrophy and dilation of the left chamber. Severe chronic serofibrinous pericarditis, so-called cor villosum and hydropericardium (800 ml). Heart 1220 g! Moderate hypertrophy and dilation of the right ventricle. Congestion of liver, spleen, kidneys, gastrointestinal tract.

Kidneys: Enlarged, severely congested (420 g). Moderate siderosis of some proximal convoluted tubules, intense siderosis of Henle's loops (Fig. 2), considerable siderosis of several distal convoluted tubules (in contrast to the findings of Roberts).

4. Traumatic Hemolytic Anemia Following Implantation of Cardiac Valvular Prostheses

In 1954 Rose *et al.* reported that following implantation of a Hufnagel prosthesis into the aorta descendens immediately below the left subclavian artery all eight patients under observation showed a lowered hematocrit compared to the time before operation. The decrease amounted to 3—8, in one case 16 mm. This type of hemolysis has to be distinguished from hemolysis produced by extracorporal circulation during the operation (Cahill and Kolff, 1959; Stewart and Sturridge, 1959; Keith *et al.*, 1961; Osborn *et al.*, 1962; Nunn *et al.*, 1963; Radochova *et al.*, 1967; Shaw, 1967).

Evidence for hemolysis caused by cardiac prosthesis was first obtained by Stohlman *et al.* (1955, 1956). These authors implanted a lucite conduit containing a Hufnagel valve between the left ventricular apex and thoracic aorta in 15 dogs. In all animals red cell destruction took place and was associated with hemoglobinemia, hemoglobinuria, anemia, reticulocytosis and renal siderosis. The hematocrit began to fall 7 to 10 days after the operation and reached values of 20 to 50% of the hematocrit before the operation. The reticulocyte count began to increase 3 to 5 days postoperatively up to $150^0/_{00}$. Initial Hb values in blood serum were 180—800 mg-%, and even several months after the operation levels of 75—280 mg-% were observed. Each animal showed hemosiderinuria. Erythrocyte life span was markedly reduced. The kidneys of four animals dying during the experiment showed intense hemosiderosis, predominantly of the proximal convoluted tubules.

α) *Clinical Aspects*

Since the first report by Sayed *et al.* in 1961 on two cases of traumatic hemolytic anemia following cardiac surgery more than 80 cases have been published to date (Table). In addition, traumatic hemolysis caused by surgery of heart valves was observed by the following authors whose papers were either not obtainable or contain no exact description of the individual cases: SARNOFF et al. (1955); McGOON et al. (1963); DE CESARE et al. (1964); DENNIS et al. (1964); LARSON and KIRKLIN (1964); ANDERSEN et al. (1965); GREEN (1965); TJORSTAD (1966); PEDEFERRI et al. (1967). According to GEHRMANN et al. (1966) hemolytic complications have to be anticipated in almost two thirds of patients with implantation of a valvular prosthesis. Following implantation of a Starr-Edwards prosthesis, 9 out of 201 patients (= 4.5 %) developed a manifest hemolytic anemia (PEDEFERRI et al., 1967).

Hemoglobinemia was markedly present in many cases (Table). Sometimes values of up to 1 g-% were measured (REED and DUNN, 1964), values above 200 mg-% are no rarity (VERDON et al., 1963, case 2; SAYED et al., 1961, case 1; PIROFSKY et al., 1965, case 6). Consequently, *hemoglobinuria* is frequent (Table). In a few patients, precise levels are given (SAYED et al., 1961: 2.6 to 6.0 g/24 hr.; PIROFSKY et al., 1965: 156 mg-%).

Methemalbuminemia was observed by several authors (SAYED et al., 1961; SIGLER et al., 1963; MARSH, 1964, 1966; REED and DUNN, 1964; BUCHER et al., 1965; VINER and FROST, 1965). This is well understandable in view of the high Hb levels in blood plasma which by far exceed the binding capacity of haptoglobin for Hb (see p. 101).

In many cases *haptoglobin* could not be found in the blood serum (SAYED et al., 1961; SIGLER et al., 1963; MARSH, 1964, 1966; STEVENSON and BAKER, 1964; DE CESARE et al., 1965; YENKO et al., 1965) or it was considerably diminished (DE CESARE et al., 1965; PETZ et al., 1966; REYNOLDS et al., 1967). In some cases haptoglobin levels rose following surgery (SAYED et al., 1961; SIGLER et al., 1963).

The *serum iron level* (normal value: 50—200 µg-%, VAHLQUIST, 1959) was frequently normal (SIGLER et al., 1963; DE CESARE et al., 1965; BRODEUR et al., 1965, 1966; RUBINSON et al., 1966; REYNOLDS et al., 1967), sometimes decreased (SIGLER et al., 1963; VERDON et al., 1963; BRODEUR et al., 1965; FURUHJELM et al., 1964; SANYL et al., 1964; YENKO et al., 1965; RUBINSON et al., 1966; REYNOLDS et al., 1967) or elevated (SAYED et al., 1961; VINER and FROST, 1965; PETZ et al., 1966: 376 µg-%). These deviations from the normal state are well known in hemolytic anemias and explained by increased erythrocyte destruction or a high rate of regeneration (VAHLQUIST, 1959).

The *iron-binding capacity* (normal value: 250—400 µg; LAURELL, 1959) is mostly normal (BRODEUR et al., 1965, 1966; BUCHER et al., 1965; DE CESARE et al., 1965; YENKO et al., 1965; RUBINSON et al., 1966; REYNOLDS et al., 1967) or elevated (VERDON et al., 1963; case 1: 457 µg; FURUHJELM et al., 1964: 543 µg; PETZ et al., 1966, case 1: 410 µg; SANYL et al., 1964; VINER and FROST, 1965). Higher values than normal may be explained by a state of iron deficiency (LAURELL, 1959).

Daily *urinary excretion of iron* is described as too high (SIGLER et al., 1963, case 1: 56—390 µg-%; case 2: 1,200 µg-%; case 3: 380—520 µg-%; REYNOLDS et al., 1967, case 2: 1,000 µg-%) or normal (YENKO et al., 1965: 3.6 µg-%).

Table. *Traumatic hemolytic anemia*

Authors	Age, Sex	Time before operation			Surgery Type of prosthesis
		Type of vitium	Ht (%)	Hb (g-%)	
Sayed et al. (1961) Case 1	25, ♂	Ost. I Def.	—	15.1	Teflon patch
					bare teflon, reoperation after 6 mths.
Case 2	no details given				
Sigler et al. (1963) Case 1	5, ♀	ASD/VSD	38,4	12	Teflon patch
					Excision of bare teflon
Case 2	16, ♀	Ost. I Def.	42	—	Teflon patch
Case 3	8, ♂	ASD/VSD	34	—	Teflon patch
Verdon et al. (1963) Case 1	17, ♂	ASD	48	15.7	Teflon patch correction
Case 2	11, ♀	Complete AV Canal	—	—	Teflon patch
Furuhjelm et al. (1964)	15, ♂	ASD/VSD	—	—	Suture Teflon patch
Gehrmann et al. (1964) Case 1	33, ♂	Ao Ins.	—	16.1	3 Hufnagel valves Fixation of disrupted valve
Case 2	26, ♂	Ao Ins.	—	15.8	3 Hufnagel valves

following cardiac surgery. Case reports

Time interval	Ht (%)	Hb (g-%)	Reti (%)	Schistocytes Poikilocytes Fragmento- cytes (%)	Hb-emia (mg-%)	Hemo- globin- uria	Hemo- siderin- uria
?	—	6.5	7.7	S, B	150 to 316	2.6 to 6.0 g/day	+++
?	—	norm.	< 1	Ø	4	—	+++
3 w.	27	—	14—22	—	43—57	—	++++
6 m.	23	6.1	17	P	—	—	—
11 m.	17.5	4.4	—	P	—	—	—
4 m.	43 to 51	—	< 3	Ø	(+)	Ø	(+)
2 w.	20	<10	~40	—	—	—	++++
5 m.	25	6	11	P	—	—	—
2 m.	32	10	—	—	—	—	—
8 m.	24	7.7	↑	P	—	—	—
16 m.	37.5	12	↑	—	13—50	—	++++
14 d.	32	11	—	—	—	—	—
4 m.	29	8.4	5—10	—	19	—	—
2 m.	—	12	8	—	—	—	—
9 d.	↓	—	—	—	250	3 mg/ min	—
4 m.	—	—	20—30	P, F	+	+	—
8 m.	—	8	—	—	—	—	—
4 d.	—	8.9	—	—	—	—	—
1 w.	—	—	—	—	—	—	—
?	25 to 30	<10	5—20	P, F	—	—	—
20 m.	—	9.3	7.1	—	—	—	+++
6 w.	—	13.8	—	Ø	—	—	—
9 m.	—	10	8.2	S, P	—	+	—
6 m.	—	10.6	6.1	S, P	—	—	—
6 w.	—	14.8	—	Ø	—	—	—
2 m.	—	15.0	—	Ø	—	—	—
10 m.	—	10.9	6.4	S, P	—	—	—

Table

| Authors | Age, Sex | Time before operation | | | Surgery |
		Type of vitium	Ht (%)	Hb (g-%)	Type of prosthesis
MARSH *et al.* (1964)					
Case 1	48, ♂	Ao Sten.	—	14.2	Starr-Edwards
Case 2	47, ♂	Ao Vit.	—	12.5	Starr-Edwards
REED *et al.* (1964)	32, ♂	Ao Sten.+Ins.	—	—	Starr-Edwards
					Valve re-attached
SANYL *et al.* (1964)	15, ♀	Ost. I+II Def.	n.	n.	Teflon patch
STEVENSON *et al.* (1964)					
Case 1	16, ♂	Ao Ins.	n.	n.	Starr-Edwards
Case 2	39, ♂	Ao Vit.	—	—	Starr-Edwards
BRODEUR *et al.* (1965)					
Case 2	50, ♂	Ao Ins.	—	—	Starr-Edwards
Case 3	43, ♂	Ao Sten.+Ins.	—	—	Starr-Edwards
Case 10	45, ♂	Ao Sten.+Ins.	—	—	Starr-Edwards
Case 24	57, ♀	Ao Sten.	—	—	Starr-Edwards
Case 25	51, ♂	Ao Sten.+Ins.	—	—	Starr-Edwards
Case 31	39, ♂	Ao+Mit. Ins.	—	—	Starr-Edwards
Case 38	50, ♂	Sten.+Ins.	—	—	Starr-Edwards
Case 45	53, ♀	Ao Sten.+Ins.	39	—	Starr-Edwards
Case 47	38, ♀	Ao Sten.+Ins.	37	—	Starr-Edwards
BUCHER *et al.* (1965)					
Case 1	40, ♀	Sept. I Def.	41	13.6	Teflon patch
Case 2	18, ♀	VSD	—	—	Teflon patch
DE CESARE *et al.* (1965)					
Case 1	35, ♂	Ao Vit.	44	—	Dacron prosthesis Disk valve

(continued)

Time after operation							
Time interval	Ht (%)	Hb (g-%)	Reti (%)	Schistocytes Poikilocytes Fragmentocytes (%)	Hb-emia (mg-%)	Hemoglobinuria	Hemosiderinuria
6 w.	—	5.2	14.6	F ++	42—98	—	++
3 w.	—	7.8	12.0	F ++	26—32	—	++
4 d.	~26	~ 8.5	—	—	4	—	—
12 d.	~32	~10	—	—	>100	++	—
30 d.	~18	~ 7	—	—	>450	—	—
4 h.	—	—	—	—	50	Urine clear	—
8 h.	—	—	—	—	>850	++	—
4 d.	~16	~ 5	—	—	>750	—	—
7 w.	—	7	—	—	—	—	—
7 m.	17	5	—	F, P	—	—	+
2 m.	—	8	3—8	20—27	5.6—18	+	—
4 m.	—	12.4	8.3	P	18	—	—
5 m.	25	7.7	1—9	17—21 P	1.5	+	—
7 m.	35	—	3.8	—	—	—	—
23 m.	27	10	7.1	S	—	—	++++
12 m.	38	—	1.3	—	—	—	—
10 m.	42	—	1.8	—	—	—	—
11 m.	30	—	2.9	—	—	—	—
6 m.	37	—	0.6	—	—	—	—
6 m.	44	—	0.8	—	—	—	—
13 m.	29	—	4.5	—	—	—	—
4 m.	39	—	2.7	—	—	—	—
8 m.	36	—	2.1	—	—	—	—
14 d.	12	4.8	6.9	P, F, S	+	+	—
3 a.	—	10.6	3.4	(P, F, S)	Ø	Ø	—
26 m.	25	—	12	7 F	39	—	++++
?	35	—	2—4	3—4	—	—	—
?	34	—	2—3	Ø	—	—	—

Table

| Authors | Age, Sex | Time before operation | | | Surgery |
		Type of vitium	Ht (%)	Hb (g-%)	Type of prosthesis
De Cesare et al. (1965) Case 2	23, ♂	Ao Vit.	—	—	3 Dacron valves
Case 3	35, ♂	Ao Sten. + Ins.	42	—	correction 3 Dacron valves
Pirofsky et al. (1965) Case 1	32, ♂	Ao, Mi, Tri Vit.	—	—	Starr-Edwards (Mi, Ao, Tri) Fix. of Mi. + Tri. prosth.
Case 2	37, ♀	Mi + Ao Vit.	—	—	Starr-Edwards
Case 3	24, ♀	Ao Sten.	—	—	Starr-Edwards
Case 4	42, ♂	Ao Sten.	—	—	Starr-Edwards
Case 5	28, ♂	Ao + Mi Vit.	47	—	Starr-Edwards
Case 6	35, ♂	Ao Sten.	—	—	Starr-Edwards
Case 7	34, ♂	Ao + Mi + Tri Vit.	—	—	Starr-Edwards Ao, Mi, Tri
Viner et al. (1965)	45, ♀	Ao Vit.	—	15.2	Teflon valve
Yeh et al. (1965)	38, ♂	Ao Sten.	47	15.6	Bahnson-Teflon cusps Starr-Edwards

(continued)

| Time after operation | | | | | | | |
Time inter- val	Ht (%)	Hb (g-%)	Reti (%)	Schistocytes Poikilocytes Fragmento- cytes (%)	(Hb-emia mg-%)	Hemo- globin- uria	Hemo- siderin- uria
6 m.	43	—	—	—	—	—	—
23 m.	34	—	7.1	—	—	—	—
29 m.	25	—	17	11 F	—	—	++++
37 m.	27	—	14	—	—	—	—
1 m.	n.	—	n.	—	n.	—	—
2 w.	36	—	—	—	—	—	—
8 m.	28 to 32	—	10	—	—	—	—
12 m.	35	—	7	11 F	—	—	—
16 m.	40	—	1	—	—	—	—
9 d.	30	—	4	—	—	—	—
18 d.	18	5.3	5	—	—	—	—
6 m.	n.	—	n.	—	—	—	—
9 d.	34.5	—	0.7	—	—	—	—
12 d.	26	—	6.5	—	—	—	—
10 d.	34	—	2.5	—	—	—	—
13 d.	30	—	5.5	—	—	—	—
67 d.	39	14	0.9	—	—	—	—
3 d.	32.5	—	—	—	—	—	—
14 d.	22	—	2.0	—	—	—	—
27 d.	17	—	6.0	—	—	—	—
3 m.	35	12.4	3.4	—	—	—	—
5 d.	35	—	0.8	—	—	—	—
12 d.	35	—	3.5	—	—	—	—
36 d.	34	—	2.9	—	—	—	—
6/7 d.	33	—	2.3	—	420	156	—
44 d.	23	—	20.1	—	—	—	—
7 m.	32.5	—	6.4	—	—	—	—
8 d.	32	—	3.6	—	—	—	—
28 d.	29	—	9.2	—	—	—	—
51 d.	34	11.8	4.0	—	—	—	—
14 m.	—	7	13	—	—	—	—
15 m.	—	—	28	F	—	—	—
20 m.	—	4	16	P, F, B*	—	—	—
18 m.	30	9.8	—	—	—	—	—
20 m.	24	8.0	11.9	—	—	—	—
22 m.	23	6.4	—	—	—	—	—
10 m.	41	13.8	4.2	—	—	—	—

* B = Burr cells

Authors	Age, Sex	Time before operation			Surgery
		Type of vitium	Ht (%)	Hb (g-%)	Type of prosthesis
Yenko et al. (1965)					
Case 1	8, ♂	Mi Ins.	47	14.7	Teflon bolster
Case 2	8, ♂	Ost. I + II Def.	36	11.8	Teflon patch
Brodeur et al. (1966)					
Case 1	34, ♀	Mi Vit. + Ao Ins. —		—	Starr-Edwards
Case 3	38, ♂	Mi Vit. + Ao Ins. —		—	Starr-Edwards
Case 6	47, ♀	Mi Vit. —		—	Starr-Edwards
Case 9	32, ♀	Mi Vit. + Ao Sten. —		—	Starr-Edwards
Brodeur et al. (1966)					
Case 1	31, ♂	Ao, Mi, Tri	—	—	Starr-Edwards
Case 2	39, ♂	Ao + Mi Ins.	—	—	Starr-Edwards
Case 5	52, ♀	Ao, Mi	—	—	Starr-Edwards
Case 6	29, ♂	Ao, Mi	—	—	Starr-Edwards
Case 7	36, ♂	Ao, Mi	36	—	Starr-Edwards
Case 8	36, ♀	Ao, Mi	—	—	Starr-Edwards
Case 9	48, ♀	Ao, Mi, Tri	—	—	Starr-Edwards
Case 10	25, ♀	Ao, Mi, Tri	—	—	Starr-Edwards
Gehrmann et al. (1966)					
Case 1	28, ♂	Ao Sten.	—	16.4	Starr-Edwards
Case 3	37, ♂	Ao Sten.	—	14.6	Starr-Edwards
Case 6	34, ♂	Ao Sten. + Ins.	—	14.6	Starr-Edwards
Case 7	30, ♂	Ao Ins.	—	14.1	Starr-Edwards
Case 8	32, ♂	Ao Ins.	—	15.1	Starr-Edwards
Case 9	29, ♀	Mi Ins.	—	13.1	Starr-Edwards
Case 10	27, ♀	Mi Ins.	—	13.0	Starr-Edwards
Case 11	39, ♂	Ao Ins.	—	16.1	Hufnagel
Case 12	26, ♂	Ao Ins.	—	15.8	Hufnagel
Case 13	36, ♀	Ao Sten.	—	15.2	Bahnson
Marsh et al. (1966)	57, ♀	Mi Ins.	—	—	Hammersmith prosthesis

(continued)

Time after operation							
Time inter-val	Ht (%)	Hb (g-%)	Reti (%)	Schistocytes Poikilocytes Fragmento-cytes (%)	Hb-emia (mg-%)	Hemo-globin-uria	Hemo-siderin-uria
12 d.	27	8.5	5.1	—	—	—	—
5 w.	29	8.8	6.2	—	—	—	—
6 w.	28	—	—	—	—	—	—
8 m.	27 to 34	8.7 to 10.8	2.8 to 5.9	—	20.8	—	0 to ++++
8 m.	39	—	1.2	—	—	—	—
23 m.	43	—	2.1	—	—	—	—
37 m.	36	—	2.3	—	—	—	—
8 m.	38	—	0.4	—	—	—	—
3 m.	28	—	4.3	—	—	—	—
9 m.	41	—	2.3	F	—	—	—
6 m.	33	—	3.1	F, H, S	—	—	—
13 m.	30	—	3.6	F, H, S	—	—	++
3 m.	37	—	1.3	—	—	—	—
4 m.	37	—	1.8	—	—	—	—
13 m.	36	—	0.2	—	—	—	—
5 m.	37	—	1.5	—	—	—	—
3 m.	37	—	0.6	—	—	—	—
5 m.	—	11.5	5.3	0.9 S	25.1	—	—
6 w.	—	12.9	5.6	2.7 S	—	—	—
3 m.	—	11.6	7.5	2.9 S	25.4	—	—
4 m.	—	8.3	14.1	13.7 S	55.4	—	—
4 m.	—	13.4	3.9	2.9 S	12.5	—	—
3 m.	—	12.0	2.2	1.4 S	17.3	—	—
2 m.	—	12.0	2.9	3.2 S	11.3	—	—
16 m.	—	10.6	6.1	18.9 S	25.9	—	—
10 m.	—	10.9	6.4	11.2 S	—	—	—
18 m.	—	12.8	1.9	0.6 S	1.2	—	—
12 w.	—	8.7	—	—	—	—	+
19 w.	—	6.4	14.0	P, F	18—26	—	+

Authors	Age, Sex	Time before operation			Surgery
		Type of vitium	Ht (%)	Hb (g-%)	Type of prosthesis
McGarvey et al. (1966)	56, ♂	Ao Vit.	—	—	Starr-Edwards
Petz et al. (1966) Case 1	42, ♂	Ao Sten.	42	13.2	Starr-Edw.
Case 2	32, ♀	Ao Ins.	36.5	12.2	Reoperation Starr-Edwards Dacron patch
Rubinson et al. (1966) Case 1	48, ♂	Ao Sten.	43	—	Müller-Teflon prosthesis
Case 2	44, ♀	Ao, MI, Vit.	49	—	Starr-Edwards Müller-Teflon prosthesis
Case 3	37, ♂	Ao Vit.	44	—	Müller-Teflon prosthesis
Case 4	33, ♀	Ao Sten.	43.5	—	2 Teflon cusps
Case 5	38, ♂	Ao Sten.	48	—	Starr-Edwards
Westring et al. (1966)	20, ♀	Ao Vit.	31	10	Starr-Edwards Fix. of prost.
Forshaw et al. (1967) Case 1	28, ♂	Mi Sten.	—	14.8	Starr-Edwards
Case 2	37, ♀	Ao Mi.	—	—	Mi. Ao pr.
Reynolds et al. (1967) Case 1	30, ♀	Mi Vit.	—	—	Starr-Edwards
Case 2	30, ♀	Mi Sten.	—	14.2	Starr-Edwards
Case 3	33, ♂	Ao Ins.	—	—	

(continued)

Time after operation							
Time interval	Ht (%)	Hb (g-%)	Reti (%)	Schistocytes Poikilocytes Fragmentocytes (%)	Hb-emia (mg-%)	Hemoglobinuria	Hemosiderinuria
7 d.	32	9.2	6.2	S	>40	+	+
18 d.	27	8.3	9.8	S	>40	+	+
33 d.	26	7.8	11.6	S	>40	+	+
3 m.	24	8.4	6.5	10	—	—	+++
8 m.	21	—	17.6	20 S	65	—	—
6 m.	30	—	4.7	8 S	26	—	—
6 w.	39	12.6	—	—	—	—	—
8 m.	17.5	5.7	14.8	16 S	81	—	+
18 m.	32	9.9	7.2	S	—	+	+
?	43	—	n.	—	—	0	—
23 m.	36	—	7.4	—	—	+	+
29 m.	36	—	6.2	—	95	—	—
2 a.	32.5	—	7.9	—	—	0	+
10 m.	30	9.8	3.2	—	—	—	—
14 m.	30	8.0	—	—	—	—	—
2 w.	32	—	—	—	—	—	—
14 m.	39	—	2.4	S	—	0	0
6 m.	21	6.8	6.8	S	37.8	—	+
1 m.	—	6.5—8	5—25	S	—	—	+
9 d.	—	5.9	18	P, S, B	—	—	—
26 d.	—	12.6	3	n.	—	—	—
39 d.	—	12.7	5	—	—	—	—
?	—	8.3	14	P, S, B	—	—	+
3 m.	—	8.8—7	14	P, 20 S	—	—	+
10 to 11 m.	—	9.6 to 11.4	6.4	15 S	34	—	—
11 w.	—	5.9	9.6	4 S	60	—	—
20 m.	36	12	5.7	—	—	—	—
ca. 2 w.	—	10	7	5 S	61.6	—	++++

Changes of erythrocyte morphology and function are of special interest. In many cases the blood smear is characterized by the appearance of so-called *fragmentocytes, schistocytes, pyknocytes* or *helmet cells*. Some authors describe the presence of *"burr cells"* in the blood smears of patients following cardiac surgery.

Schistocytes (fragmentocytes, pyknocytes) are desintegrated erythrocytes (EHRLICH, 1886) which on a blood smear appear "as if they had burst or, at times, as if a wedge had been removed" (MIALE, 1962). They are the result of abnormal cellular destruction in hemolytic processes.

If these cells assume the shape of hemispheres they are often called *"helmet cells"* (possible German translation: "Hauben"- or "Stahlhelm"-Zellen). DAMESHEK (1954) in his first publication on traumatic hemolysis in chronic valvular disease describes them as follows: "Helmet cells assume different shapes and might be specified as Germanic, British or American".

Burr cells were first described by SCHWARTZ and MOTTO in 1949. These are erythrocytes with a diameter of 7.5 μ or below and one or more spiderlike processes. They are found predominantly in uremia but also in patients with cancer of the stomach and bleeding ulcers of the stomach (SCHWARTZ and MOTTO, 1949) and in children with acute hemolytic anemia (AHERNE, 1957; ALLISON, 1957; SHUMWAY and MILLER, 1957; LOCK and DORMANDY, 1961). At least some cases of the hemolytic uremic syndrome appear to be equivalent to the generalized Sanarelli-Shwartzman phenomenon (see case No. 11, p. 135).

Fragmentocytes, helmet cells and burr cells are frequently observed in the blood of patients with cardiac valvular prostheses (Table). The normal blood contains up to 0.3 % (mean: 0.28 %) schistocytes (WESTRING, 1966). In children higher values are found (up to 1.9 % in full term infants and 1.3—5.6 % in premature infants: TUFFY *et al.*, 1959). In patients with valvular prostheses more than 25 % schistocytes were observed (STEVENSON and BAKER, 1964).

The *erythrocyte life span* is frequently diminished (SAYED *et al.*, 1961; SIGLER *et al.*, 1963; VERDON *et al.*, 1963; FURUHJELM *et al.*, 1964; MARSH, 1964, 1966; STEVENSON and BAKER, 1964; BUCHER *et al.*, 1965; DE CESARE *et al.*, 1965; VINER and FROST, 1965; YEH, 1965; YENKO *et al.*, 1965; McGARVEY *et al.*, 1964; PETZ *et al.*, 1966; RUBINSON *et al.*, 1966; REYNOLDS *et al.*, 1967; BRODEUR *et al.*, 1965; GEHRMANN *et al.*, 1966).

Bone marrow hyperplasia with predominance of the erythroid series was observed by many authors (VERDON *et al.*, 1963; GEHRMANN *et al.*, 1964; REED and DUNN, 1964; STEVENSON and BAKER, 1964; DE CESARE *et al.*, 1965; VINER and FROST, 1965; YEH, 1965; PETZ *et al.*, 1966; RUBINSON *et al.*, 1966; REYNOLDS *et al.*, 1967). PETZ *et al.* (1966) furthermore observed occasional sideroblasts. Electronmicroscopically, hemosiderin deposits were found in the mitochondria of erythroblasts and reticulocytes.

β) Pathology

Renal siderosis was found by several authors. Sometimes it was localized in the proximal convoluted tubules (SIGLER *et al.*, 1963; YENKO *et al.*, 1965), in one other case in the distal part of the tubular system (REED and DUNN, 1964: "lower nephron nephrosis with deposits of hemoglobin pigment in all tissues"). No precise localization is given by VINER and FROST (1965) or by WESTRING (1966). Seven cases published in 1966 by ROBERTS and MORROW showed hemosiderin deposits mainly in the proximal convoluted tubules (epithelial cells and lumina), in Bowman's space, in the epithelial cells of the glomerulum and in the epithelial cells of Henle's loops.

We observed renal siderosis in two cases following cardiac surgery. One of them offered the aspect of a marked "blue kidney".

Case No. 8

42 y. old man.

Clinical history: 1942 rheumatoid fever. 1954 diagnosis of aortic insufficiency. 1962 replacement of the aortic valve by a teflon prosthesis with 3 leaflets. 1963 second operation because a tear in the prosthesis had developed. Since then the patient developed the symptoms of a traumatic hemolytic anemia with Hb values of 35—45%. He expired in Sept. 1965 under the symptoms of global cardiac insufficiency.

Autopsy (S 797/65): Large defects were found at the site of contact between the leaflets of the artificial valve. Both ventricles were severely hypertrophied (left chamber 22 mm, right chamber 12 mm, weight 900 g). The lungs showed chronic congestion and a severe edema, the liver a cirrhose cardiaque, spleen and kidneys the signs of chronic congestion.

Kidneys: Markedly enlarged and congested (490 g). Brown color on surface and cut surface. Microscopically *"blue kidney"* (Fig. 3 and 4): Extremely severe siderosis of the proximal convoluted tubules with desquamation of epithelial cells into the lumina. Severe siderosis of Henle's loops. Moderate to slight siderosis of some distal convoluted tubules and collecting tubules. Focal interstitial siderosis in cortex and medulla. Slight siderosis of some epithelial cells of Bowman's capsules. Diffuse light blue staining of the plasma in several large vessels.

Case No. 9

38 y. old man.

Clinical history: 1964 replacement of the insufficient aortic valve by a Starr-Edwards ball prosthesis. The patient was now hospitalized because of fever (39° C), accelerated sedimentation rate, erythrocyturia, diastolic murmur over the aortic areal. Therapy with penicillin. June 12th hemiparesis on the right side. The patient died on June 17th, 1967, in pulmonary edema.

Autopsy (S 444/67): A fresh endocarditis was found in the region of the sutures where the prosthesis had been fixed to the aortic wall. The left ventricle was hypertrophied and dilated. The dorsal wall of the left chamber showed a 12:6 cm area of granulation tissue, the apex and septum a 9:4 cm myocardial infarction. The lungs were congested and edematous, bronchopneumonia was present in both lungs. The brain showed an apoplectic hemorrhage in the left hemisphere.

Kidneys: Markedly enlarged (450 g) and congested. Sharp demarcation between the pale cortical tissue and the dark red medulla. Microscopically subacute extra-capillary and intracapillary diffuse glomerulonephritis. Diffuse moderate to severe siderosis of the proximal convoluted tubules. Focal siderosis of the distal convoluted tubules and of the loops of Henle. Siderosis of the endothelial cells of several vessels at the corticomedullary junction. Protein casts gave a positive Prussian blue reaction in many tubules (Fig. 5).

The *morphology of renal siderosis* following implantation of cardiac valvular prostheses may be summarized as follows: Hemosiderin is found predominantly inside the epithelial cells of the proximal convoluted tubules (Fig. 6). This corresponds with the site of hemosiderin deposition in PNH (see p. 105)

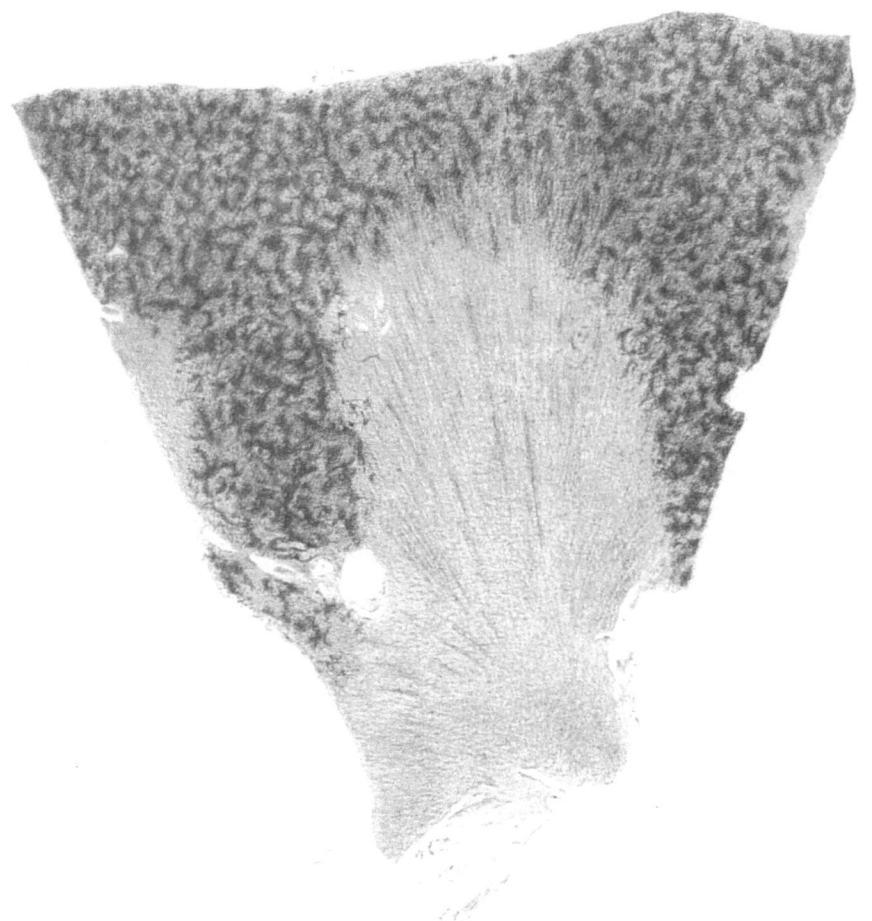

Fig. 3. Renal siderosis following implantation of an aortic teflon prosthesis. "Blue kidney". Case No. 8. Prussian blue reaction. Microscopic slide, low magnification

and in chronic cardiac valvular disease (see p. 109). In addition, the plasma within the blood vessels may show a diffuse light blue staining with Prussian blue (see case no. 8). It may be concluded that *renal siderosis is the result of intense intravascular hemolysis*. The same picture is observed following repeated injections of hemoglobin into rabbits (Muir and Young, 1932). In contrast to the kidney, spleen and liver are essentially free of iron in hemolytic anemia following chronic cardiac valvular disease and cardiac surgery.

If only small amounts of Hb are liberated in the blood stream they are bound to haptoglobin. Since the high molecular Hp-Hb complex cannot be

Fig. 4a—c. Renal siderosis following implantation of an aortic teflon prosthesis. Hemosiderin is found predominantly within the epithelial cells of the proximal convoluted tubules while the distal convoluted tubules are essentially free of hemosiderin. Case No. 8 ("blue kidney"). Prussian blue reaction. a 50×. b and c 280×

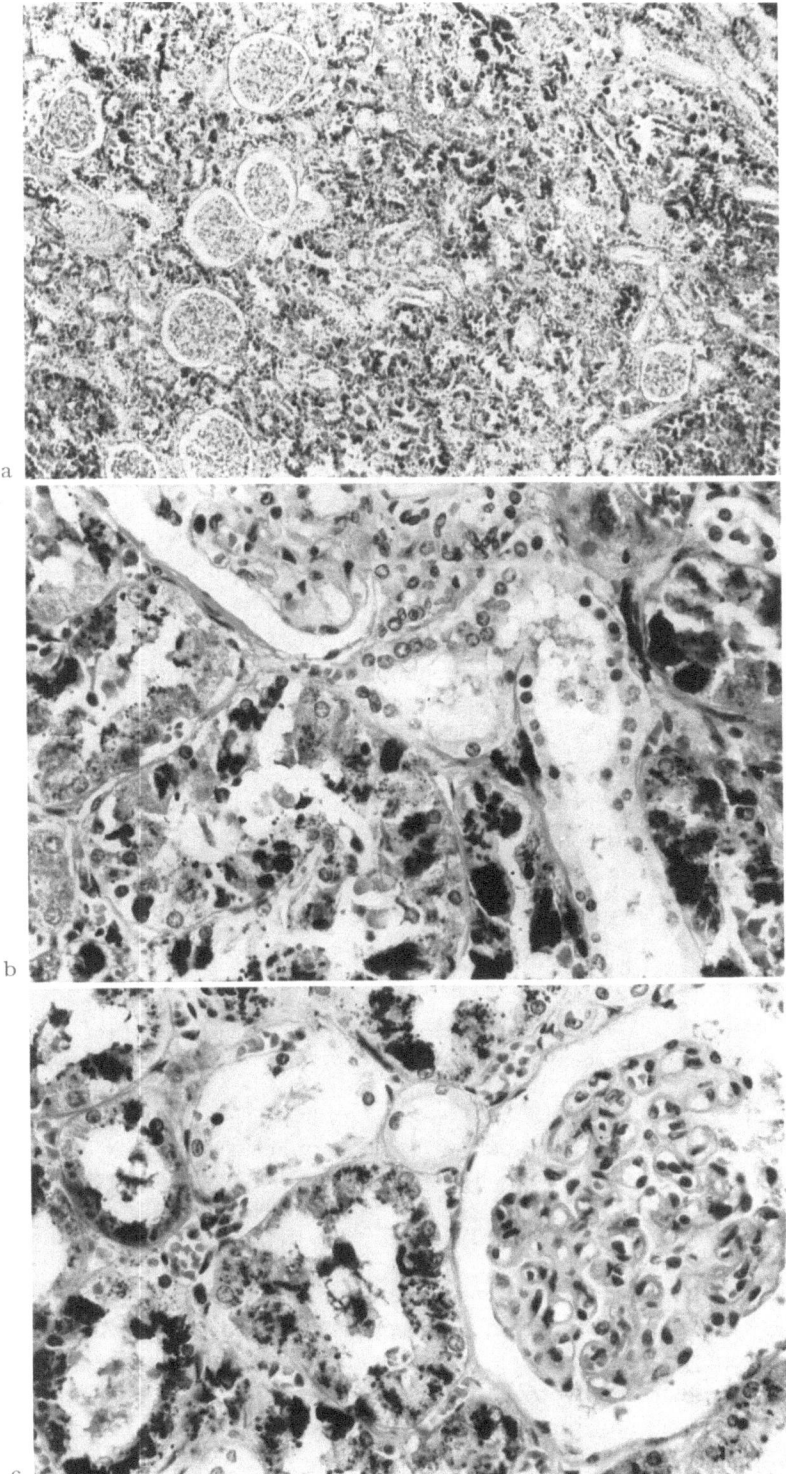

Fig. 4a—c

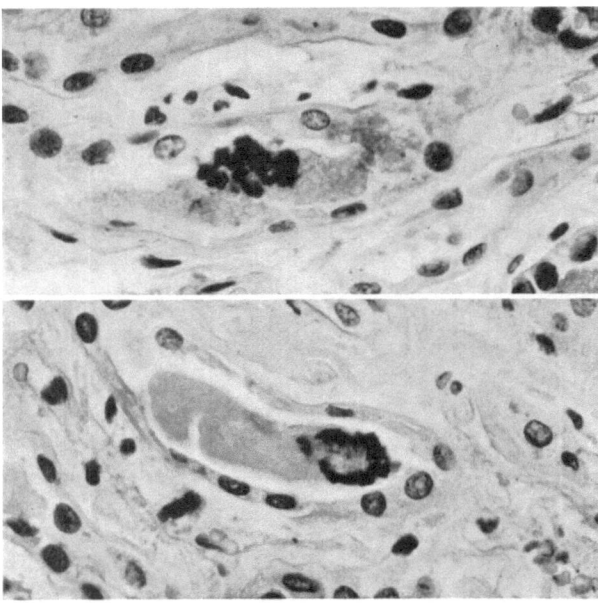

Fig. 5. Deposition of pigmented casts containg hemosiderin in the lumina of the loops of Henle. Implantation of a Starr-Edwards ball prosthesis 3 years prior to death. Case No. 9. Prussian blue reaction. 550 ×

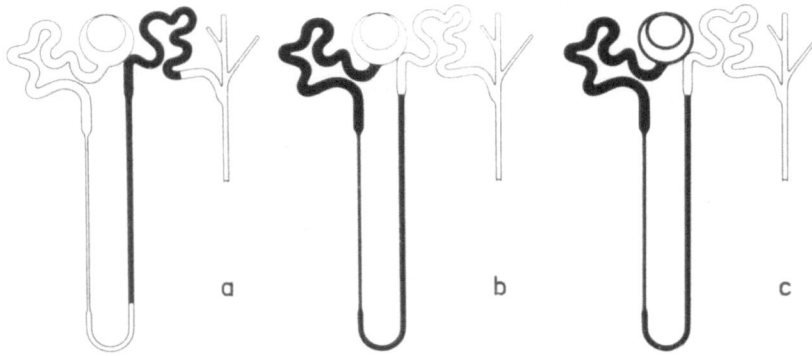

Fig. 6a—c. Renal siderosis in primary and secondary hemochromatosis (a), paroxysmal nocturnal hemoglobinuria (b) and following chronic cardiac valvular disease and implantation of cardiac valvular prostheses (c). Parts of the nephron with predominant siderosis are drawn black

eliminated by the kidney renal siderosis does not occur. The Hp-Hb complex is removed instead by the RES in liver, spleen and bone marrow, and the heme molecule is broken down via the chain of bile pigments. Part of it, however, is transformed into hemosiderin. This raises the question as to why siderosis of the spleen, liver and bone marrow is missing in traumatic hemolytic conditions and siderosis is restricted to the kidneys. One possible explanation is that iron turnover in spleen and liver is much greater than in the kidneys and that enhanced turnover of hemosiderin in connection with increased utilization of iron by the hyperplastic bone marrow causes breakdown of hemosiderin and reutilization of the iron by the bone marrow via transport in blood stream.

γ) Pathogenesis

Several factors have been discussed which might provoke hemolysis in patients with valvular prostheses.

Erythrocyte antibodies could not be demonstrated by many authors (SAYED *et al.*, 1961; MARSH, 1964, 1966; PIROFSKY *et al.*, 1965; PETZ *et al.*, 1966; GEHRMANN *et al.*, 1964, 1966; REYNOLDS *et al.*, 1967; SIGLER *et al.*, 1963; FURUHJELM *et al.*, 1964; REED and DUNN, 1964; STEVENSON and BAKER, 1964; BUCHER *et al.*, 1965; DE CESARE *et al.*, 1965; VINER and FROST, 1965; YEH *et al.*, 1965; YENKO *et al.*, 1965; McGARVEY, 1966; RUBINSON *et al.*, 1966). HJELM *et al.* (1964), BRODEUR *et al.* (1965), PIROFSKY *et al.* (1965) and PEDEFERRI *et al.* (1967), however, observed a positive Coombs test in a few cases. In 2 patients the Coombs test was still positive at the end of the period of investigation (42 and 146 days after the operation; PIROFSKY *et al.*, 1965, case 1 and 3).

There is no substantial evidence in favor of the hypothesis that the hemolysis might be caused by a *direct chemical effect* of the material forming the prosthesis (PIROFSKY *et al.*, 1965; for ref. see VINER and FROST, 1965).

Unquestionably the *regurgitation of the blood* through the opening of the prosthesis plays an important role. SCHADE *et al.* (1967) observed the highest LDH values in those patients who at auscultation had the most severe degree of regurgitation. Regurgitation has also been used to explain the hemolysis occurring 1. in Hufnagel prostheses following insufficiency of the sutures and 2. if in operated ostium I defects the blood stream is directed by the coexisting mitral insufficiency to parts of the teflon patch which are not endothelialized (GEHRMANN *et al.*, 1966; SAYED *et al.*, 1961; SIGLER *et al.*, 1963). BRODEUR *et al.* (1965) also assume that regurgitation of the blood under high systolic pressure is the main pathogenic factor of traumatic hemolysis. RUBINSON *et al.* (1966) calculated that the single erythrocyte has to pass the aortic valve 5.7 times until it finally enters the aorta if regurgitation amounts to 70% of the stroke volume (e.g. in aortic insufficiency). The chance for traumatic fragmentation is thereby considerably increased (see Fig. 7).

The *transvalvular pressure gradient* apparently influences hemolysis since it is highest in aortic stenosis without prosthetic replacement (GEHRMANN *et al.*, 1966). According to GEHRMANN *et al.* (1966) it is not the decisive factor, since patients with mitral insufficiency usually fail to develop hemolysis. The gradient is, however, important since turbulence of the blood around the prosthesis increases with the size of the pressure gradient (GEHRMANN *et al.*, 1966).

Many authors emphasize the influence of *turbulence* on traumatic hemolysis (SIGLER *et al.*, 1963; REED and DUNN, 1964; MARSH, 1964; BRODEUR *et al.*, 1965; DE CESARE *et al.*, 1965; VINER and FROST, 1965; PETZ and GOODMAN,

1966). According to GEHRMANN *et al.* (1966) transition of laminar into turbulent current occurs if Reynold's number (970 ± 80 for blood) is exceeded. Reynold's number is defined by the quotient of V (velocity of blood stream) times D (diameter of blood vessels) and n (viscosity of blood). Since n may be considered to be constant in all cases, V and D appear to determine the size of Reynold's number. If turbulence occurs, shear forces which develop at the interface between layers moving at different velocities rupture the erythro-

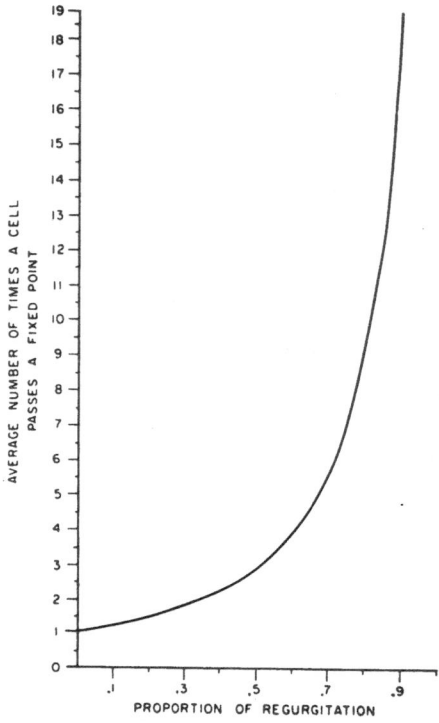

Fig. 7. The relationship of the magnitude of regurgitant blood flow to the average frequency with which a cell is traumatized (Tp). The proportion of regurgitation (p) is the fraction of total forward stroke volume which regurgitates in the succeeding diastole. (From RUBINSON *et al.*, 1966)

cytes' membranes and produce hemolysis (VINER and FROST, 1965; see further PO-TUN FOK and SCHUBOTHE, 1960). Turbulence may be of such extent that cavitation occurs, i.e. the development of spaces filled with gas which collapse. High quantities of energy are liberated by this procedure and destroy the erythrocytes (GEHRMANN *et al.*, 1966, 1968).

The *rough surface* of the prosthesis may also attribute to mechanical hemolysis (VINER and FROST, 1965). This is supported by the observation that in extracorporal circulation hemolysis produced in tubes with smooth inner surface is much less than in tubes with rough surface (STEWART and STURRIDGE, 1959). The same mechanism is effective in the collision of blood with the rigid calcified valves during systole (VINER and FROST, 1965) and also when the erythrocytes are damaged by the force of impact of blood against the artificial heart valve (VINER and FROST, 1965; MARSH, 1964, 1966). Mechanical hemolysis further occurs when erythrocytes are squashed between the plastic ball and the steel basket of the Starr-Edwards prosthesis (GEHRMANN et al., 1966).

A special mechanism of hemolysis has been discussed by BUCHER et al. (1965). They suppose that the specific hemodynamic conditions in anemias following implantation of valvular prostheses favor the *activation of phosphatidase A* in blood plasma and by this the liberation of lysolecithin from the erythrocyte membrane. This is supported by their observation that erythrocyte sedimentation rate is inhibited by plasma following mechanical hemolysis in vitro.

If the many theories concerning the mechanism of hemolysis produced by valvular prostheses are summarized it appears most probable that *mechanical hemolysis is the predominant pathogenic factor*. One of the chief arguments in favor of this is the existence of fragmented erythrocytes in the blood of these patients combined with the lack of substantial evidence in favor of hemolysis due to chemical or immunological factors.

Two additional factors may favor the development of mechanical hemolysis:

1. Hemolysis is enhanced by physical exercise. On the other hand, it improves markedly if the patients are kept in bed (DE CESARE et al., 1965; MILLER et al., 1966).

2. Hemosiderosis of the kidneys leads to hemosiderinuria (see below, p. 136). The loss of iron is the cause of iron deficiency anemia developing in these patients which is frequently aggravated by insufficient dietary intake of iron. The state of iron deficiency decreases the erythrocyte life span. Thus anemia is favored. Furthermore, anemia is followed by an increase of heart frequency, stroke and minute volume, and through this the chance for mechanical fragmentation of erythrocytes is increased (SANYL et al., 1964; REYNOLDS et al., 1967). In this way circuli vitiosi are produced which aggravate iron deficiency as well as hemolysis.

5. Traumatic Hemolytic Anemia in Microangiopathy (Microangiopathic Hemolytic Anemia)

α) *Thrombotic Thrombocytopenic Purpura* (MOSCHCOWITZ)

In 1953 MONROE and STRAUSS supposed that the fragments of erythrocytes observed in blood vessels and tissues of patients with thrombotic thrombocytopenic purpura (TTP) might be the result of mechanical destruction in the obturated small vessels and that the hemolytic anemia common in this disease might be explained in this way. This was confirmed by ADELSON et al. (1954) in three cases. These authors observed numerous helmet cells, other types of

9*

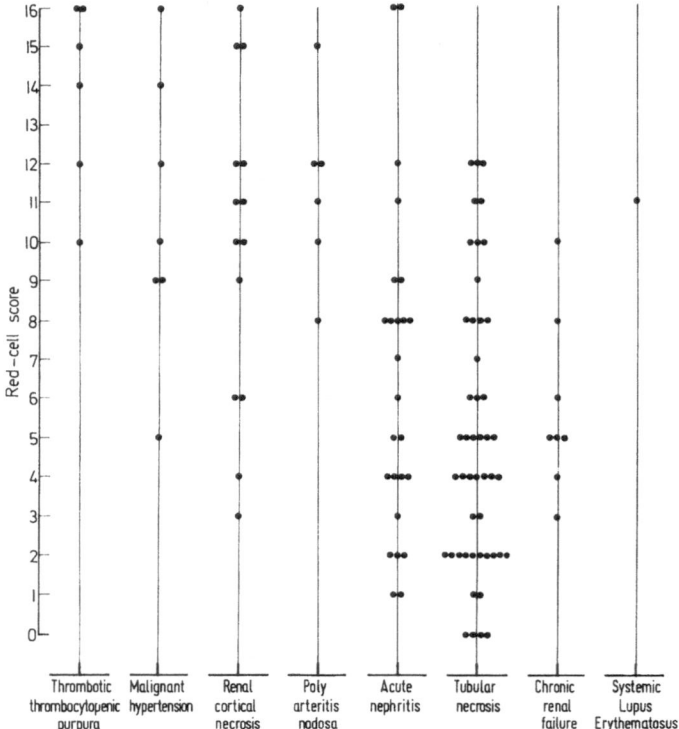

Fig. 8. Relationship between red-cell score and histological diagnosis in patients with microangiopathic hemolytic anemia. (From BRAIN et al., 1962)

poikilocytes and spherocytes in the blood smear of patients with TTP. No data are given concerning hemosiderinuria or renal siderosis.

A traumatic pathogenesis of the hemolytic anemia in TTP is also assumed by DAMESHEK (1964), VINER and FROST (1965), McGARVEY et al. (1966) and STEVENSON and BAKER (1964). BRAIN et al. (1962) described 6 cases with typical fragmentocytes and helmet cells (Fig. 8). It is not clear whether hemosiderinuria or renal siderosis was present in these patients or not.

Our own series of cases of TTP comprises three patients in whom the kidneys could be investigated for the presence of hemosiderin. In 1 case hemosiderin was found.

Case No. 10

R. K., 45 y. old man.

Clinical diagnosis: Intense intravascular hemolysis with numerous schistocytes. Thrombocytopenia (10,000 platelets/mm³). Normal plasma coagulation factors and fibrinogen (83%), no evidence of consumption coagulopathy. Coombs test negative. Clinical diagnosis: Thrombotic thrombocytopenic purpura? Evans-Duane syndrome (acquired hemolytic anemia + immunothrombocytopenia)?

Autopsy (S 317/68): Numerous petechiae in the skin of the thorax, abdomen and extremities. Purpura cerebri. Petechiae in the mucous membranes of the stomach, ileum, colon, urinary bladder, right renal pelvis, subendocardial fatty tissue, endo- and myocardium. Microscopically microthrombi predominantly composed of plate-

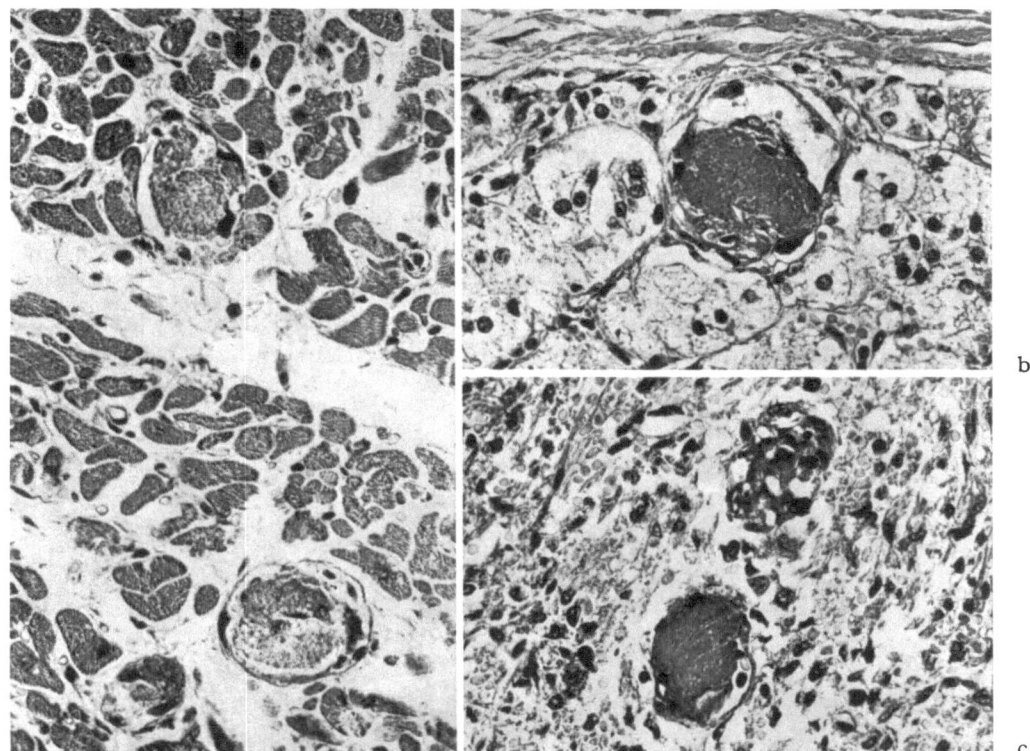

Fig. 9a—c. Obturation of small vessels in the myocardium (a) adrenal gland (b) and pituitary gland (c) in thrombotic thrombocytopenic purpura. Case No. 10. a Hematoxylin-eosin. b and c Ladewig. 300 ×

lets in numerous organs incl. brain, heart, liver, kidney, adrenal glands and pituitary gland (posterior lobe), see Fig. 9.

Kidneys: Normal size (300 g). Hemorrhages and microthrombi see above. Very slight diffuse hemosiderosis of some epithelial cells of the proximal convoluted tubules near the surface. No granular siderosis of the proximal convoluted tubules or other parts of the nephron.

To our knowledge this is the first case of TTP with renal siderosis published so far. Unquestionably the low degree of siderosis is explained by the short duration of the illness. In addition, the hemolysis might have been too small to produce significant hemoglobinuria. Haptoglobin was not estimated in this patient but it may be assumed that it was not completely saturated by the Hb appearing in the blood serum as a result of intravascular hemolysis.

β) Microangiopathic Hemolytic Anemia in other Diseases

The relations between microangiopathy including TTP and hemolysis were thoroughly studied by BRAIN *et al.* (1962) who introduced the term "microangiopathic hemolytic anemia" for these conditions.

Hemolytic anemia was found in 25 out of 120 patients with microangiopathy (acute or chronic renal failure: 113, TTP: 2, metastatic cancer: 5).

In these 25 cases the following diagnoses had been made: TTP (6), malignant hypertension (5), renal cortical necrosis (4), polyarteriitis nodosa (2), acute glomerulonephritis (2), disseminated lupus erythematodes (1), metastatic cancer (5). Changes of erythrocyte morphology were graded from 0 to 16. The type of vascular lesions was furthermore determined (arteriolar fibrinoid necrosis, necrotizing arteriitis, hyaline thrombi in arterioles and capillaries). Erythrocyte morphology was little disturbed in patients without vascular lesions, and the most severe alterations of the red blood cells were observed in the patients with prominent vascular changes.

The results of Brain et al. show that traumatic hemolysis may be caused by vascular lesions of different origin and nature. Meanwhile they have been

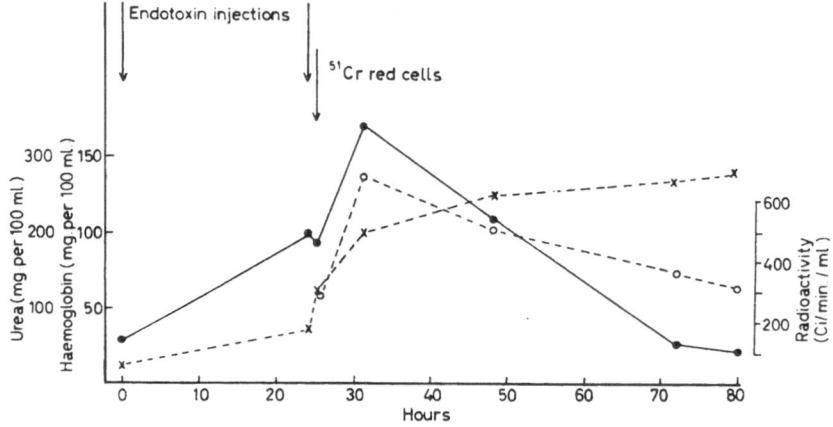

Fig. 10. Plasma haemoglobin (•), urea (×) and radioactivity (○) during a generalized Shwartzman reaction resulting in renal cortical necrosis. 51 Cr labelled red cells transfused 90 minutes after second endotoxin injection. (From Brain and Hourihane, 1967, Fig. 5)

confirmed by Landaw (1964, for ref. see there) and by Forshaw and Harwood (1966) in numerous cases. Among 327 cancer patients 17 (6%) had marked poikilocytosis (Forshaw and Harwood, 1966). In 50% of the positive cases cancer of the stomach and intestine was present.

Schistocytosis and plasma Hb-emia may be observed in rabbits with generalized Sanarelli-Shwartzman phenomenon (Brain and Hourihane, 1967, Fig. 10). The authors consider that although the means by which intra-vascular hemolysis might be brought out remain uncertain, the experiments provide further evidence in support of the hypothesis that changes in small vessels may lead to hemolytic anemia.

The papers cited above do not contain data concerning the hemosiderin content of the kidneys.

It could be anticipated from the results mentioned above that renal siderosis might occur in human cases of generalized Sanarelli-Shwartzman phenomenon and also in cases of peripheral circulatory failure with disseminated intravascular coagulation (REMMELE and HARMS, 1968). Among 19 cases studied now, 1 child was found who demonstrated renal siderosis.

Case No. 11

S. B., 11 months old girl.

Clinical diagnosis: Hemolytic-uremic syndrome following infection? Pleuropneumonia? Evans-Fisher syndrome? Fever of 40°C for 5 days. Macrohematuria, oliguria. Thrombocytes 5,000/mm^3.

Autopsy (S 233/65): Severe bronchopneumonia of the right upper lobe with pulmonary gangrene in the 2nd segment. Septic thrombophlebitis of the pulmonary vein with so-called white pulmonary infarction. Hemorrhagic effusion in the left pleural cavity. Dilatation of both ventricles. Numerous thrombi rich in fibrin within the capillaries of the glomerular tuft and pulmonary capillaries. Consumption coagulopathy ("Verbrauchskoagulopathie") with petechiae in the urinary bladder, urethra, renal cortex and medulla and capsule of the adrenal glands. — Diagnosis was either TTP or generalized SSP. The age of the infant and the clinical history may be considered to speak in favor of the assumption that the child died from generalized SSP.

Kidneys: Apart from the changes caused by the coagulopathy itself (fibrin thrombi, hemorrhages) the kidneys show numerous casts within the tubules which give a diffuse positive Prussian blue reaction. The epithelial cells of the proximal convoluted tubules are tinged pale blue near the lumina. No granular siderosis of the epithelial cells.

Three facts are suggested by this case: 1. Generalized SSP may be accompanied by renal siderosis; 2. The hemolytic-uremic syndrome of childhood may be due to generalized SSP. 3. Bacterial endotoxin may cause anemia not only by suppression of bone marrow erythropoiesis (FRUHMAN, 1966) but also by peripheral destruction of erythrocytes.

We have also tried to find hemosiderin in the kidneys of patients who died from metastatic cancer of the gastrointestinal tract, but we were not successful.

c) Other Hemolytic Anemias

Renal siderosis has been described in *paroxysmal cold hemoglobinuria*. SUSSMAN and KAYDEN (1948) observed a siderosis of the tubular contents as well as of the tubular epithelial cells. Siderosis was found predominantly within the epithelial cells of the distal convoluted tubules and Henle's loops. Another case has been reported by LEONARDI and RUOL (1960). The localization of hemosiderin within the tubular apparatus is not given.

Patients with hemoglobinuria due to *cold hemagglutinins* usually demonstrate no hemosiderinuria (STATS *et al.*, 1948). In contrast to these authors SCHUBOTHE and ALTMANN (1950) found hemosiderin within the epithelial cells of the proximal convoluted tubules, the thick part of Henle's loops, the distal convoluted tubules and the cells of the glomerular tuft while the thin part of Henle's loops did not contain any hemosiderin (Fig. 11).

LEONARDI and RUOL (1960) describes renal siderosis in some cases of *chronic and acute autoimmune hemolytic anemia, thalassemia minor and hereditary spherocytosis*. The precise localization of hemosiderin is not given.

Fragmentocytes were observed in a case of *hemolytic anemia following treatment with sulfapyridine* (STATS *et al.*, 1948). It is not known whether the kidneys contained hemosiderin or not.

A case of "*hemolytic anemia coexistent with osteomyelosclerosis*" with renal siderosis was described by SCHAUER (1961). Hemosiderosis was present in the proximal convoluted tubules and parts of Henle's loops while the glomeruli and the collecting tubules were free of hemosiderin.

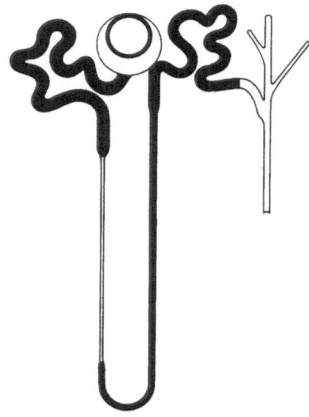

Fig. 11. Renal siderosis in hemoglobinuria due to cold hemagglutinins. (According to the description given by SCHUBOTHE and ALTMANN, 1950)

E. Effects of Renal Siderosis

1. Hemosiderinuria

Normal blood plasma does not contain hemosiderin since hemosiderin is storage iron and not transport iron. If hemosiderin is found in the urine this is evidence for renal siderosis. Hemosiderin is demonstrated in urine by performing the Prussian blue reaction with the urinary sediment. At microscopical examination hemosiderin appears as blue-stained granules within renal epithelial cells, as amorphous sediment and, occasionally, as blue-pigmented tubular casts (CROSBY and DAMESHEK, 1951).

Hemosiderinuria is usually found in chronic Hb-emia (CROSBY, 1955). CROSBY and DAMESHEK (1951) observed hemosiderinuria in every case showing hemoglobinemia. In general, the amount of hemosiderin in the urine varied with the concentration of plasma Hb.

The only conditions without Hb-emia in which hemosiderinuria exists are primary and secondary hemochromatosis (CROSBY and DAMESHEK, 1951).

It therefore seems clear that each cause of renal siderosis may simultaneously lead to hemosiderinuria. Hemosiderinuria is fundamentally different from Hb-uria in so far as it is the result and not the cause of renal siderosis.

2. Renal Function

The majority of authors agrees that renal function is not impaired by renal siderosis (STATS et al., 1948; LEONARDI and RUOL, 1960; ROBERTS and MORROW, 1966; REYNOLDS et al., 1967). This is true even for the cases with a "blue kidney" (ROBERTS and MORROW, 1966; personal observation). It is difficult, of course, to differentiate the effects of Hb-uria and renal siderosis. If Hb-emia and Hb-uria continue to exist, impairment of renal function may well be produced by hemoglobinuria and not by renal siderosis.

When hemolysis ceases hemosiderinuria may persist for some time. This observation strongly suggests that the urinary route of iron excretion is much more important than the possible route via the blood of the peritubular capillaries (ROBERTS and MORROW, 1966).

References

ADDIS, T.: Glomerular nephritis, diagnosis and treatment. New York: Macmillan 1948. Cit. by RANDERATH and BOHLE, 1959.

ADELSON, E., HEITZMAN, E. J., FENNESSEY, J. F.: Thrombohemolytic thrombocytopenic purpura. Arch. intern. Med. 94, 42—60 (1954).

AHERNE, W. A.: The "burr" red cell and azotaemia. J. clin. Path. 10, 252—257 (1957).

ALLEN, A. C.: The kidney. Medical and surgical diseases. New York: Grune & Stratton 1951.

ALLISON, A. C.: Acute haemolytic anaemia with distortion and fragmentation of erythrocytes in children. Brit. J. Haemat. 3, 1—18 (1957).

— Haptoglobins. Blut 5, 201—204 (1959).

ALTHOFF, H.: Wirkung des Desferrioxamin B auf Gewebsschnitte einer Nieren-haemosiderose. Arzneimittel-Forsch. 16, 768—771 (1966).

— Nierenhämosiderose und hämoglobinurische Nephrose als Spätkomplikation einer paroxysmalen nächtlichen Hämoglobinurie (Marchiafava-Micheli-Syndrom). Mat. med. Nordmark 19, 299—311 (1967).

ANDERSEN, M. C., GABRIELI, E., ZIZZI, J. A.: Chronic hemolysis in patients with ball-valve prosthesis. J. thorac. cardiovasc. Surg. 50, 501—510 (1965).

BELL, E. T.: Renal diseases. Philadelphia. Lea & Febiger 1947. Cit. by RANDERATH and BOHLE, 1959.

BLACKSHEAR, P. L., JR., FORSTROM, R., WATTERS, CHR., DORMAN, F. D.: Effects of flow and turbulence on the formed elements of blood. In: Prosthetic heart valves. Ed. by L. A. BREWER, p. 52—67. Springfield (Ill.): Thomas 1969.

BOONE, A. W., HALTIWANGER, E., CHAMBERS, R. L.: Football hematuria. J. Amer. med. Ass. 158, 1516—1517 (1955).

BRAIN, M. C., DACIE, J. V., O'B. HOURIHANE, D.: Microangiopathic hemolytic anemia: the possible role of vascular lesions in pathogenesis. Brit. J. Haemat. 8, 358—374 (1962).

— O'B. HOURIHANE, D.: Microangiopathic haemolytic anaemia: The occurrence of haemolysis in experimentally produced vascular disease. Brit. J. Haemat. 13, 135—142 (1967).

BRANDT, J. L., FRANK, N. R., LICHTMAN, H. C.: The effect of hemoglobin solutions on renal functions in man. Blood 6, 1152—1158 (1951).

BRODEUR, M. T. H., KOLER, R. D., STARR, A., GRISWOLD, H. E.: Red cell survival in patients with mitral valvular disease and mitral valve prostheses. Circulation, Suppl. I to 33 and 34 (1966).

Brodeur, M. T. H., Sutherland, D. W., Koler, R. D., Griswold, H. E.: Hemolytic anemia and valvular disease. New Engl. J. Med. 272, 104—105 (1965).

— — — Starr, A., Kimsey, J. A., Griswold, H. E.: Red blood cell survival in patients with aortic valvular disease and ball-valve prostheses. Circulation 32, 570—581 (1965).

Bucher, U., Gurtner, H. P., Kummer, H.: Gesteigerte Hämolyse nach Herzoperationen. Schweiz. med. Wschr. 95, 1508—1511 (1965).

Cahill, J. J., Kolff, W. J.: Hemolysis caused by pumps in extracorporal circulation. J. Appl. Physiol. 14, 1039—1044 (1959).

Cartwright, G. E., Gubler, C. J., Wintrobe, M. M.: J. clin. Invest. 33, 685 (1954). Cit. by Frick, 1964.

Cleton, F. J., Blok, A. P. R.: Post-transfusional hemosiderosis. In: Iron metabolism, p. 347—358. Berlin-Göttingen-Heidelberg-New York: Springer 1964.

Cooley, T. B.: A severe type of hereditary anemia with elliptocytosis. Interesting sequence of splenectomy. Amer. J. med. Sci. 209, 561—568 (1945).

Croizat, P., Guichard, A., Revol, L., Creyssel, R., Meunier: Etude anatomoclinique et chimique d'un cas de maladie de Marchiafava-Micheli. Sang 19, 218—228 (1948).

Crosby, W. H.: Paroxysmal nocturnal hemoglobinuria. Relation of the clinical manifestations to underlying pathogenetic mechanisms. Blood 8, 769—812 (1953).

— The metabolism of hemoglobin and bile pigment in hemolytic disease. Amer. J. Med. 18, 112—122 (1955).

— Dameshek, W.: The significance of hemoglobinemia and associated hemosiderinuria, with particular reference to various types of hemolytic anemia. J. Lab. clin. Med. 38, 829—841 (1951).

— Sheehy, T. W.: Hypochromic iron-loading anaemia: Studies of iron and haemoglobin metabolism by means of vigorous phlebotomy. Brit. J. Haemat. 6, 56—65 (1956).

Dacie, J. V., Smith, M. D., White, J. C., Mollin, D. L.: Refractory normoblastic anaemia: A clinical and haematological study of seven cases. Brit. J. Haemat. 5, 56—82 (1959).

Dameshek, W., Castleman, B. J.: Case records of the Massachusetts General Hospital. Case 52-1964. New Engl. J. Med. 271, 898—905 (1964).

DeCesare, W., Rath, C., Hufnagel, C.: Hemolytic anemia following aortic valvuloplasty. X. Congr. Internat. Soc. Hematol. Stockholm 1964.

— — — Hemolytic anemia of mechanical origin with aortic-valve prosthesis. New Engl. J. Med. 272, 1045—1050 (1965).

Dennis, E. W., Johnson, P. C., Kinard, Jr., S. A., McCall, B. W., Pitzele, S., DeBakey, M. E.: The pattern of red blood cell survival after prosthetic ball valve replacement. Cardiovasc. Res. Cent. Bull. 3, 62—68 (1964).

Dreyfus, J.-C., Schapira, G.: The metabolism of iron in hemochromatosis. In: Iron metabolism, p. 296—325. Berlin-Göttingen-Heidelberg-New York: Springer 1964.

Ehrlich, P.: Über einen Fall von Anämie mit Bemerkungen über regenerative Veränderungen des Knochenmarks. Charité-Ann. 1886. Zit. nach F. Himmelweit: Paul Ehrlich. Gesammelte Arbeiten. Erster Band: Histologie, Biochemie und Pathologie, p. 160—165. Berlin-Göttingen-Heidelberg: Springer 1956.

Feit, J., Belusa, M.: Hypochrome hypersiderämische Anämie mit Hämochromatose. Zbl. allg. Path. path. Anat. 103, 227—234 (1961).

Finch, C. A.: Physiopathologic mechanisms of iron excretion. In: Iron metabolism, p. 452—460. Berlin-Göttingen-Heidelberg-New York: Springer 1964.

Finny, C. M.: Functional haemoglobinuria. Brit. med. J. 1926 II, 685.

Förster, A.: Über Marschhämoglobinurie. Münch. med. Wschr. 66, 554—557 (1919).

Forshaw, J., Harwood, L.: Poikilocytosis associated with carcinoma. Arch. intern. Med. 117, 203—205 (1966).

FORSHAW, J., HARWOON, L.: Red blood cell abnormalities in cardiac valvular disease. J. clin. Path. **20**, 848—853 (1967).

FRICK, P. G., BRUNNER, H. E.: Megaloblastäre Folsäuremangel-Anämie bei Hämochromatose. Schweiz. med. Wschr. **93**, 1502—1505 (1963).

FRUHMAN, G. J.: Bacterial endotoxin: Effects on erythropoiesis. Blood **27**, 363—370 (1966).

FURTH, F. W.: Unpublished studies. Cit. by CROSBY, 1955.

FURUHJELM, U., LANDTMAN, B., LAUNIALA, K., NEVANLINNA, H. R., SULAMAA, M., TUUTERI, L.: Hemolytisk anemi efter tillslutning av ostium-primum-defekt. Nord. Med. **72**, 1446—1448 (1964).

GAITHER, J. C.: Paroxysmal nocturnal hemoglobinuria: A successful imposter. New Engl. J. Med. **265**, 421—430 (1961).

GASSER, C., GAUTIER, E., STECK, A., SIEBENMANN, R. E., OECHSLIN, R.: Hämolytisch-urämische Syndrome: Bilaterale Nierenrindennekrosen bei akuten erworbenen hämolytischen Anämien. Schweiz. med. Wschr. **85**, 905—909 (1955).

GEHRMANN, G.: Personal communication (1968).

— BLEIFELD, W., KAULEN, D.: Herzklappenfehler und Hämolyse. Klin. Wschr. **44**, 1229—1235 (1966a).

— — LOOGEN, F.: Mechanische Hämolysen nach Implantation künstlicher Herzklappen. Z. Kreisl.-Forsch. **55**, 25—33 (1966b).

— LOOGEN, F.: Mechanische hämolytische Anämie nach Implantation künstlicher Aortenklappen. Dtsch. med. Wschr. **89**, 625—630 (1964).

Geigy-Tables 1960, p. 548.

GELPI, A. P., ENDE, N.: An hereditary anemia with hemochromatosis. Studies of an unusual hemopathic syndrome ressembling thalassemia. Amer. J. Med. **25**, 303—314 (1958).

GERHARTZ, H.: Sideroachrestic anaemia in reticuloses. Proc. 9th Cong. Europ. Soc. Haemat. Lisbon 1963, p. 319—324.

GILLIGAN, D. R., ALTSCHULE, M. D., KATERSKY, E. M.: Studies of hemoglobinemia and hemoglobinuria produced in man by intravenous injection of hemoglobin solutions. J. clin. Invest. **20**, 177—187 (1941).

— — — Physiological intravascular hemolysis of exercise. Hemoglobinemia and hemoglobinuria following cross-country runs. J. clin. Invest. **22**, 859—869 (1943).

— BLUMGART, H. L.: March hemoglobinuria. Studies of the clinical characteristics, blood metabolism and mechanism with observations on three new cases and review of literature. Medicine (Baltimore) **20**, 341—395 (1941).

GISINGER, E., PUXKANDL, H.: Die Beeinflussung der renalen Eisen- und Kupferausscheidung. Wien. Z. inn. Med. **36**, 491—497 (1955).

GLASER, R. J.: Hemoglobinuria and cardiovascular-renal disease. Amer. J. Med. **4**, 594—605 (1948).

GOLDISH, R. J., AUFDERHEIDE, A. C.: Secondary hemochromatosis. II. Report of a case not attributable to blood transfusions. Blood **8**, 837—844 (1953).

GREEN, R. A.: Hemolytic anemia and open heart surgery. Minn. Med. **48**, 1545—1547 (1965).

GUINAND, S., TONNELAT, J., BOUSSIER, G., JAYLE, M. F.: Propriétés physiques de l'haptoglobine, séromucoide et de sa combinaison hémoglobinique. Bull. Soc. Chim. biol. (Paris) **38**, 329—341 (1956).

HAM, T. H.: Hemoglobinuria. Amer. J. Med. **18**, 990—1006 (1955).

HEDINGER, C.: Zur Pathologie der Hämochromatose. Hämochromatose als Syndrom. Helv. med. Acta **20**, Suppl. 32, 5—109 (1953).

HEILMEYER, L.: Die sideroachrestischen Anämien. Folia haemat. (Frankfurt), N.F. **6**, 9—18 (1961).

HEITZMAN, E. J., CAMPBELL, J. S., STEFANINI, M.: Paroxysmal nocturnal hemoglobinuria with hemosiderin nephrosis. Amer. J. clin. Path. **23**, 975—986 (1953).

Hesse, E., Filatov, A.: Experimentelle Untersuchungen über das Wesen des hämolytischen Schocks bei der Bluttransfusion und die therapeutische Beeinflussung desselben. I. Die Nierenfunktionsstörungen im akuten Experiment. Z. exp. Med. **86**, 211—230 (1933).

Hjelm, M., Högmann, C. F., Finnson, M., Malers, E.: Transient auto-antibody formation in case of open heart surgery with no signs of increased red cell destruction. Vox Sang. (Basel) **9**, 505 (1964). Cit. by Pirofsky, 1965.

Hutt, M. P., Reger, J. F., Neustein, H. B.: Renal pathology in paroxysmal nocturnal hemoglobinuria. An electron microscopic illustration of the formation and disposition of ferritin in the nephron. Amer. J. Med. **31**, 736—747 (1961).

Jacquet, P., Dérobert, L., Plas, F., Hadengue, A.: Apropos d'un cas de maladie de Marchiafava-Micheli. Sem. Hôp. Paris **25**, 2143—2146 (1949).

Jundell, I., Fries, K. A. E.: Die Anstrengungsalbuminurie. Eine Studie über die Einwirkung maximaler Körperanstrengungen (des Sports und des Trainings) auf die Nieren. Nord. med. Arkiv 1911, Afd. II, Häft 1. N: R 2, 44. Cit. by Gilligan and Blumgart, 1941.

Keith, H. B., Ginn, E., Williams, G. R., Campbell, G. S.: Massive hemolysis in extracorporal circulation. J. thorac. cardiovasc. Surg. **41**, 404—407 (1961).

Koszewski, B. J.: The occurrence of megaloblastic erythropoiesis in patients with hemochromatosis. Blood **7**, 1182 (1952). Cit. by Muggia and Olivetti, 1967.

Landaw, S. A.: Hemolytic anemia as a complication of carcinoma. Case report and review of the literature. J. Mt Sinai Hosp. N.Y. **31**, 167 (1964). Cit. by Forshaw and Harwood, 1966.

Larson, R. E., Kirklin, J. W.: Early and late results of partial and total replacement of the aortic valve with individual teflon cusps. J. thorac. cardiovasc. Surg. **47**, 720—724 (1964).

Lathem, W.: The renal excretion of hemoglobin: regulatory mechanisms and the differential excretion of free and protein-bound hemoglobin. J. clin. Invest. **38**, 652—658 (1959).

— Worley, W. E.: The distribution of extracorpuscular hemoglobin in circulating plasma. J. clin. Invest. **38**, 474—483 (1959).

Laurell, C.-B.: Serumproteine und Eisentransport. In: Eisenstoffwechsel, hrsgg. von W. Keiderling, p. 103—111, Stuttgart: Thieme 1959.

— Nyman, M.: Studies on the serum haptoglobin level in hemoglobinuria and its influence on renal excretion of hemoglobin. Blood **12**, 493—506 (1957).

Lennert, K., Oerkermann, H.: Pathologische Anatomie der sideroachrestischen Anämie (Untersuchung von 4 Fällen). Beitr. path. Anat. **136**, 34—57 (1967).

Leonardi, P., Ruol, A.: Renal hemosiderosis in the hemolytic anemias: diagnosis by means of needle biopsy. Blood **16**, 1029—1038 (1960).

Lichty, J. A., Jr., Havill, W. H., Whipple, G. H.: I. Renal thresholds for hemoglobin in dogs: Depression of threshold due to frequent hemoglobin injections and recovery during rest periods. J. exp. Med. **55**, 603—615 (1932).

Lock, S. P., Dormandy, K. M.: Red-cell fragmentation syndrome: A condition of multiple aetiology? Lancet **1961 I**, 1020—1024.

MacDonald, R. A.: Hemochromatosis and hemosiderosis. Springfield (Ill.): C. C. Thomas 1964.

— Mallory, G. K.: Hemochromatosis and hemosiderosis; autopsy study of 211 cases. Arch. intern. Med. **105**, 686—700 (1960).

Mähr, G., Wuketich, S.: Erythroblastosis maligna sideroblastica. Dtsch. Arch. klin. Med. **207**, 154—176 (1961).

Maier, C.: Megaloblastäre Vitamin-B_6-Mangelanämie bei Hämochromatose. Schweiz. med. Wschr. **87**, 1234—1235 (1957).

Marchiafava, E., Nazzari, A.: Nuovo contributo allo studio degli itteri cronici emolitici. Policlinico, Sez. med. **18**, 241—254 (1911).

MARSH, G. W.: Intravascular haemolytic anaemia after aortic-valve replacement. Lancet 1964 II, 986—988.
— Mechanical haemolytic anaemia after mitral-valve replacement. Brit. med. J. 1966 II, 31—32.
MASON, J. B., MANN, F. C.: The effect of hemoglobin on volume of the kidney. Amer. J. Physiol. 98, 181—185 (1931).
McGARVEY, J. F., SPITZER, S., SEGAL, B. L., BRODSKY, I.: Hemolytic anemia with aortic ball-valve prosthesis. Report of a case. Dis. Chest 50, 97—100 (1966).
McGOON, D. C., MANKIN, H. T., KIRKLIN, J. W.: Results of open-heart operation for acquired aortic valve disease. J. Thorac. Cardiovasc. Surg. 15, 47—66 (1963).
MENGEL, C. E., KANN, H. E., Jr., MERIWETHER, W. D.: Studies of paroxysmal nocturnal hemoglobinuria erythrocytes: increased lysis and lipid peroxide formation by hydrogen peroxide. J. clin. Invest. 46, 1715—1723 (1967).
MERLISS, R. R.: Paroxysmal nocturnal hemoglobinuria. New Engl. J. Med. 246, 642—646 (1952).
MIALE, J. B.: Laboratory medicine-hematology, 2nd ed. St. Louis: C. V. Mosby 1962.
MILLER, D. S., MENGEL, C. E., KREMER, W. B., GUTTERMANN, J., SENNINGEN, R.: Intravascular hemolysis in a patient with valvular heart disease. Ann. intern. Med. 65, 210—215 (1966).
MILLS, H., LUCIA, S. P.: Familial hypochromic anemia associated with postsplenectomy erythrocyte inclusion bodies. Blood 4, 891—904 (1949).
MONROE, W. M., STRAUSS, A. F.: Intravascular hemolysis; morphologic study of schistocytes in thrombotic purpura and other diseases. Sth. med. J. (Bgham, Ala.) 46, 837—842 (1953).
MOORE, C. V., DUBACH, R.: Physiology of iron metabolism: resorption, conservation, elimination, and physiological iron losses. In: Eisenstoffwechsel, hrsg. von W. KEIDERLING, S. 112—127. Stuttgart: Thieme 1959.
MOSTOFI, F. K., VORDER BRUEGGE, C. F., DIGGS, L. W.: Lesions in kidneys removed for unilateral hematuria in sickle-cell disease. Arch. Path. 63, 336—351 (1957).
MUGGIA, F. M., OLIVETTI, R. G.: Megaloblastic anemia associated with parenchymal hemosiderosis. N. Y. State J. Med. 67, 444—451 (1967).
MUIR, R., DUNN, J. S.: The retention of iron in the organs in haemolytic anaemia. J. Path. Bact. 19, 417—428 (1914/15).
— YOUNG, J. S.: The relation of the liver to the disposal of hemoglobin. J. Path. Bact. 35, 113—126 (1932).
NAJEAN, Y.: Discussion to FRICK 1964. In: Iron Metabolism, p. 461. Berlin-Göttingen-Heidelberg-New York Springer 1964.
NEWMAN, W. V., WHIPPLE, G. H.: IV. Hemoglobin injections and conservation of pigment by kidney, liver and spleen. The influence of diet and bleeding. J. exp. Med. 55, 637—652 (1932).
NUNN, D. B., BARILA, T. G., ATWOOD, E. L.: Hemolysis studies on three types of artifical heart pump valves. Trans. Amer. Soc. artif. intern. Org. 9, 253—261 (1963).
NYMAN, M.: Serum haptoglobin, methodical and clinical studies. Scand. J. clin. lab. Invest. 2, Suppl. 39 (1959).
OSBORN, J. J., COHN, K., HAIT, M., RUSSI, M., SALEL, A., HARKINS, G., GERBODE, F.: Hemolysis during perfusion. Sources and means of reduction. J. thorac. cardiovasc. Surg. 43, 459—464 (1962).
PEDEFERRI, G., CHARON, P., DUBOST, CH.: Anemia emolitica dopo sostituzione dell' apparato valvolare aortico con protesi di STARR-EDWARDS. Minerva med. 58, 2155 (1967).
PETZ, L. D., GOODMAN, J. R.: Ringed sideroblasts and intramitochondrial iron in cases of mechanical hemolytic anemia. Ann. intern. Med. 64, 635—643 (1966).

Pirofsky, B.: Aortic valve surgery and autoimmune hemolytic anemia. Amer. Heart J. 70, 426—428 (1965).
— Sutherland, D. W., Starr, A., Griswold, H. E.: Hemolytic anemia complicating aortic-valve surgery. An autoimmune syndrome. New Engl. J. Med. 272, 235—239 (1965).
Plötner, K., Petzel, H.: Über die Höhe der renalen Eisenausscheidung und zur Frage der Harneisenbestimmung. Klin. Wschr. 32, 821—822 (1954).
Porges, O., Strisower, R.: Über Marschhämoglobinurie. Dtsch. Arch. Klin. Med. 117, 13—25 (1914).
Po-Tun-Fok, F., Schubothe, H.: Studies on various factors influencing mechanical hemolysis of human erythrocytes. Brit. J. Haemat. 6, 355—361 (1960).
Radochova, D., Chrobák, L., Šmid, A., Dvořák, K.: Der Anteil der Hämolyse an der Anämie nach Anwendung der Herz-Lungen-Maschine. Thoraxchir. u. vask. Chir. 15, 195—198 (1967).
Randerath, E., Bohle, A.: Die Pathomorphologie der Nierenausscheidung. Handbuch der allgemeinen Pathologie, Bd. V/2, S. 140—293. Berlin-Göttingen-Heidelberg: Springer 1959.
— Krückemeyer, K.: Experimentelle Untersuchungen zur Frage der Hämoglobinausscheidung durch die Niere. Zbl. allg. Path. path. Anat. 85, 313—325 (1949).
Reed, W. A., Dunn, M.: Fatal hemolysis following ball valve replacement of the aortic valve. J. thorac. cardiovasc. Surg. 48, 436—442 (1964).
Reid, W. L.: Effect of intravenous injections of distilled water on the kidney. Amer. J. Physiol. 90, 168—171 (1929).
Remmele, W., Harms, D.: Zur pathologischen Anatomie des Kreislaufschocks beim Menschen. I. Mikrothrombose der peripheren Blutgefäße. Klin. Wschr. 46, 352—357 (1968).
Reynolds, R. D., Coltman, Ch. A., Beller, B. M.: Iron treatment in sideropenic intravascular hemolysis due to insufficiency of Starr-Edwards valve prostheses. Ann. intern. Med. 66, 659—666 (1967).
Roberts, W. C.: Renal hemosiderosis (blue kidney) in patients with valvular heart disease. Amer. J. Path. 48, 409—419 (1966).
— Morrow, A. G.: Renal hemosiderosis in patients with prosthetic aortic valves. Circulation 33, 390—398 (1966).
Rose, J. C., Hufnagel, C. A., Freis, E. D., Harwey, W. P., Partenope, E. A.: The hemodynamic alterations produced by a plastic valvular prosthesis for severe aortic insufficiency in man. J. clin. Invest. 33, 891—900 (1954).
Ross, J. F.: Hemoglobinemia and the hemoglobinurias. New Engl. J. Med. 233, 691—696, 732—737, 766—772 (1945).
Rubinson, R. M., Morrow, A. G., Gebel, P.: Mechanical destruction of erythrocytes by incompetent aortic valvular prostheses. Amer. Heart J. 71, 179—186 (1966).
Sanyl, S. K., Polesky, H. F., Hume, M., Browne, M. J.: Spontaneous partial remission of postoperative hemolytic anemia in a case with ostium primum defect. Circulation 30, 803—807 (1964).
Sarnoff, S. J., Case, R. B., Stohlman, F., Jr.: Intravascular hemolysis following insertion of the Hufnagel Lucite ball valve in the circulation and comparative observations with an elastic silicone valve. Read before Ann. Soc. artif. intern. Org. (1955). Cited by Stohlman et al., 1956.
Sayed, H. M., Dacie, J. V., Handley, D. A., Lewis, S. M., Cleland, W. P.: Haemolytic anaemia of mechanical origin after open heart surgery. Thorax 16, 356—360 (1961).
Schade, S. G., Rowe, G. G., Young, W. P., Lockey, S. D., Clatanoff, D. V.: Intravascular hemolysis with the Gott-Daggett valve. J. thorac. cardiovasc. Surg. 53, 605—612 (1967).

SCHAUER, A.: Zur Pathogenese der Siderosen. Frankfurt. Z. Path. **71**, 334—341(1961).

SCHUBOTHE, H., ALTMANN, H. W.: Kältehämagglutinine als Ursache chronischer hämolytischer Anämien. Z. klin. Med. **146**, 428—479 (1950).

SCHULTZE, H. E., HEREMANS, J. F.: Molecular biology of human proteins. Vol. 1. Nature and metabolism of extracellular proteins. Amsterdam-London-New York: Elsevier 1966.

SCHUMACHER, G., SCHLUMBERGER, H. D.: Eigenschaften, Bestimmung und klinische Bedeutung von Haptoglobin. Klin. Wschr. **40**, 67—71 (1962).

SCHWARZMANN: Cit. by DREYFUS, J. C., SHAPIRA, G., 1964.

SCHWARTZ and MOTTO (1949). Cit. by MIALE, 1962.

SHAW, S.: Simple method for estimating plasma haemoglobin during open heart surgery. J. clin. Path. **20**, 95 (1967).

SHELDON, J. H.: Haemochromatosis. London: Oxford Univ. Press 1935. Cit. by MACDONALD, 1964.

SHINOWARA, G. Y.: Spectophotometric studies on blood serum and plasma. The physical determination of hemoglobin and bilirubin. Amer. J. clin. Path. **24**, 696—710 (1954).

SHUMWAY, C. N., Jr., MILLER, G.: An unusual syndrome of hemolytic anemia, thrombocytopenic purpura and renal disease. Blood **12**, 1045—1060 (1957).

SIGLER, A. T., FORMAN, E. N., ZINKHAM, W. H., NEILL, C. A.: Severe intravascular hemolysis following surgical repair of endocardial cushion defects. Amer. J. Med. **35**, 467—480 (1963).

STATS, D., WASSERMANN, L. R., ROSENTHAL, N.: Hemolytic anemia with hemoglobinuria. Amer. J. clin. Path. **18**, 757—777 (1948).

STEVENSON, T. D., BAKER, H. J.: Haemolytic anemia following insertion of Starr-Edwards valve prosthesis. Lancet **1964 II**, 982—985.

STEWART, J. W., STURRIDGE, M. F.: Hemolysis caused by tubing in extracorporal circulation. Lancet **1959 I**, 340—342.

STOHLMAN, F., Jr., SARNOFF, S. J., CASE, R. B.: Hemolytic syndrome following insertion of a lucite ball valve prosthesis in the vascular system. Clin. Res. Proc. **3**, 96 (1955).

— STANLEY, J., SARNOFF, S. J., ROBERT, B., CASE, R. B., NESS, A. T.: Hemolytic syndrome following the insertion of a lucite ball valve prosthesis in the cardiovascular system. Circulation **13**, 586—591 (1956).

STURGEON, P., SHODEN, A.: Mechanisms of iron storage. In: Iron metabolism, p. 121—146. Berlin-Göttingen-Heidelberg-New York: Springer 1964.

SUSSMAN, R. M., KAYDEN, H. J.: Renal insufficiency due to paroxysmal cold hemoglobinuria. Arch. intern. Med. **82**, 598—610 (1948).

TJORSTAD, K. O.: Mechanical hemolytic anemia after plastic surgery of the mitral valve. Norsk laegeforening **86**, 1104—1106 (1966).

TUFFY, P., BROWN, A. K., ZUELZER, W. W.: Infantile pyknocytosis. J. Dis. Child. **98**, 227—241 (1959).

VAHLQUIST, B.: Plasma iron. Transport iron: Circulating plasma or serum iron. In: Eisenstoffwechsel, hrsg. von W. KEIDERLING, S. 93—101. Stuttgart: Thieme 1959.

VERDON, T. A., Jr., FORRESTER, R. H., CROSBY, W. H.: Hemolytic anemia after open-heart repair of ostium primum defects. New Engl. J. Med. **269**, 444—446 (1963).

VERLOOP, M. C.: Les anémies sidéro-achrestiques. Nouv. Rev. franc. Hémat. **5**, 201—208 (1965).

— BIERENGA, M., DIEZERAAD-NJOO, A.: Primary or essential sideroachrestic anemias. Acta haemat. (Basel) **27**, 129—145 (1962).

VEYRAT, R., MAURICE, P. A.: Anémie hypochrome mégaloblastique grave, avec hypersidérémie et hémochromatose, corrigée par la pyridoxine. Schweiz. med. Wschr. **91**, 1215—1217 (1961).

Viner, E. D., Frost, J. W.: Hemolytic anemia due to a defective teflon aortic valve prosthesis. Ann. intern. Med. 63, 295—301 (1965).

Walthard, B.: Zur pathologischen Anatomie der endogenen Pigmentierung. Schweiz. Z. Path. 9, 711—714 (1946).

Westring, D. W.: Aortic valve disease and hemolytic anemia. Ann. intern. Med. 65, 203—209 (1966).

Witts, L. J.: The paroxysmal haemoglobinurias. Lancet 1936 II, 115—120.

Yates, J. L., Thalhimer, W.: Treatment of pernicious anemia. A patient who received one hundred and thirteen transfusions. J. Amer. med. Ass. 87, 2156—2157 (1926).

Yeh, T. J., Ellison, R. G., Wright, Cl.-S.: Hemolytic anemia due to a ruptured prosthetic aortic cusp. J. thorac. cardiovasc. Surg. 49, 963—967 (1965).

Yenko, N. R., Hartmann, J. R., Stamm, S. J.: Hemolytic anemia following open heart repair of congenital defects. Northw. Med. (Seattle) 64, 493—495 (1965).

Zingg, W., Zollinger, H. U.: Experimentelle Haemoglobin- und Haemosiderin-speicherung in den Nierenmitochondrien. Mikroskopie 6, 72—82 (1951).

Ziperovich, S., Paley, H. W.: Severe mechanical hemolytic anemia due to valvular heart disease without prosthesis. Ann. intern. Med. 65, 342—346 (1966).

Department of Pathology, Dartmouth Medical School,
Hanover, New Hampshire 03755, U.S.A.

Morphogenesis of Anencephaly and Related Malformations *

Miguel Marin-Padilla

With 10 Figures

Table of Contents

I. Introduction

Anencephaly (cranioschisis) is the most representative example of a large heterogeneous group of developmental malformations characterized by abnormalities of the central nervous system and surrounding mesodermal structures. Many of these malformations have been known since ancient times and today many can be reproduced experimentally either by the administration of various teratogens or by mechanical means. Some of these malformations, *e.g.* anencephaly (cranioschisis) and complete cranio-myeloschisis (craniorhachischisis) represent the most severe abnormalities known to man; others, *e.g.* localized open myeloschisis (rhachischisis) and meningomyelocele (cystic rhachischisis), although compatible with life, require extensive surgical and medical management; while still others, *e.g.* occult spina bifida (occult rhachischisis), characterized by localized vertebral defects, often escape

* This work has been supported by Grant GM 10210 from U.S.P.H.S.

clinical detection. This review does not presume to cover a complete classification of these malformations since there are many intermediate morphological variations which are difficult to classify in one or the other group. It includes, however, the most representative examples of these malformations; furthermore, it points to the extraordinary structural differences existing among them and, it indicates the extremes of severity and the extent of the defects which can occur. This communication, which deals with the analysis of only these malformations, assumes that a clear understanding of their basic defects will help to comprehend better the defects which characterize the entire group.

The morphological complexity, the structural diversity and the different connotation which these malformations have to different investigators (embryologists, anatomists, pathologists, teratologists, surgeons and other clinicians) have resulted in abundant, confusing and often contradictory literature. A survey of this literature or a discussion of the numerous theories advanced about the origin of these malformations and the reasoning behind them is a difficult taks beyond the scope of the present communication. It is hoped here to present a detailed analysis of the basic defects of the central nervous system and of the surrounding mesodermal structures which characterize these malformations, since once the nature of these defects is understood and the defects defined, one will be better prepared to discuss their origin and morphogenesis.

Two facts common to all malformations of this group should be emphasized. First, the primary "injury" leading to them occurs very early in embryonic life, and second, this injury appears not to interfere with the subsequent intrauterine development, to maturity, of the affected embryo. Therefore, several developmental stages in the evolution of these malformations can be recognized and they must be considered in the evaluation of their basic defects. In the present study three main developmental stages are recognized in the embryonic evolution of these malformations: the early, the intermediate and the terminal stage. The early developmental stage follows, soon after the injury, occurs very early in embryonic life, and it coincides with the establishment of the mesodermal skeleton of the affected embryo. This stage is the least understood and is the stage around which most controversies and discussions concerning these defects are centered. It is referred to as the "dysrhaphic" or the "mesodermal stage" in the evolution of these malformations. The intermediate developmental stage, of which little information is available, coincides with the establishment of the cartilaginous skeleton of the affected embryo. It is referred to as the "exencephalic" or the "cartilaginous stage" in the evolution of these malformations. The terminal developmental stage coincides with the establishment of the osseous skeleton of the affected embryo and is perhaps the best known, for material is more readily available from both human and experimentally induced malformations. It is referred to as the "anencephalic" or the "osseous stage" in the evolution of these malformations.

For the analysis of the basic defects I propose a reverse developmental approach. In other words: a) to start with the investigation of the terminal stage which is better known and its defects are better defined and established; b) to continue with the investigation of the intermediate stage, and to discuss some new material; and c) to conclude with the investigation of the less defined and poorly understood changes of the early stages.

Preceding the analysis of the embryonic evolution of these malformations it will be necessary to a) outline the status of our present knowledge on the origin of these malformations, and b) present some embryological considerations on the sequence of events leading to the closure of the neural folds in the mammalian embryo.

II. Analysis and Critique of the Main Theories on the Origin of These Malformations

Most of the theories expressed on the origin of these malformations, with few exceptions, could be grouped into one of two basic concepts. Either these malformations are the result of a reopening of a previously closed neural tube; or they are the result of a primary failure of closure of the neural tube. These two basic concepts, which are in a way opposing, were the first to be expressed. In 1769, MORGAGNI expressed the idea that imbalances of the cerebrospinal fluid, causing an excessive accumulation, could cause a reopening (rupture) of a previously closed neural tube. Later in 1886, VON RECKLINGHAUSEN expressed the idea that a primary failure of closure of the neural tube could result in these malformations.

In spite of insufficient supportive experimental data, the idea of MORGAGNI still has today its ardent supporters (GARDNER, 1968; PADGET, 1968). KEEN (1962—1966), also favors the MORGAGNI interpretation of the origin of these malformations based on his analysis of the morphological defects of the skull in anencephaly. The fact that JELINEK (1960) was able to demonstrate that mechanical reopening of a closed neural tube *can* cause anencephaly in the chick would indicate that perhaps a modified MORGAGNI opinion, namely reopening of a previously closed neural tube, should be considered as one possible cause of the origin of some of these malformations. Such a reopening could be produced by direct mechanical means or it could be the result of the rupture of a localized area of necrosis as has been suggested to be the mechanism in radiation-induced malformations (WILSON *et al.*, 1953). It should, however, be emphasized that in order to produce these severe malformations irradiation of embryos must take place very early in embryonic life and before the closure of the neural tube (HICKS and D'AMATO, 1966). These observations suggest that the necrosis described after radiation could be secondary to selective damage of certain cells affecting the embryonic tissues *before* the closure of the neural tube.

Primary failure of closure of the neural tube is today the most generally accepted concept concerning the origin of these malformations. Abundant clinical and experimental data supported it, which conclude that the injury occurs before the closure of the neural tube and interferes with the normal process of closure. The arguments and the controversies are centered around which of the embryonic tissues is primarily affected to cause this failure of closure. In this respect the most generally accepted point of view is that the neuroectoderm is the primarily affected tissue and that the mesodermal (skeletal) abnormalities are secondary defects resulting from the lack of proper induction by the anomalous nervous system. A less generally accepted point of view is that the mesoderm is the primarily affected tissue and that the abnormalities of the central nervous system are the result of exposure of the unclosed and unprotected neuroectoderm. It should be emphasized that there are observations in the literature which favor either of these two opposing points of view. A re-evaluation of some of these observations is therefore indicated.

The literature on this subject is abundant and extremely confusing and it is difficult to reconstruct from it any meaningful correlation of data. It is also difficult to find any agreement on the stage of embryonic development affected by the different teratogens or agreement on the critical periods for the induction of a given malformation. The confusion has resulted from the use, by the various investigators, of different experimental animals, different teratogens, as well as different methods and amount of teratogen administered, either once or several times during embryonic development. Likewise, because embryos were examined at different times after the teratogenic insult, it is difficult to correlate the findings reported.

In most reports on clinical and experimental anomalies of this type the defect (unclosed neural tube) was fully established. The analysis of such material is of little help in ascertaining what the primary disturbance may have been. It has not been sufficiently emphasized in the study of these malformations that alterations in the neuroectoderm and in the mesoderm can occur following the failure of closure of the neural tube, nor that they can be the consequence of exposure rather than the cause. If one enforces strictly a delay between the administration of the teratogen (preferably in a single dose of a standard amount) and observation of the results to a few hours this would enhance a careful evaluation of the data. There are observations in the literature indicating that light microscopic pathological changes are detectable from 6 to 10 hours after the administration of a single dose of vitamin A; perhaps even earlier changes could be detected with the electronmicroscope.

The nature of the so-called "primary" alterations of either the neuroectoderm or of the mesoderm which are cited in support of the two different points of view concerning the origin of these malformations should be evaluated with these ideas in mind. It should be emphasized that in the study of early developmental stages in these malformations one should be able to ascertain which are the primary targets of the insult. It is possible that these lead to secondary events, perhaps much more spectacular (e.g. failure of closure of the neural tissue) and that at some stage of development the primary and secondary alterations might overlap. It is then that a distinction of what is primary and secondary may be difficult.

The fact that JELINEK has been able to produce anencephaly by mechanical reopening of a previously closed neural tube would indicate that neither primary alterations in the neuroectoderm nor in the mesoderm were necessary to induce the malformation. Furthermore, his study indicates that the defects of the central nervous system and of the mesodermal structures encountered later in the evolution of the malformations, induced in this manner, are best explained as the consequences of the reopening of the neural tube. I would like to point out, however, that the malformations induced by mechanical means differ fundamentally in their origin and morphogenesis from those considered here.

In view of the observations just reviewed one can conclude the following: a) the exposure of the neuroectoderm and of the mesoderm which result either from the reopening of a previously closed neural tube, or from a primary failure of closure leads to early alterations in these tissues; b) these alterations of the neuroectoderm and of the mesoderm might explain some of the basic defects of the central nervous system and skeletal structures seen; c) these alterations are perhaps not the cause of the primary failure of closure of the neural tube; and d) the cause of the primary failure of closure of the neural tube, remains unknown.

III. Embryological Considerations on the Closure of the Neural Tube

One of the most important events in the development of the embryo is the closure of the neural tube. We have seen that primary failure of closure or a secondary reopening of it can lead to various types of malformations characterized by defects in the central nervous system and in the surrounding mesodermal structures. A clear understanding of the sequence of events leading to the closure of the neural tube and of the participation of the different cellular components is a necessary prerequisite for the comprehension of these malformations. The closure of the neural tube proper (neuroectoderm) represents only one of the events of a complex embryonic process in which other cellular structures participate. This complex process begins with the approximation and the fusion of the neural folds and includes the closure of the surface ectoderm, the neuroectoderm and the mesoderm. During this time the neural crest cells begin to appear, to proliferate, and to migrate. The sequence of events beginning with the apposition of the neural folds to the complete closure of all cellular components have been investigated in the golden hamster (Fig. 1). It consists, at a given time and embryonic region, of the following steps: a) fusion of the neural folds at the level of the presumptive neural crest cells which are not yet morphologically recognizable; b) active proliferation of the neural crest cells (now morphologically recognizable) with their forming a wedge between the lips of the partially closed neural folds; c) fusion and

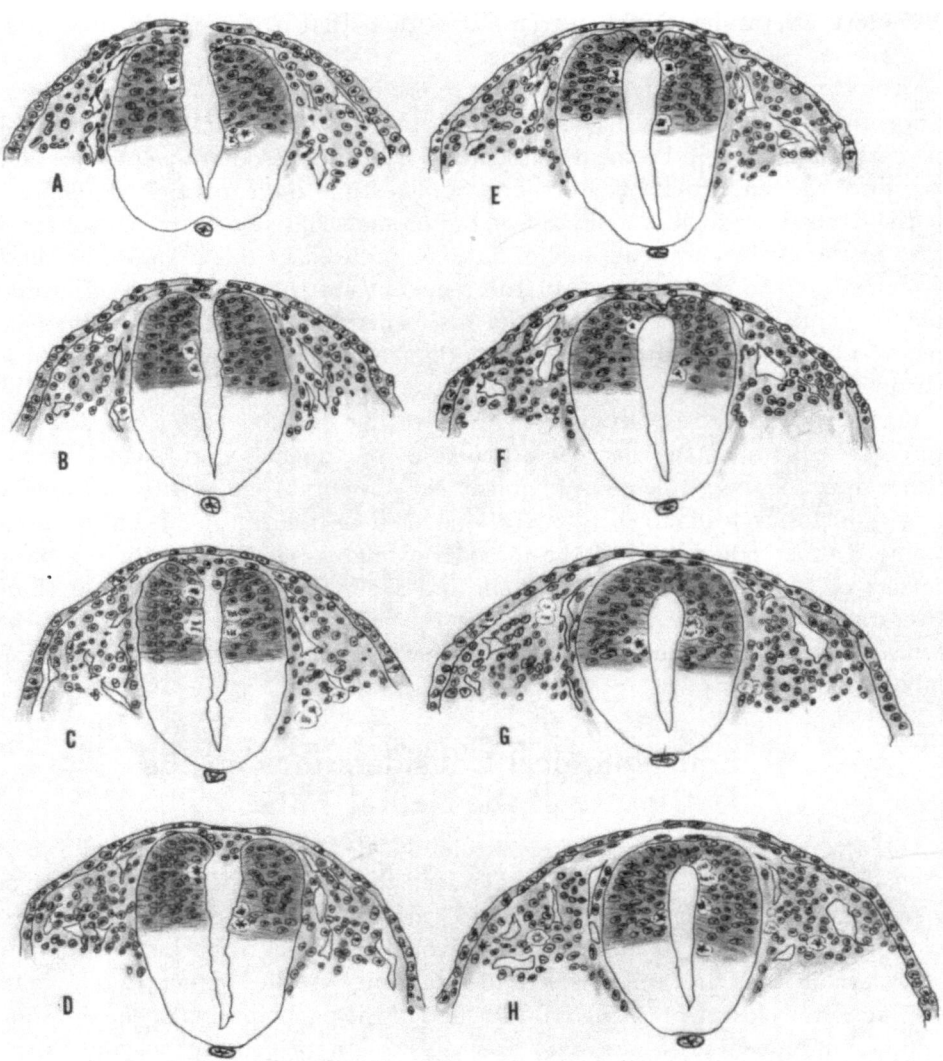

Fig. 1 A—H. Camera lucida drawings of the sequence of events in the closure of neural folds in the golden hamster. The drawings were made from eight selected cuts of a serially sectioned embryo. The embryo was 8 days and 5 hours old. A Approaching neural folds. B Contact of the neural folds at the level of the presumptive neural crest cells. C Fusion and closure of the surface ectoderm. D and E Active proliferation of neural crest cells forming a distinctive wedge. F Fusion of the neuroectoderm beginning at the ependymal surface and progressing dorsally (G) until its complete closure. The fusion and closure of the neuroectoderm coincides with a diminution in the number of neural crest cells in the region. H Terminal stage of the process of closure with the formation of a space between the ectoderm and the neuroectoderm occupied by migrating mesodermal cells. Preceding the process of closure the neural folds must undergo a progressive growth (elevation) up to the point of apposition and fusion. A failure in the formation of the neural folds or a failure to achieve the required elevation will result in primary failure of closure

closure of the surface ectoderm establishing a continuous layer; d) progressive diminution of the number of neural crest cells due to their active migration to the periphery; e) fusion of the neuroectoderm beginning at the ependymal surface and progressing dorsally until its complete closure; and f) formation of a space between the surface ectoderm and the closed neuroectoderm, soon to be occupied by migrating mesodermal cells. In the hamster there is a great deal of variation from one region of the embryo to another in the time required to complete this process, the amount of embryonic tissue involved in it, the number of neural crest cells formed, and the separation between the closures of the ectoderm from that of the neuroectoderm. It is quite possible that species differences may also exist among the different animals. These differences should be determined and considered in the study and analysis of experimentally-induced malformations.

All the cellular components of the neural folds (neural crest cells, surface ectoderm, neuroectoderm and mesoderm) participate in the process of closure. The concept that failure of closure of the neural tube involves only the failure of the neuroectoderm (neural tube proper) is erroneous. This concept should be exchanged for a more general one, namely that the process of closure is a complex phenomenon in which all the cellular components of the neural folds actively participate, resulting not only in the closure of the neuroectoderm (neural tube proper) but also in the closure of the ectoderm and mesoderm. Also, that important and reciprocal inductive functions exist between all the cellular components, and that one cannot consider any of them without reference to the others. In view of the notochordal alterations described in these malformations the interrelationship between it and the process of closure should also be considered.

One more aspect to be considered in the process of closure which is seldon analysed or discussed is the formation of the neural folds themselves. The neural folds become apparent late in the presomite and early in the somite stages of the embryo as slightly elevated structures marking the lateral boundaries of the neural groove. They grow rapidly by continuous elevation and a progressive increase in the number of their supporting mesodermal cells. The growth (elevation) of the neural folds progresses until apposition, fusion and closure occur. The supporting mesodermal cells of the neural folds proliferate in situ but many derive from the chordomesodermal system. If the neural folds fail to develop of if they fail to grow progressively because of an insufficient number of mesodermal cells, they will not reach the stage for apposition and fusion which then results in a primary failure of closure. In such a case, it would not be necessary to postulate neuroectodermal or *late* mesodermal alterations to explain the primary failure of closure, although these alterations in the neuroectoderm and in the mesoderm are necessary to explain the basic defects of the central nervous system and of the skeletal structures which characterize these malformations. These alterations could be the direct consequences of the failure of closure, namely exposure of these tissues to amniotic fluid. The reduction of mesodermal cells and the notochordal alterations described in the early stages of these malformations give support to this idea of primary chordomesodermal alterations causing the primary failure of closure. A clear understanding of this important embryonic phenomenon will help considerably in a better understanding of the origin and nature of these malformations.

IV. Analysis of the Developmental Stages of the Embryonic Evolution of these Malformations

The basic defects of the central nervous system and of the surrounding mesodermal (skeletal) structures will be analyzed and described separately starting with the terminal stages of these malformations.

1. Anencephalic or Osseous Stage

Central Nervous System (CNS) Defects. Little need be said about the basic defects of the CNS at this developmental stage. All the exposed areas of the CNS (the brain in anencephaly, the brain and the spinal cord in complete myeloschisis and the spinal cord in localized myeloschisis) depict the end result of a progressive degenerative process which started earlier during embryonic development. The exposed tissues of the CNS are transformed into the so-called areas cerebro- or medullo-vasculosa (Figs. 2c and 7). These amorphous areas consist of hemorrhagic masses of fibrovascular tissue with scattered nervous elements. The latter are composed mainly of glial cells with an occasional, but rare, recognizable neuron. There are no recognizable anatomical structures, the focal areas of surviving nervous elements having escaped degeneration perhaps due to the development of some vascular independence.

A striking feature of these anomalies is that regardless of their type, those CNS structures that are exposed tend to undergo extensive degenerative

Fig. 2a and b. Anterior and posterior views of human exencephaly with cervical and high dorsal myeloschisis (intermediate or cartilaginous stage in the evolution of these malformations). This 14 week old fetus was the product of a spontaneous abortion. Notice the low set ears, the prominent and elevated nose and maxilla (monkey's face), the protruding tongue and the short neck (retarded longitudinal growth of the affected vertebral region). The brain is prominent, protruding, apparently overdeveloped and covered by fragments of meningeal tissue. The failure of closure of the brain occurs somewhere between the III ventricle and the acqueduct both of which communicate with the exterior (see Fig. 9). The cortex (everted), the thalamus, the cerebellum and the mid-brain structures were recognizable and their development and histological differentiation was considered to be within normal limits. The holes in the back of the specimen were accidentally produced. (Compare with Fig. 2c)

Fig. 2c. Posterior view of human anencephaly with cervico-dorso-lumbar myeloschisis (terminal or osseous stage in the evolution of these malformations). Compare with Fig. 2a and b. It illustrates the areas cerebro- and medullo-vasculosas. Notice the short neck and the lordotic position of the affected vertebral column (retarded longitudinal growth). The severity of the vertebral defects suggests a failure in the formation of the neural folds

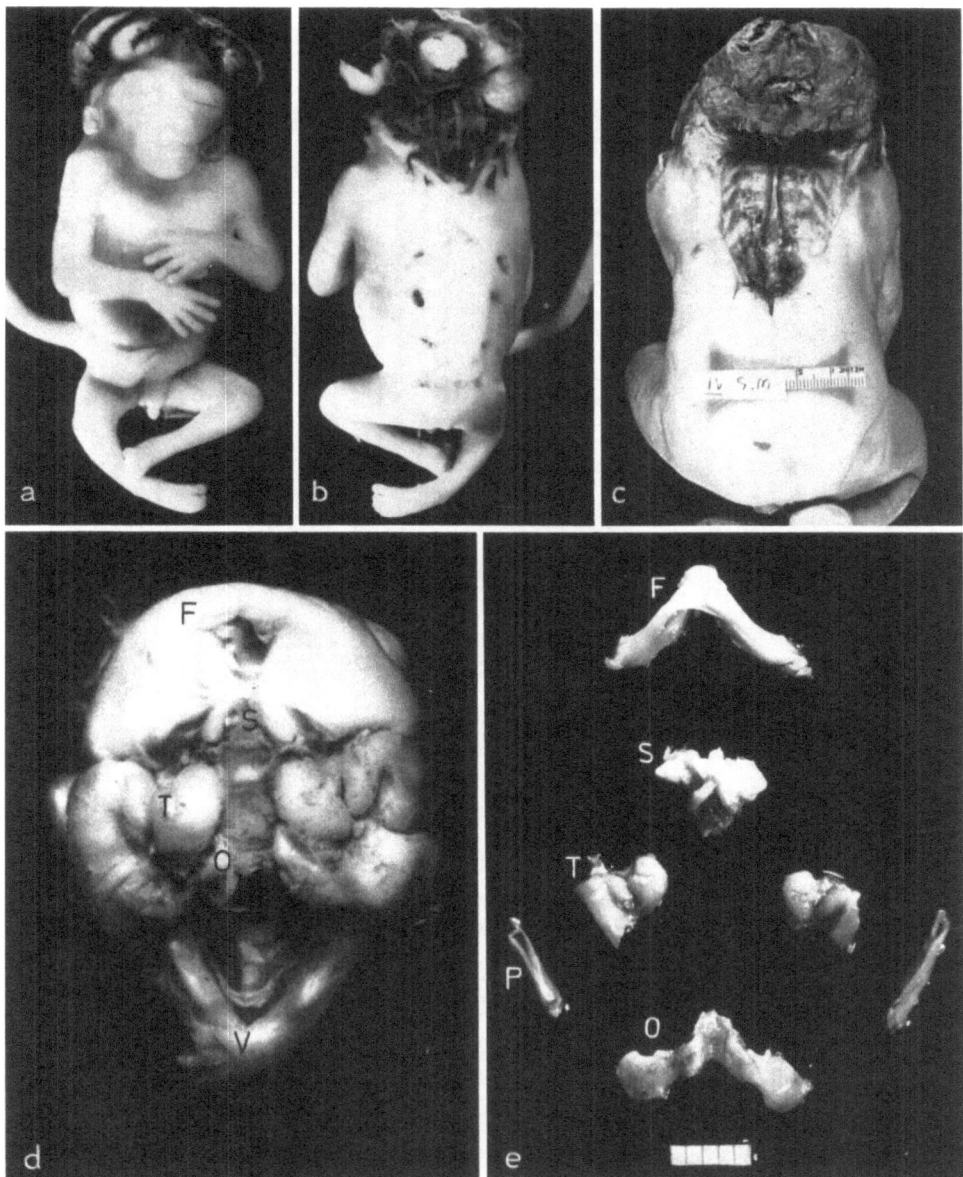

Fig. 2d. Superior view of the cartilaginous skeleton of the base of the skull from the case shown in Fig. 2a and b. It illustrates the failure of closure of the neurocranium, the absence of a cranial cavity and of a foramen magnum. Note also the cervical schisis. Notice the reduction of the antero-posterior diameter of the base of the skull. (Key: *F* Frontal, *S* Sphenoid, *T* Temporal, *O* Occipital, *V* Vertebral arches of the dorsal region)

Fig. 2e. Detail of some of the cartilaginous "bones" of the skull of human exencephaly (Fig. 2d). *F* Frontal bone which is represented only by its orbital portions. *S* Sphenoid bone showing rudimentary lesser wings, stunted greater wings, marked reduction of its transverse diameter, and large pterygoid processes (not visible but which are deviated anteriorly). *T* Temporal bones with stunted petrous portions and rudimentary squamas. *O* Occipital bone composed of a basilar portion and two lateral ones with rudimentary squamas. *P* Rudimentary parietals bones

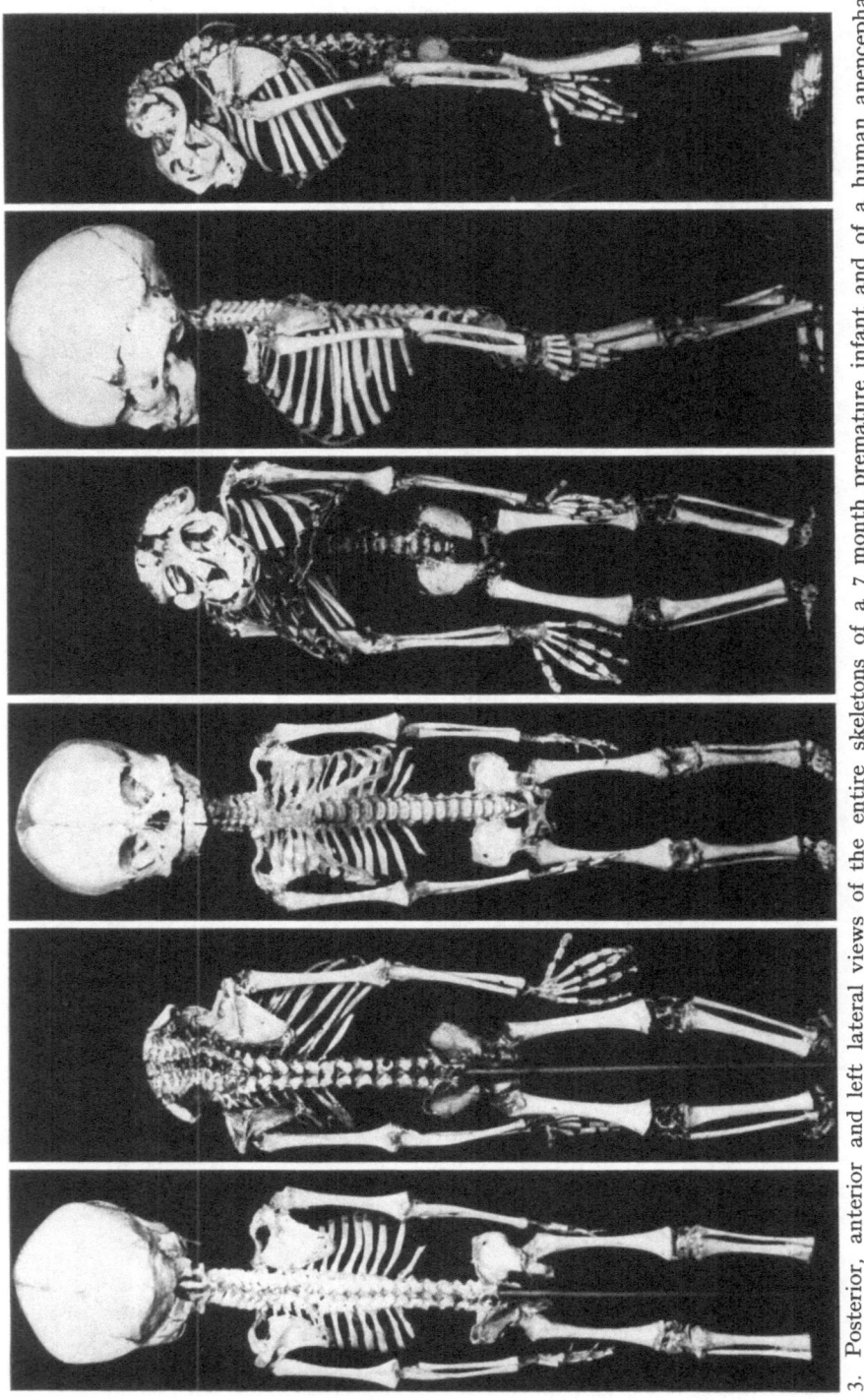

Fig. 3. Posterior, anterior and left lateral views of the entire skeletons of a 7 month premature infant and of a human anencephalic with cervical myeloschisis. Note the severity of the skeletal defects which characterize these malformations, and the marked deviation from normal of the skull and the affected vertebral column. The anomalous position of the facial bones, the lordosis and shortness of the cervical column, the absence of a cranial cavity and the abnormal base of the skull are also illustrated. From a reconstructed skeleton like this, one can analyse and determine the basic differences among the defects of the neurocranium, the viscerocranium and the chondrocranium. The basic defects of the vertebral column can be analysed in a similar manner

changes, while those that are enclosed and protected by mesoderm are generally normally formed. In cases of simple anterior anencephaly in which the foramen magnum and the planum nuchale of the squama occipitalis are formed, the cerebellum and the mid-brain structures are protected and intact, while the remainder of the brain is destroyed. In complete anencephaly in which the foramen magnum is not formed the cerebellum and the midbrain structures are totally destroyed. Cases of anencephalic human monsters have been reported with small defects (GAMPER, 1926) in which large portions of the brain are protected and therefore intact, thus permitting a longer survival (weeks) of these infants. In such cases the intact areas of the brain appear to be well developed and function normally. In anencephaly the peripheral portions of the cranial nerves which are well protected distal to the cranial cavity are "intact" but their proximal, intracranial and unprotected portions are totally destroyed. The eyes in anencephaly are usually normal, or show minor changes, and the optic nerves are intact up to the point of entrance into the cranial cavity where they are no longer recognizable. In craniorhachischisis (anencephaly with partial or complete myeloschisis) the peripheral portions of the spinal nerves which are protected are "intact" while the proximal unprotected portions are destroyed. It should be pointed out that the peripheral portions of the cranial and spinal nerves can easily be dissected out and one can demonstrate their normal anatomical distributions. Although the peripheral portions of these nerves are usually considered as "intact", they are composed only of their afferent elements. The efferent portions have degenerated as a result of the destruction of their nucleus of origin in the exposed brain or spinal cord. The spinal ganglia are frequently intact and their neurons remain recognizable perhaps because of their origin from neural crest cells which, as a rule, are not affected in these malformations. In summary then the basic defects of the CNS at the anencephalic stage are characterized by destruction of exposed areas and preservation of the protected structures with indications that the protected areas are well developed and apparently function normally.

Skeletal Defects. In anencephaly the skull as a whole (Fig. 6) is characterized by the lack of a proper cranial cavity and by reduction of its transverse diameter and marked reduction of the antero-posterior or longitudinal diameters. These skulls are incompetent to lodge and protect the developing brain. It is important to recall the embryological differences of origin and of evolution between the bones of the face (viscerocranium), the bones of the cranial vault (membranous neurocranium) and the bones of the base of the skull (chondrocranium). These differences help to explain the different behavior of these bones in these malformations.

At this late stage in the evolution of these malformations the skeletal defects are well established and can be readily investigated. These prominent and characteristic skeletal defects (Fig. 3) have not received sufficient attention, for they have generally been considered to be secondary to the anomalous CNS. Study of these skeletal defects indicates, however, that perhaps some

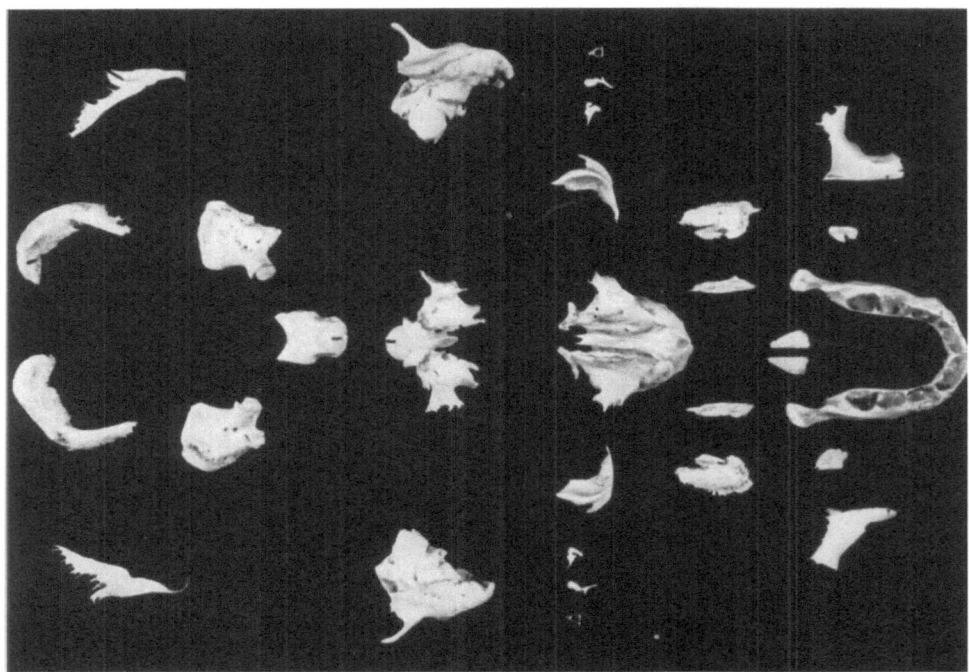

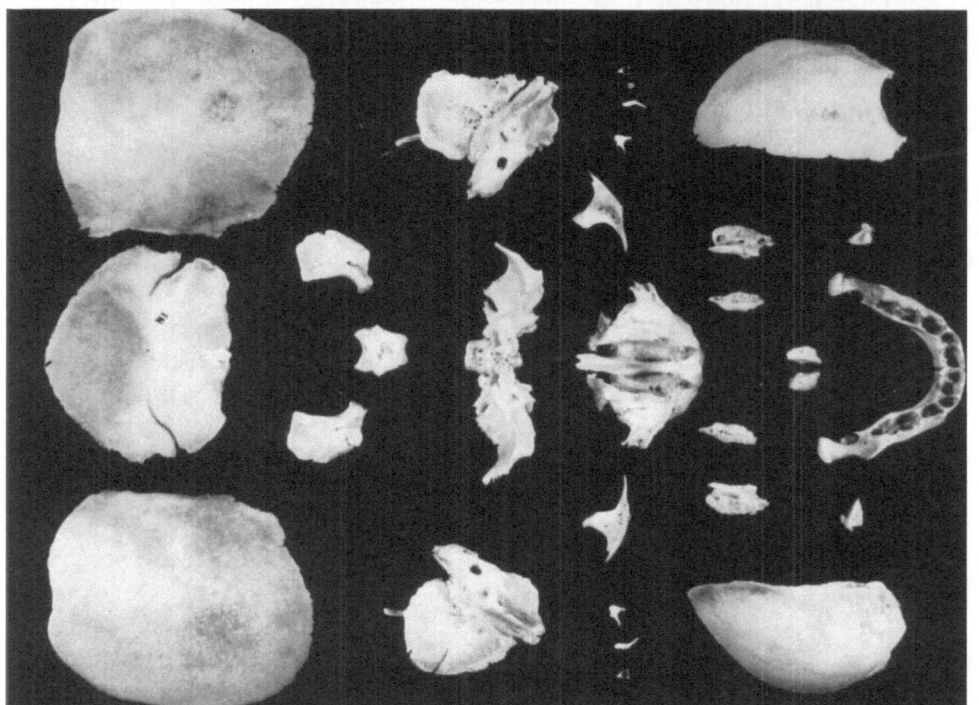

Fig. 4

could be the result of early mesodermal alterations. Analysis of the skeletal defects of the head in these malformations (Figs. 3, 4 and 6) has demonstrated that all the bones are not equally affected. Some are abnormal in position, others are rudimentary, while still others are fundamentally abnormal. The bones of the face (Fig. 4) depict only anomalous positions (slight posterior rotation) and reduction of their transverse diameter. This is well represented by the defects of the maxilla and mandible. The reconstruction demonstrates that their defects are the result of their articulation with the more basically abnormal sphenoid and temporal bones of the base of the skull. The typical facial appearance of human (Fig. 2A and B) and of experimentally-induced anencephaly (Fig. 8), i.e. elevated and pointed nose, shortness and elevation of the maxilla and protruding tongue, are the result of these defects of the facial bones. The bones of the calvarium (cranial vault) (Fig. 4), the frontal, the parietals and the squamae of the temporals and of the occipital, are all present but represented by small or rudimentary bony fragments. Since no completely formed membranous neurocranium ever existed on these malformations, the defects of these bones appear to be the result of the primary schisis. The rudimentary size of these bones represent the "amount" of membranous neurocranium left behind by the primary schisis and they reflect indirectly its size. In some of these malformations there appears to be some degree of secondary collapse of the membranous neurocranium which indicates that the size of the bones of the calvarium is perhaps smaller than the amount of membranous neurocranium available primarily. These bones also show anomalous positions resulting from their articulation with the abnormal bones of the base of the skull. In some cases of anencephaly the frontal bone is rotated posteriorly and collapsed, which is typical only of the terminal stage of the malformation. This anomalous position appears to be the result of secondary collapse following the destruction of the brain.

The bones of the base of the skull (Fig. 4) are fundamentally abnormal in these malformations. The morphological differences between the structure of these and normal bones is indeed remarkable. The petrous portions of the temporal bones in anencephaly are stunted structures in which it is difficult to identify anatomical features. The ossicles inside the otic cavities on the

Fig. 4. Reproduction of the entire skeleton of the heads of a normal (left) and of an anencephalic (complete form) infant (right) to illustrate and to compare the basic skeletal defects of these malformations. The following bones, starting from the left upper corner, are shown: the parietals and the squama of the occipital which in anencephaly is represented by two fragments; the basilar portion of the occipital with its two lateral portions; the temporals with rudimentary squamas in anencephaly and the sphenoid; the ossicles, the zygomatics and the maxilla with the vomer and the palatines; the lateral masses of the ethmoid and the turbinate bones; and the frontals, the lacrimals, the mandible and the two nasals. The rudimentary size of the bones of the cranial vault (neurocranium), the normal but narrow bones of the facial skeleton (viscerocranium), and the fundamental defects of the bones of the base of the skull (chondrocranium) are illustrated. The teeth in anencephaly are normal

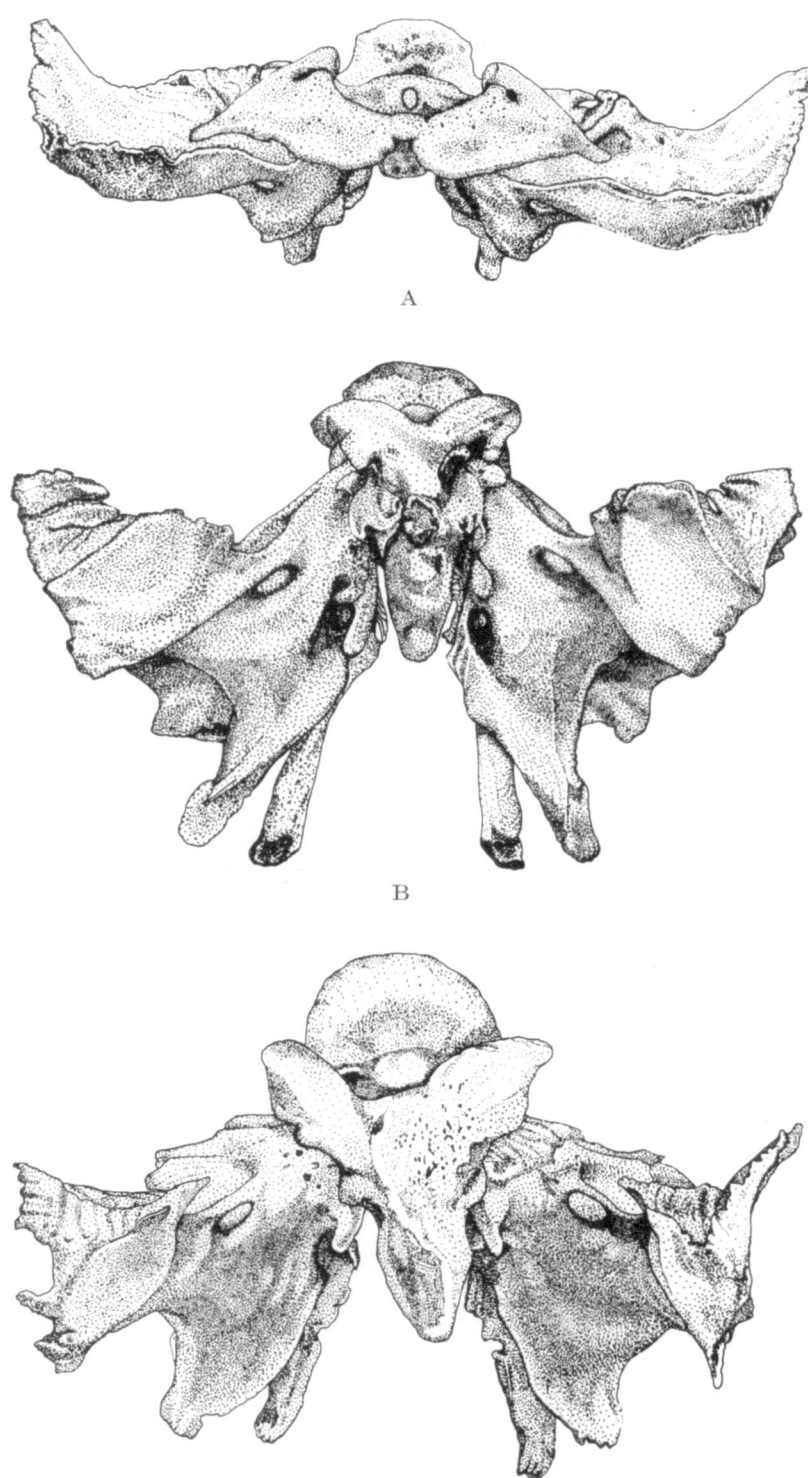

A

B

C

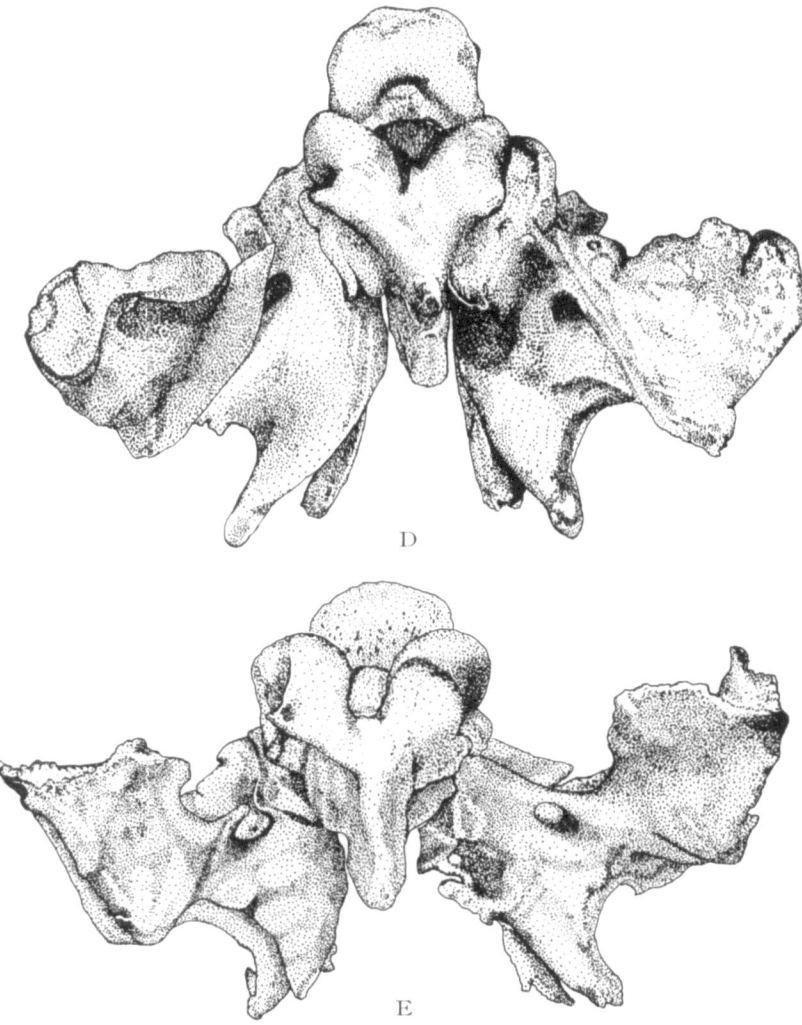

Fig. 5A—E*. Reproduction (india-ink drawing) of the sphenoid bones of: A Normal infant to use for comparison. B Simple anterior anencephaly. C Complete anencephaly. D Anencephaly with partial myeloschisis; and E Anencephaly with complete myeloschisis. These illustrate the structural similarity of these bones in the various forms of this malformation. The fundamental defects consist of: rudimentary lesser wings, stunted and contracted greater wings, long pterygoid processes deviated anteriorly and obliquely, prominent and ossified rostrum, and marked reduction of the transverse diameter of the bone

other hand, are normal, perhaps because they have a different embryonic origin related more to the viscerocranium than to the chondrocranium, being the former not basically affected. The structural defects of the sphenoid bone in the various forms of anencephaly (Fig. 5) are the best examples of the

* *Acknowledgement.* I wish to express my sincere gratitude to Mrs. VALMA PAGE for contributing the illustrations used for Figures 5 A—E.

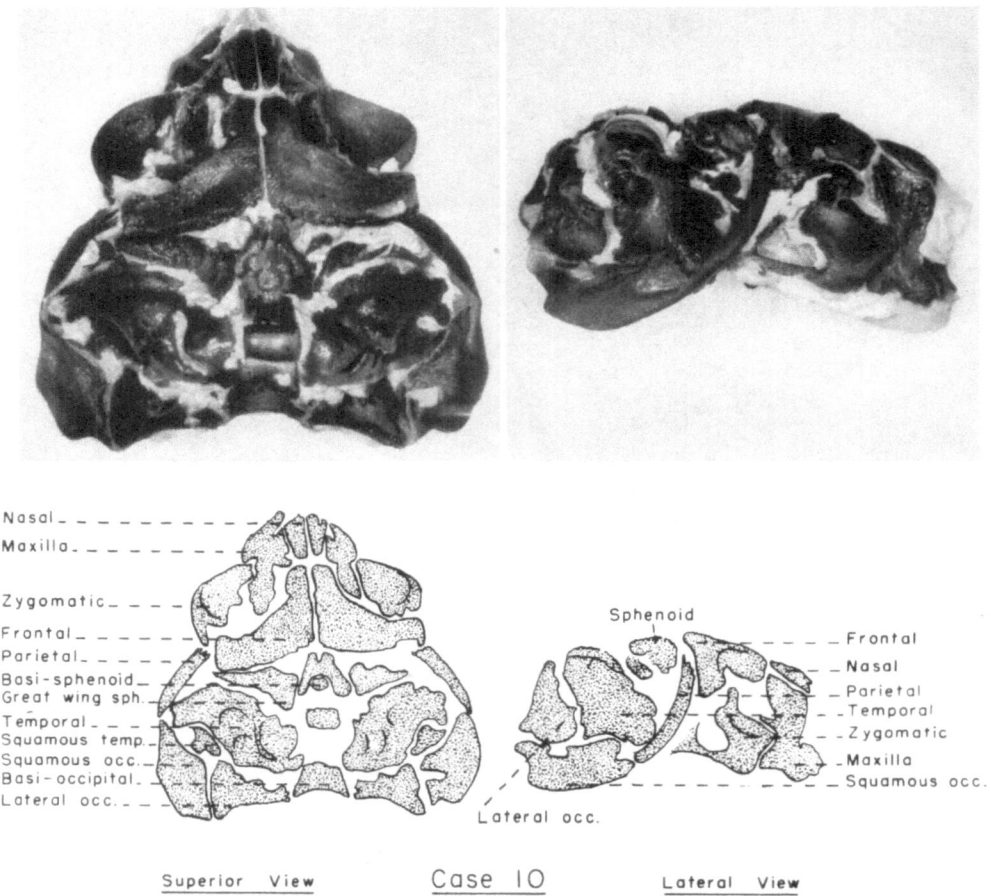

Fig. 6. Skeleton of the head of a human complete anencephaly similar to the one reproduced in Fig. 4. The mandible is absent. It illustrates the anomalous position of the
facial bones, the abnormal configuration of the base of the skull, the lack of a cranial
cavity and reduction of the antero-posterior diameter of the base of the skull. The cartilaginous sphenoid-occipital articulation has been removed for study of notochordal
abnormalities. [From MARIN-PADILLA, M.: Study of the skull in human cranioschisis.
Acta anat. **62**, 1—20 (1965), reproduced with permission]

Fig. 7. Three examples of vertebral defects of human craniorhachischisis (anencephaly
with partial or complete myeloschisis). The first two illustrate the area medullo vasculosa
the intact spinal ganglia (arrows), and the defects of the vertebral neural arches. The
last vertebrae represent a severely affected one. It has two centers of ossification, two
notochordal rests (arrows) and severe antero-lateral deviation of its neural arches.
[From MARIN-PADILLA, M.: Study of the vertebral column in human craniorhachischisis.
The significance of the notochordal alterations. Acta anat. **63**, 32—48 (1966), reproduced
with permission]

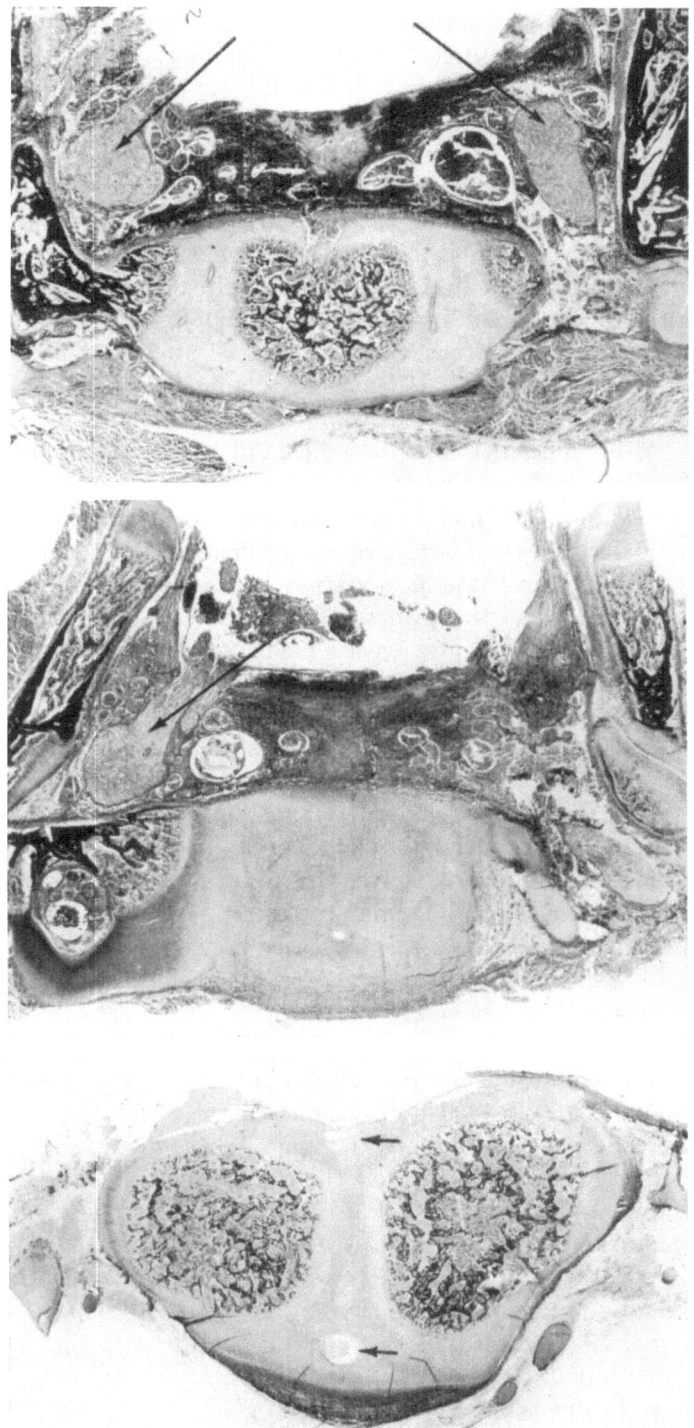

Fig. 7

severe deviation from the normal encountered in these malformations. Analysis
of the sphenoid bones of simple anterior anencephaly, of complete anencephaly, of anencephaly with partial myeloschisis and of anencephaly with
complete myeloschisis have demonstrated the extraordinary similarity of their
basic defects in spite of the great dissimilarity of the associated CNS defects.
It is difficult to explain the structural similarities of these sphenoid bones as
secondary to such varied anomalous states of the CNS (lack of proper induction). This observation has suggested the possible existence of early,
perhaps chordomesodermal alterations which affect the formation of the
chondrocranium in these malformations. The defects of the temporal and
occipital bones are similar in the various forms of anencephaly.

The analysis of the vertebral defects in craniorhachischisis (Fig. 7) (anencephaly with partial or complete myeloschisis) has demonstrated that there
are significant differences between the defects of the neural arches and those
of the vertebral bodies (vertebral axis). The neural arches are separated, with
lateral or antero-lateral deviation; they are small and rudimentary in most
instances. The defects of the neural arches are believed to be the result of the
primary schisis. Their size, lateral deviation and separation reflect indirectly
the size and the extent of the primary schisis. The defects of the vertebral
bodies appear to me to be more basic. They consist of abnormally shaped
bodies containing irregular centers of ossification which are often duplicated
or in anomalous positions. Notochordal abnormalities are frequently encountered in association with the abnormal vertebral bodies in craniorhachischisis.
The most frequently described notochordal abnormalities are: anomalous
location (anterior, posterior or lateral) of notochordal rests in the vertebral
bodies, and anomalous branches of notochordal tissue simulating partial or
localized duplications. The origin and the nature of these notochordal abnormalities in craniorhachischisis remain unknown. However, their association
with the defects of the vertebral axis has been considered to be an indication
of the possible existence of early, perhaps chordomesodermal, alterations
affecting the formation of the axial skeleton. The vertebral column in craniorhachischisis (Fig. 7) is characterized by the lack of a proper spinal cavity
and, therefore, it is considered to be incompetent to lodge and protect the
developing spinal cord. It is also characterized by a reduction of the longitudinal diameter (growth) of affected regions.

In summary, the skeletal defects at the terminal stages of these malformations are of various types, some are directly related to the primary schisis,
others appear to be the result of their articulation with basically abnormal
bones, while still others appear to be primarily affected as a result of possible
early chordomesodermal alterations.

In experimental animals with a short gestation like the hamster, the
terminal or anencephalic stages of these malformations are practically never
seen. In the rat, however, having a longer gestation, anencephaly is frequently
found at the time of birth. GIROUD and MARTINET (1957) have described in
great detail the CNS defects of exencephaly and anencephaly in the rat. They

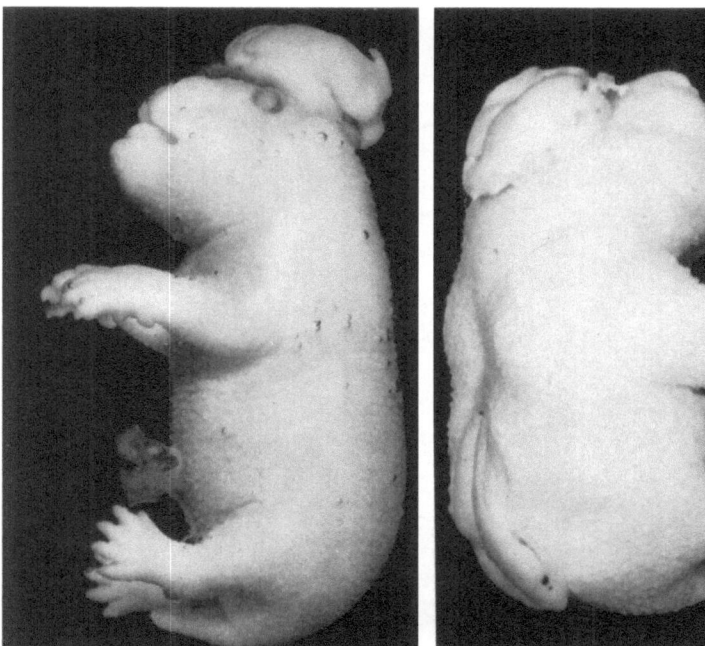

Fig. 8. Examples of vitamin A induced exencephaly and exencephaly with lumbo-sacral myeloschisis in the hamster. To illustrate the typical facial features: elevation of the nose and the maxilla, and protruding tongue. The brain and spinal cord are unclosed and prominent

have demonstrated the relationship of these defects as two stages in the evolution of the same basic abnormality. In experimentally induced anencephaly all exposed areas of the CNS are destroyed and the protected ones are not only intact, but considered normal. The development of the CNS in spite of the lack of closure is considered to be normal and the degeneration secondary to exposure.

The analysis of the skeletal structures of the head in experimentally induced anencephaly in hamsters (Fig. 9) has demonstrated that the skull as a whole lacks a proper cranial cavity and its transverse, and particularly its anteroposterior diameters, are markedly reduced. It is, therefore, primarily incompetent to lodge and protect the developing brain which protrudes prominently (exencephaly) (Fig. 8) and depicts superficial but progressive degeneration. Analysis of the facial bones discloses posterior rotation causing the anterior elevation of the snout which is so typical for the affected hamsters. The facial bones also depict a slight reduction of the transverse diameter resulting from their articulation with the narrow base of the skull. The bones of the calvarium are small and rudimentary, but all are identifiable. Their size reflects the extent of the primary schisis. The cartilaginous nature of the skeleton of the hamster at the time of birth makes it very difficult to analyze the individual bones. However, the overall skeletal defects appear to be

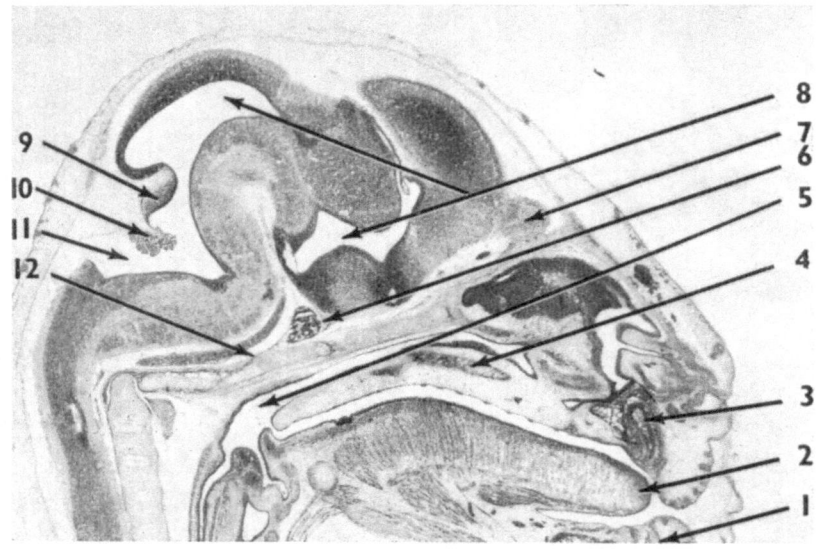

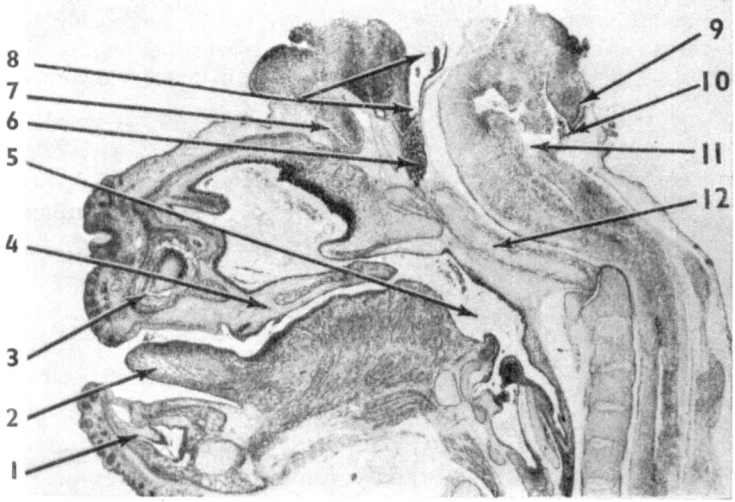

Fig. 9. Sagittal section of the heads of a normal (above) and of an exencephalic hamster (below) induced experimentally with vitamin A (the normal hamster is a newborn and the abnormal one was obtained one day prior to delivery). To illustrate the abnormal elevation of the nose and the maxilla, the marked reduction of longitudinal diameter of the base of the skull, the protruding brain squeezed out of the incompetent cranial cavity and the site of the failure of closure located somewhere between the III ventricle and the acqueduct. (Key: *1* Mandible, *2* Tongue, *3* Maxilla, *4* Palate, *5* Pharynx, *6* Pituitary gland, *7* Olfactory bulb under the everted neocortex, *8* The III ventricle and the acqueduct (both of which communicate with the exterior indicating the site of primary failure of closure), *9* Cerebellum, *10* Choroid plexus, *11* IV ventricle, *12* Basilar portion of the sphenoid

similar to those described in the human malformations (Figs. 3, 4 and 9). Analysis of experimentally induced (vitamin A) lumbo-sacral myeloschisis (Figs. 8 and 10) has demonstrated identical skeletal defects to those described in human craniorhachischisis (Fig. 7).

2. Exencephalic or Cartilaginous Stage

These malformations, in spite of the extent and the severity of the fundamental defects, are perfectly compatible with intrauterine life. The majority of human cases described are encountered at the time of birth and they are, therefore, at the terminal or anencephalic stage of the malformations. Few cases have been reported in the literature of the intermediate or cartilaginous stages of the malformations in man. HUNTER (1935) described a case of simple exencephaly recovered from a tubal pregnancy. A case of exencephaly with cervical and high dorsal myeloschisis (Fig. 2A and B) obtained from a spontaneous abortion, is discussed and analyzed here. Human exencephaly is characterized by an unclosed skull with protruding, partially everted and apparently overdeveloped brain and by severe skeletal defects of the head and of the affected vertebral regions. Exencephaly thus represents an earlier developmental stage of anencephaly.

CNS Defects. The analysis of the brain and the spinal cord (when affected) in human exencephaly has demonstrated that in spite of the failure to close it has undergone a normal development. Anatomical structures are recognized, and are reported as histologically normal or having only minor variations. The thalamus, the cranial and spinal nerves and their nuclei or origin, the cerebellum and the mid-brain structures are reported as normal. The optic cups, nerves, chiasm and tracts, as well as the cochlear and vestibular portions of the otic system are also reported as normal anatomically and histologically. However, some abnormalities in the lamination of the neocortex (reversion of the order) and superficial focal degeneration have been reported in human exencephaly. The brain is partially covered by fragments of meningeal tissue

Fig. 10A—H. Selected sections from a single hamster (13 days old) with vitamin A induced lumbo-sacral myeloschisis (rhachischisis). A Section above the defect showing normal spinal cord, normal closure of the vertebral neural arches, but an abnormal vertebral body with a large notochordal rest deviated toward the left side. B Section above but closer to the defect showing normal spinal cord, abnormal separation of the vertebral neural arches (occult spina bifida) and abnormal vertebral body with a large notochordal rest deviated toward the right side. C and D Sections closer to the defect showing occult spina bifida and meningocele, vertebral and notochordal defects (arrow) and the beginning of the failure of closure (D). E and F Section through the defect showing open myeloschisis and rhachischisis. G Section through the defects showing complete absence of the vertebrae and notochordal duplication. H Enlargement of the enclosed area of G to illustrate the notochordal duplication (arrows). These sections illustrate the severity of the defects of the vertebral axis and the notochordal alterations which are considered to be the result of early chordomesodermal disturbances affecting the formation of the axial skeleton in these malformations and not the consequenc of the CNS defects (H.E × 10; H. × 40)

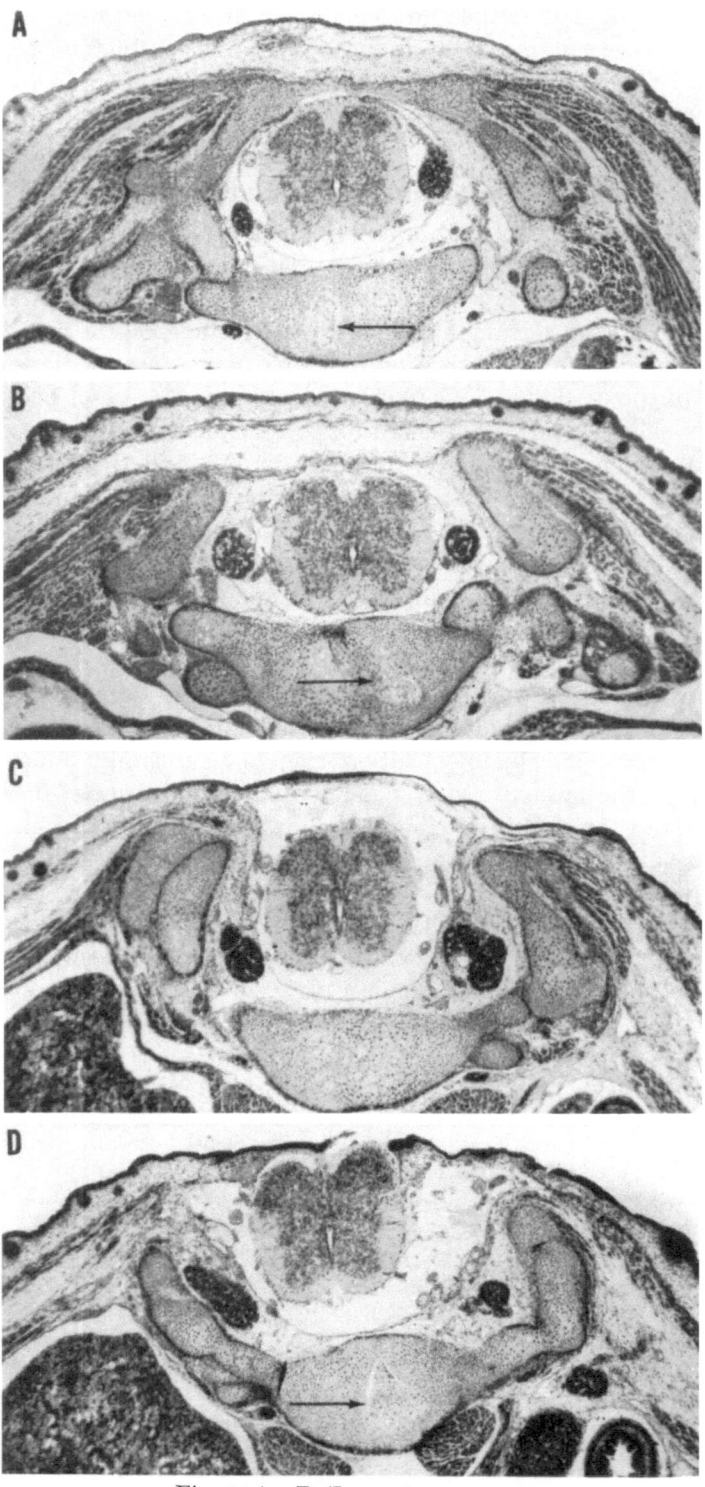

Fig. 10A—D (Legend see p. 165)

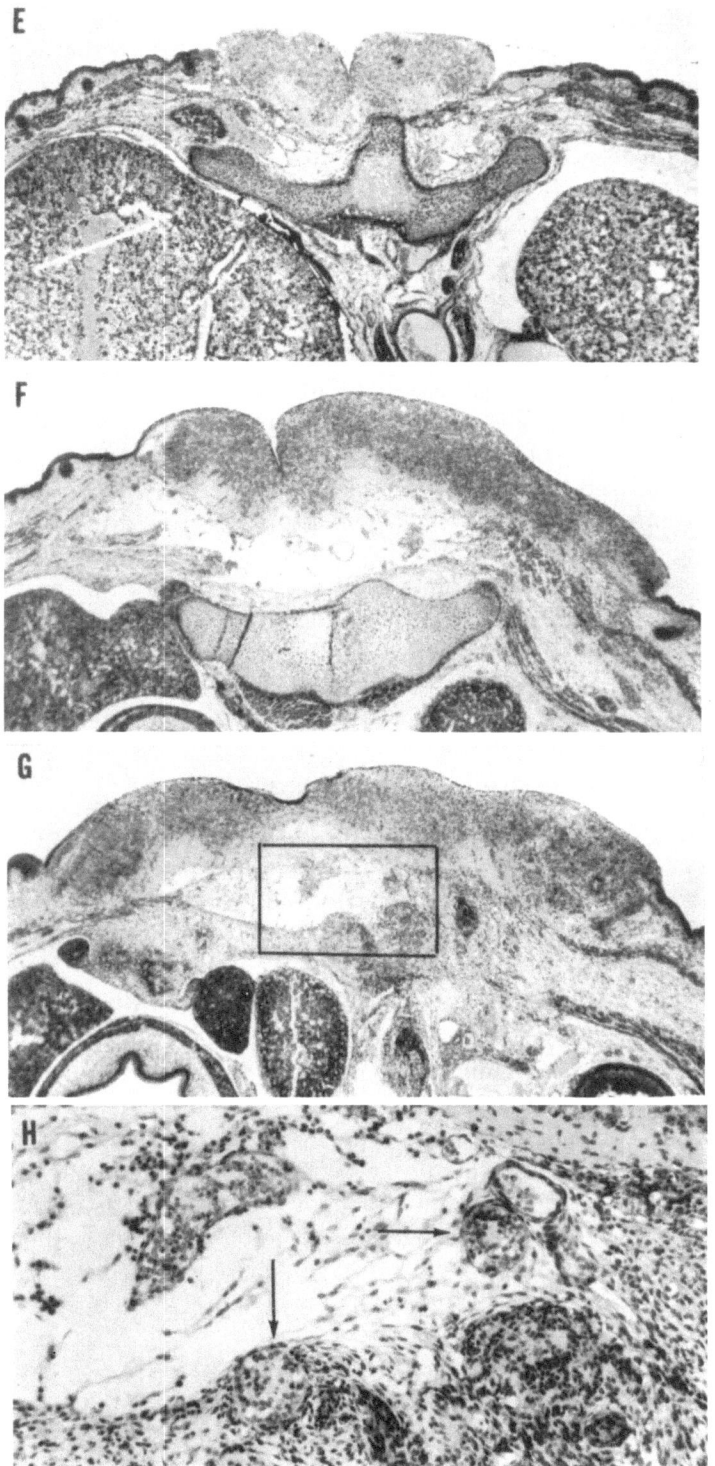

Fig. 10 E—H (Legend see p. 165)

(Fig. 2A and B). The typical protrusion and apparent overdevelopment of the brain in exencephaly (Fig. 2A and B) appear to be due to the lack of a suitable cranial cavity to lodge it (Fig. 2D). It is the result of the brain being progressively squeezed out of the incompetent cranial cavity during its own progressive development.

Skeletal System. Analysis of the defects of the cartilagenous skeleton of the head in exencephaly (Fig. 2D and E) has demonstrated the same type of basic abnormalities encountered in anencephaly. This is not surprising since the osseous skeleton of anencephaly may be considered as an ossified replica of the cartilaginous skeleton of exencephaly. The facial bones in exencephaly depict only anomalies of position and reduction of the transverse diameter. The bones of the calvarium are small and rudimentary but all can be identified. The bones of the base of the skull are fundamentally abnormal and of these, the defects of the sphenoid bone are noteworthy (Fig. 2D and E). This bone is characterized by small stunted lesser wings, contracted and small greater wings, prominent and long pterygoid processes in an antero-oblique position and by a prominent rostrum. These defects are identical to those of the sphenoid bone in anencephaly and they are considered as a prominent and distinct feature of these malformations. The skull in exencephaly lacks a suitable cranial cavity and its transverse and antero-posterior diameters are greatly reduced. The analysis of the affected vertebrae has demonstrated the same basic defects encountered in the terminal stages of these malformations.

3. Dysrhaphic or Mesodermal Stage

The early stages of these malformations in both human and experimental animals are characterized by an unclosed neuroectoderm (Dysrhaphism) and by mesodermal alterations affecting primarily the unsegmented mesoderm. The dysrhaphic defect may be localized in the cephalic or in the caudal region, or it may involve the entire dorsal aspect of the embryo.

CNS Defects. The unclosed, slightly everted neuroectoderm of very young affected embryos shows normal development and histological differentiation. In somewhat older embryos it might depict some degree of folding and an apparent over-development. These changes must be evaluated in relation to the surrounding mesodermal structures which already begin to show some degree of underdevelopment and collapse, especially noticeable in the cephalic region of the embryos. These changes become more accentuated as the affected embryo grows, and marked apparent overgrowth and folding have then been described. Cellular hypoplasia and focal superficial areas of degeneration have also been reported in the unclosed neuroectoderm, more frequently in older embryos.

Skeletal System. Mesodermal alterations have been described in the early dysrhaphic stages in both human and experimentally induced malformations. In young embryos alterations are found usually in the unsegmented mesoderm, especially in the cephalic region, while in older embryos the somites also show alterations. The alterations described in the unsegmented mesoderm consist of a loose arrangement of cells as well as a reduction in their number. These changes are invariably accompanied by the accumulation of extracellular fluid (edema). In older embryos the rarefication of the mesodermal cells and the amount of accumulated extracellular fluid increase and collapse of the mesodermal tissue becomes apparent. In older embryos a reduction in the number of somitic cells and focal somite necrosis have been reported. Also, in older embryos, notochordal alterations (anomalies of position, anomalous branches, localized or partial duplication) are frequently found. It should once more be emphasized that all of these changes have been reported both in human and in experimentally induced malformations.

Some final coments should be made about the less severe form of these malformations, the spina bifida occulta or occult rhachischisis. In essence this malformation is characterized by a normally closed neural tube and by vertebral defects which are related structurally to those encountered in the most severe forms of the malformations here discussed. Several clinical types of spina bifida are known, those with normal spinal cord, with ectodermal sinuses, with meningocele, with meningomyelocele, to mention only the most common. In all these cases vertebral defects are found which gives further support to the idea that there are early mesodermal alterations in these malformations which are considered primary and not secondary to the CNS defects as in generally believed. A sequential analysis of an experimentally induced myeloschisis illustrating the evolution, extent, types of defects and notochordal alterations is depicted in Fig. 10. The fact that in spina bifida occulta (Fig. 10B), the spinal cord is closed and normal, but the vertebra affected are abnormal is perhaps the strongest argument in favor of the existance of early chordomesodermal alterations in these malformations.

V. Discussion

The present analysis has attempted to indicate that in the malformations under discussion there are characteristic defects in both the CNS and the skeletal (mesodermal) structures throughout their entire embryonic development. The primary defect of the CNS is the failure of closure of the neuroectoderm, which necessarily also involves the failure of closure of the dorsal ectoderm and of the mesoderm. The unclosed neuroectoderm, although apparently capable of normal development and histological differentiation, undergoes a progressive degenerative process leading eventually to the total destruction of all its exposed and unprotected areas. From the very early stages on and through the entire evolution of these malformations the CNS is not properly lodged in a suitable cranial or spinal cavity. This fact explains the apparent overdevelopment and folding of the CNS which is so characteristic of the early and intermediate stages of these malformations. There are indications that the protected and unexposed structures of the CNS are functionally and histologically normal. This gives support to the idea that there are no primary alterations of the neuroectoderm but that the CNS anomalies are secondary due to failure of closure. It is concluded that there are various and distinct types of skeletal (mesodermal) defects in these malformations, some of which are very unlikely the result of the lack of proper induction by the anomalous CNS.

Three distinct types of skeletal (mesodermal) defects characterize these malformations: 1) The primary failure which involves the neuroectoderm, the ectoderm and the mesoderm which could explain the defects of the bones of the calvarium and of the neural arches of the vertebrae since a completely formed membranous neurocranium never existed in these malformations. The rudimentary size of these bones reflects the size of the primary schisis. 2) The facial bones (viscerocranium) are not primarily affected, they are not structurally abnormal and only depict anomalous position resulting from their adaptation to the abnormal bones of the base of the skull. The reduction of the transverse diameter of the facial bones results from their adaptation to the abnormally narrow base of the skull. 3) The bones of the chondrocranium and of the vertebral axis (vertebral bodies) are severely affected. They not only show structural anomalies but fail to develop suitable cranial and spinal cavities for the lodging of the developing CNS. The chondrocranium shows slight reduction of its transverse diameter from the early stages and marked reduction of its longitudinal diameter. A reduction of the longitudinal growth of the affected vertebral column is also a distinct feature. The pronounced lordosis of the head and vertebral column are the result of the retarded longitudinal growth of these structures in relation to the normal growth of the remainder of the embryonic body. The skeletal defects of the chondrocranium and of the vertebral axis are considered to be related to the early mesodermal alterations in affected embryos. These, so far the earliest detectable changes seen to date, consist mainly of a reduction in the number of mesodermal cells and in the accumulation of extracellular fluid in the unsegmented mesoderm. A reduction in the number of available mesodermal cells could explain the anomalous size of the base of the skull and the failure of the axial skeleton to achieve a normal longitudinal growth.

While accumulation of extracellular fluid and mesodermal collapse, which have also been described in the secondary reopening of a previously closed neural tube (KLIKA and JELINEK, 1961), could be explained as being secondary to the exposure of the mesoderm which follows the primary failure of closure; the reduction, shrinkage and rarefication of cells in the unsegmented mesoderm may well be the result of even earlier undefined disturbances in the chordomesodermal system. The fundamental defects of the axial skeleton (chondrocranium and vertebral axis) and the notochordal alterations encountered in these malformations support this concept. Furthermore, such chordomesodermal disturbances could in themselves explain the primary failure of closure of the neural folds.

The earliest mesodermal alterations described in vitamin A induced anencephaly (MARIN-PADILLA, 1966) were encountered in embryos at a developmental stage in which the closure of the neural tube was still in progress and not yet concluded. In these embryos reduction, shrinkage and rarefication of the mesodermal cells were already present (as well as some accumulations of extracellular fluid). The fact that the mesodermal alterations are encountered in very young embryos and before any detectable changes in the neuroectoderm makes it unlikely that they are the result of exposure. On the other hand, these mesodermal alterations together with the notochordal changes appear to be an indication of chordomesodermal disturbances which subsequently affect the embryonic axiation and the normal development of the neural folds. Primary, very early chordomesodermal disturbances will explain: on one hand, the fundamental defects of the axial skeleton and the notochordal alterations encountered in these malformations and, on the other hand, the failure of the formation (platyneuria) or in the progressive growth (elevation) of the neural folds such causing primary failure of closure.

Significant differences should exist, therefore, between anencephaly induced by the reopening of a previously closed neural tube and anencephaly caused by primary failure of closure. The former should not have the fundamental defects of the chondrocranium and the notochordal alterations which would distinguish them from the latter forms of the malformations. Both types should be characterized by similar defects in the CNS, since these are the result of the exposure of the neuroectoderm which follows either the primary failure of closure or its reopening. The morphogenesis of these two types of malformations are thus fundamentally quite different and, therefore, they should be considered as different entities. As far as we can ascertain, the human malformations are the result of a primary failure of closure of the neural tube and due to early chordomesodermal disturbances. Also, some of the experimentally induced malformations share with the human cases the same origin and morphogenesis.

It will be perhaps desirable in conclusion to outline some of the areas which need most urgent further investigations. A detailed comparative analysis between the chondrocrania of malformations induced by reopening of a previously closed neural tube and those resulting from primary failure of closure is urgently needed. The formation and progressive growth (elevation) of the neural folds and their relation to the embryonic chordomesodermal system should be investigated. The formation and progressive growth of the neural folds should also be investigated in experimentally induced malformations in mammals. GALLERA (1959) already investigated in the chick, exposed to an atmosphere deficient in oxygen, the early chordomesodermal disturbances and the failure in the formation of the neural folds (platyneuria). Platyneuria corresponds later in development to anencephaly in both avian and mammalian embryos.

VI. Summary

An analysis of the embryonic development of the basic defects which characterize anencephaly and related malformations has been presented.

From it the following conclusions appear justifiable. A. These malformations are characterized through their entire embryonic development by distinct CNS and skeletal defects. B. The CNS defects appear to be the consequence of the failure of closure of the neuroectoderm. The unclosed neuroectoderm, although capable of "normal" development, undergoes a progressive degenerative process leading to complete destruction of all its exposed areas, while there is preservation of those areas protected and enclosed by mesodermal tissue. C. Three distinct types of skeletal defects characterize these malformations: 1) Defects of the bones of the cranial vault and of the vertebral neural arches which are partly the consequence of the primary schisis (absence of a completely formed membranous neurocranium) and also the consequence of the basic abnormalities of the axial skeleton. In occult spina bifida or occult rhachischisis, in which there is no failure of closure of the neural tube, the spinal cord is normal but the vertebral bodies and the neural arches of the affected region depict the same type of structural defects encountered in the open forms of myeloschisis or rhachischisis. 2) The facial bones (viscerocranium) only depict anomalies of position secondary to their adaptation to basically abnormal bones of the base of the skull. 3) The bones of the base of the skull (chondrocranium) and the bodies of the vertebra (vertebral axis) are fundamentally abnormal in these malformations. The fundamental defects encountered in these skeletal structures are considered to be the consequence of early chordome sodermal disturbances affecting the embryonic axiation. D. Early chordomesodermal disturbances in these malformations are believed to interfere also with the formation of or the subsequent development of the neural folds causing primary failure of closure of the neural tube.

The analysis of the morphogenesis of anencephaly and related malformations, presented here, has emphasized general concepts on the nature of the defects and their evolution as well as on the discussion of their possible origin and morphogenesis. In order to avoid confusing disgressions from this general outline many references and details on these malformations have been omitted from the text. This, in part, has been corrected by adding a list of references separated into those related to the early, the intermediate and the terminal stages of evolution of these malformations.

References

A. References Cited in the Text

Gallera, T.: Influence de l'atmosphère artificiellement modifiée sur le développement embryonnaire du poulet. Acta anat. (Basel) 11, 549—585 (1951).

Gamper, E.: Bau und Leistungen eines menschlichen Mittelhirnwesens (Arhinencephalie mit Encepholocele). Zugleich ein Beitrag zur Teratologie und Fasersystomatik. Z. ges. Neurol. Psychiat. 102, 154—235 (1926).

Gardner, W. J.: Myelocele: Rupture of the neural tube? Clin. Neurosurg. 15, 57—79 (1968).

Giroud, A., Martinet, M.: Morphogenèse de l'anencèphalie. Arch. Anat. micr. Morph. exp. 46, 247—264 (1957).

HICKS, S. P., D'AMATO, C. J.: Effects of ionizing radiation on mammalian development. In: Advances in teratology. London: Logos Press & Academic Press 1966.

HUNTER, R. H.: Extroversion of the cerebral hemiphere in human embryo. J. Anat. (Lond.) 69, 82—83 (1935).

JELINEK, R.: Development of the experimental exencephaly in the chick. Čs. Morfol. 8, 363—378 (1960).

KEEN, J. A.: The morphology of the skull in human anencephalic monsters. S. Afr. med. J. 8, 1—9 (1962).

— Morphologie du crâne chez le foetus anencéphale. Arch. Anat. (Strasbourg) 49, 233—246 (1966).

KLIKA, E., JELINEK, R.: Histogenesis of the experimental exencephaly in the chick. Čs. Morfol. 9, 162—172 (1961).

MARIN-PADILLA, M.: Mesodermal alterations induced by hypervitaminosis A. J. Embryol. exp. Morph. 15, 261—269 (1966).

MORGAGNI, J. B.: The seats and causes of diseases investigated by anatomy. (English translation by BENJAMIN ALEXANDER.) London: A. Millar & T. Cadell 1769.

PADGET, D. H.: Spina bifida and embryonic neuroschisis. — A cause relationship. Johns Hopk. med. J. 123, 233—252 (1968).

RECKLINGHAUSEN, F. VON: Untersuchungen über die Spina bifida. II. Über die Art und die Entstehung der Spina bifida, ihre Beziehung zur Rückenmarks- und Darmspalte. Virchows Arch. path. Anat. 105, 296—330 (1886).

WILSON, J. G., JORDAN, H. C., BRENT, R. L.: Effects of irradiation on embryonic development. Amer. J. Anat. 92, 153—187 (1954).

B. References to the Early Developmental Stages

DEKABAN, A. S.: Anencephaly in early human embryos. J. Neuropath. exp. Neurol. 22, 533—548 (1963).

— BARTELMEZ, G. W.: Complete dysraphism in 14 somite human embryo. A contribution to normal and abnormal morphogenesis. Amer. J. Anat. 115, 27—42 (1964).

DZIALLAS, P.: Ein Fetus von 18 mm Sitzhöhe mit Anencephalie und Craniorhachischisis. Virchows Arch. path. Anat. 293, 662—687 (1962).

ERSKINE, C. A.: Human anencephaly in early developmental stages. Acta anat. (Basel) 23, 251—258 (1955).

FELLER, A., STERNBERG, H.: Zur Kenntnis der Fehlbildungen der Wirbelsäule. I. Die Wirbelkörperspalte und ihre formale Genese. Virchows Arch. path. Anat. 272, 613—640 (1929).

GIROUD, A.: Causes and morphogenesis of anencephaly. In: Congenital malformations. Ciba Foundation Symposium. Boston: Little & Brown Co. 1960.

— DELMAS, A., MARTINET, M.: Etude morphogenetique sur des embryons anencèphales. Arch. Anat. (Strasbourg) 47, 295—311 (1963).

— MARTINET, M.: Morphogenèse de l'anencèphalie. Arch. Anat. micr. Morph. exp. 46, 247—264 (1957).

KOCHHAR, D. M., JOHNSON, E. M.: Morphological and autoradiographic studies of cleft palate induced in rat embryos by maternal hypervitaminosis A. J. Embryol. exp. Morph. 14, 223—238 (1965).

LEMIRE, R. J., SHEPARD, T. H., ALVORD, E. C.: Caudal myelochisis (lumbo-sacral spina bifida cystica) in a five millimeter (horizon XIV) human embryo. Anat. Rec. 152, 9—16 (1965).

MARIN-PADILLA, M.: Mesodermal alterations induced by hypervitaminosis A. J. Embryol. exp. Morph. 15, 261—269 (1966).

— Mesodermal alterations induced by dimethyl sulfoxide. Proc. Soc. exp. Biol. (N.Y.) 122, 717—720 (1966).

Marin-Padilla, M., Ferm, V. H.: Somite necrosis and developmental malformations induced by vitamin A in the golden hamster. J. Embryol. exp. Morph. **13**, 1—8 (1965).

Patten, B. M.: Embryological stages in the establishing of myeloschisis with spina bifida. Amer. J. Anat. **93**, 365—345 (1953).

Sternberg, H.: Über Spaltbedingungen des Medullarohres bei jungen menschlichen Embryonen, ein Beitrag zur Entstehung der Anencephalie und der Rachischisis. Virchows Arch. path. Anat. **272**, 325—373 (1929).

C. References to Intermediate Stages

Dodds, G. S., Angelis, E. de: An anencephalic human embryo 16.5 mm long Anat. Rec. **67**, 499—505 (1937).

Ford, E. H. R.: An enencephalic human embryo of 33.5 millimetres. Acta anat. (Basel) **28**, 149—155 (1956).

Fraser, J. E.: Report on an anencephalic embryo. J. Anat. (Lond.) **56**, 12—19 (1921).

Hunter, R. H.: Extroversion of the cerebral hemisphere in human embryo. J. Anat. (Lond.) **69**, 82—83 (1935).

Stroer, W. F. H., Van der Zwan, A.: Anencephaly and rhachischisis posterior with description of a human hemicephalus of 18 mm. J. Anat. (Lond.) **73**, 441—450 (1939).

Vries, E. de: Description of a young anencephalic and amyetic embryo. Anat. Rec. **36**, 293—317 (1927).

D. References to the Terminal Stages

Deppe, B.: Beiträge zur Frage der Skelettverhältnisse bei Anencephalia und Craniorhachischisis. Virchows Arch. path. Anat. **293**, 153—164 (1934).

Doskocil, M.: Configuration of the skull base in cases with pathologically developed central nervous system. Sborn. lék. **64**, 20—33 (1962).

Keen, J. A.: The morphology of the skull in human anencephalic monsters. S. Afr. med. J. **8**, 1—9 (1962).

— Morphologie du crane chez le foetu anencephale. Arch. Anat. (Strasbourg) **49**, 233—246 (1966).

Marin-Padilla, M.: Study of the skull in human cranioschisis. Acta anat. (Basel) **62**, 1—20 (1965).

— Study of the sphenoid bone in human cranioschisis and craniorhachischisis. Virchows Arch. path. Anat. **339**, 245—253 (1965).

— Study of the vertebral column in human craniorhachischisis. The significance of the notochordal alterations. Acta anat. (Basel) **63**, 32—48 (1966).

Mathis, H.: Über 9 Fälle von Kraniorachischisis (spina bifida) mit besonderer Berücksichtigung des axialen Skeletts. Virchows Arch. path. Anat. **257**, 364—391 (1925).

Saunders, R. L.: Combined anterior and posterior spina bifida in a living neonatal human female. Anat. Rec. **87**, 255—278 (1943).

Department of Veterinary Pathology (*) and the
Department of Veterinary Microbiology (**)
Washington State University, Pullman, Washington 99163

The Chediak-Higashi Syndrome:
A Comparative Review[1]

George A. Padgett*, D. V. M., James M. Holland*, D. V. M.,
William C. Davis**, Ph. D., and James B. Henson*, D. V. M., Ph. D.

With 3 Figures

Table of Contents

I. Introduction

The Chediak-Higashi syndrome (C-HS) is a rare autosomal recessive disease first described in man by Beguez-Cesar in 1943. The most prominent features of the disease are partial oculocutaneous albinism, the presence of abnormal, large membrane bound organelles in various cell types, and increased susceptibility to infection. More recently, this syndrome has been

[1] Supported in part by Grant AI 06591 and Grant AI 06477 from the National Institutes of Health, Bethesda, Maryland. Washington State University, College of Agriculture, Experiment Station, Project 1798.

reported to occur in mink, cattle, and mice. The general characteristics and clinical aspects of the disease in these animals and man have been reviewed recently and will not be considered here (Padgett, 1968a) (Fig. 1).

Although the subject of numerous investigations, the fundamental defect which gives rise to increased susceptibility to pathogenic organisms has not been delineated. The purpose of the present review has been to assemble the available data obtained from humans, cattle, mink, and mice in a manner which we believe most likely to reveal the extent of homology of the C-HS syndrome in such phylogenetically disparate groups of animals.

II. Susceptibility to Infection
A. Children

It is difficult to prove that C-HS children are more susceptible to various infections than normal children. However, every investigator concerned with the affected children has reported that they are more susceptible to infectious diseases than normal individuals. The increased susceptibility of the C-HS children to infection is also suggested by their decreased life span. The average age of the children who were dead when their case was reported was 5.4 years, while the average age of those who were alive at the time of the report was 8.4 years. Only 5 of the 47 C-HS children have lived longer than 10 years (Padgett, 1968a). The children observed had repeated bouts of upper respiratory infection, pneumonia, tonsillitis, oral ulcers, keratitis, abscesses, boils and various other pyogenic cutaneous infections, otitis externa and interna as well as diffuse petechial haemorrhages, usually on the extremities, and frank intestinal haemorrhage. Staphylococcus aureus, Streptococcus pyogenes, pneumococci, Aspergillus spp., Monilia spp. and Pseudomonas aeruginosa were demonstrated in various lesions in the children. Padgett et al. (1968b) attempted to retrospectively document the infections that 3 C-HS children had during the time they were under observation. The children were studied for 11, 24, and 15 months, respectively, and had a total of 37 separate infections and 22 separate pyrexic episodes which were not correlated with the infections. Unfortunately, adequate documentation as to the number of infections in the 3 normal siblings in the family during the same period of time was not available. However, these children were usually normal when a C-HS affected child had fever or an infection.

On the other hand, C-HS children have been reported to recover from vaccinia, varicella, measles and mumps infections without difficulty (Stein-brinck, 1948; Donohue and Bain, 1957; Maggi et al., 1957; Saraiva et al., 1959; Jannini et al., 1963; Barkve, 1967). Despite the fact that C-HS children appear to manage some viral infections without difficulty, it is not apparent that they manage all viruses (or probable viruses) equally well. There have been several reports of a high prevalence of neoplasms in C-HS children. These reports involved 5 cases and were based on clinical and pathologic features which, in many respects, resembled malignant lymphoma (Efrati and Jonas,

1958; PAGE et al., 1962; DENT et al., 1966; WHITE, 1966b). Hepatospleno-megaly, lymphadenopathy and general cellular infiltrates which occurred not only in these 5 cases, but in nearly every C-HS child were stressed in their diagnoses. In support of their conclusion, they reported the presence of virus-like particles which resembled Bernhard Type C virus in two C-HS children (WHITE, 1966b; DENT et al., 1966). Similar particles have been reported to cause lymphoma in animals. In addition, spleen cells from one of the children were maintained in tissue culture for 152 days (DENT et al., 1966). It is of interest that SUNG et al. (1969) reporting on the neurologic lesions in 2 of these 5 children, did not conclude that they were lymphomatous in nature. Further-more, DOUGLAS et al. (1969) failed to find evidence associating virus-like particles with the C-HS in general or the cellular infiltrate in particular. Several other investigators have ruled out neoplasm as a cause of the infiltrate observed in the C-HS children they examined (PADGETT et al., 1967; DONOHUE and BAIN, 1957; MAGGI et al., 1957; SARAIVA et al., 1959; HANSSON et al., 1959; IWAI and OYAKE, 1964). In several reports, it was suggested that the lesions present may have been due to infectious mononucleosis (BEGUEZ-CESAR, 1943; PADGETT et al., 1967b; IWAI and OYAKE, 1964). In another study, however, this diagnosis was ruled out on the basis of the severity of the clinical course (HANSSON et al., 1959). The descriptions of the infiltrates present in C-HS cases which were not diagnosed as malignant lymphoma were similar to those present in cases in which such a diagnosis was made. Perhaps, at present the best that can be said is that if there is a single agent or disease process causing the tissue infiltrate which has been morphologically very characteristic in the C-HS children, the evidence concerning its identity is, at best, inconclusive.

B. Cattle

The data on susceptibility of C-HS cattle is somewhat better than that available for the children, since a prospective study of the number of infections could be undertaken. In addition, adequate numbers of control cattle subject to the same extrinsic factors were housed with the C-HS cattle.

During a single year, 13 C-HS cattle had 46 distinct infections caused by various micro-organisms and 38 pyrexic episodes which were not correlated with the infections. During the same period, 18 non-C-HS cattle had 4 separate infections and 14 unassociated pyrexic episodes. Six C-HS calves died during the year, but none of the non-C-HS calves died (PADGETT et al., 1968b).

As with the C-HS children, the increased susceptibility to infection of C-HS cattle is also suggested by their shortened life span. The average age at time of death for all C-HS cattle has been 12.4 months. Four males and 2 females have lived 3 years or longer and one of these, a bull, lived to the age of 6 years (PADGETT, 1968b) (Fig. 2).

C. Mink

The best available evidence for increased susceptibility of C-HS individuals is provided by mink. Epidemiologic studies have shown them to be more

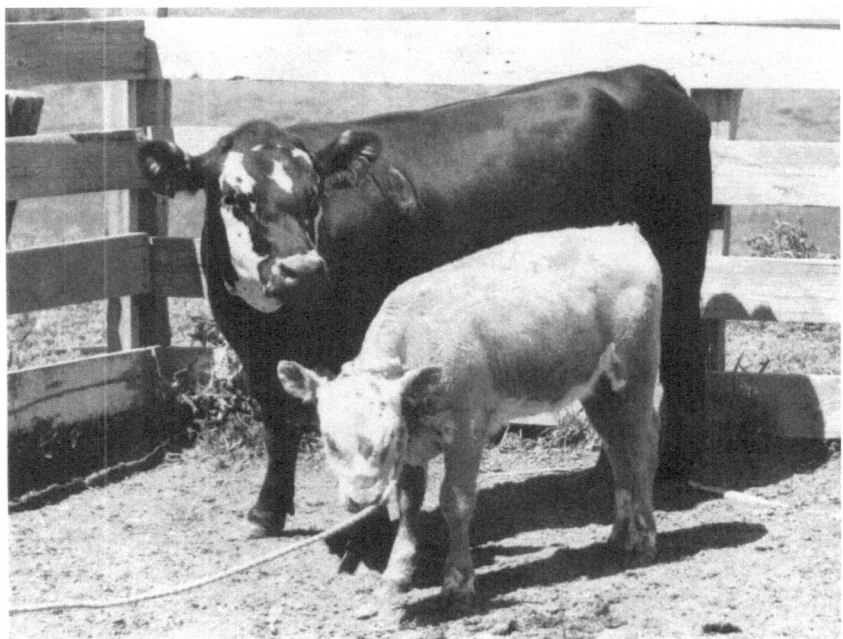

Fig. 1. Hereford X Angus cross cow and her 2 month old Chediak-Higashi calf. Notice the dilution of pigment in the calf which is light brown compared to its coal-black mother. The iris is always grey in C-HS cattle, compared to dark brown to black in normal cattle

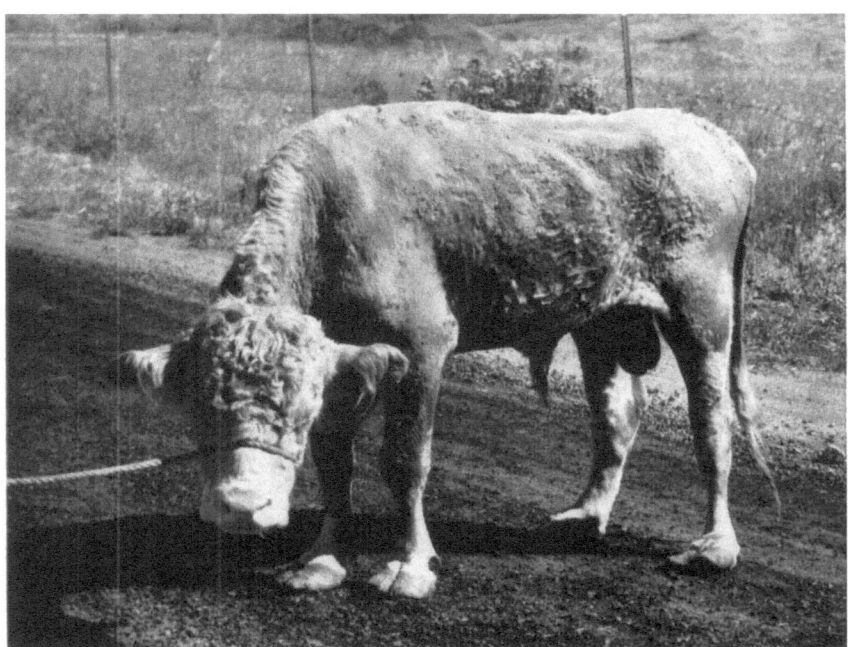

Fig. 2. Six year old Chediak-Higashi bull just prior to death. Notice the gauntness of the animal and the scruffness of its coat. At necropsy this animal had multiple pulmonary and hepatic abscesses which are characteristic in C-HS cattle. Notice the roughened and misshaped hoofs which are probably due to repeated bouts of pododermatitis

susceptible to pasteurella and corynebacterium (PADGETT *et al.*, 1968b) staphylococcal (HELGEBOSTAD, 1963) brucella (MARSH, 1968) and mycobacterium (HARTSOUGH, 1969) infections.

Probably the best single example of a disease which provides a distinct difference in susceptibility both epidemiologically and experimentally is Aleutian disease (AD).

Epidemiologic studies have shown various C-HS color phases of mink to have a 2 to 4 fold greater prevalence of AD and a 5 to 10 fold greater mortality rate than non-C-HS color phases (GORHAM *et al.*, 1965; PADGETT *et al.*, 1968b). Experimental studies have shown that C-HS mink develop the lesions of AD more rapidly than non-C-HS mink (PADGETT *et al.*, 1967b) and that they have a shorter mean time of death (GORHAM *et al.*, 1965; PADGETT *et al.*, 1968b). The latter finding has been confirmed by EKLUND *et al.* (1968). It is of considerable interest in regard to AD that the probable cause of death of C-HS and non-C-HS mink is the glomerular lesions (HENSON *et al.*, 1966). Furthermore, the glomerular lesions appear to result from the deposition of macromolecular material in the mesangial region. This macromolecular material is composed of at least complement and gamma globulin and may also contain the virus of AD, although the latter point has not been demonstrated (HENSON *et al.*, 1969).

As with the children and cattle, C-HS mink also show a shortened life span. Of 523 C-HS mink retained as breeder females, 6.1 % remained alive 3 years later and none were alive the fourth year. Whereas, 35 % of 576 non-C-HS breeder females were alive the 3rd year and 32 % were retained for the fourth breeding season.

D. Mice

At present, there is no published information which indicates that C-HS mice are more susceptible to disease than their normal counterparts. In fact, several individuals have stated that, based on general observations, there does not appear to be an increased susceptibility (CHASE, 1969; BENNETT *et al.*, 1969; PADGETT, 1969) to infection associated with the granular abnormality in mice.

III. Granulocyte Morphology, Function and Physiology

The unique pathologic feature of C-HS common to man and animals is the large membrane-bound intracytoplasmic organelles present in granule forming cells, (some of which have been shown to be lysosomes). With the exception of the mouse, large granules with pleomorphic contents have been reported to occur in cells of ectodermal, mesodermal and endodermal origin: *e.g.*, ocular pigment epithelium, skin, hair follicles, peripheral nerve, pituitary and adrenal glands, kidney, liver, stomach, muscle, leukocytes, etc. Available reports on the mouse have indicated that enlarged granules are demonstrable in leukocytes (LUTZNER *et al.*, 1967; BENNETT *et al.*, 1969). Other tissues have

12*

not been examined extensively. Although a number of descriptive studies have been conducted on the histology of C-HS granules, the developmental aspects of abnormal granule formation have not been delineated. Moreover, their relationship to the increased susceptibility to infection has not been demonstrated.

A. Granule Morphology and Histochemistry

Despite the fact that abnormal granules have been found to be distributed in various tissues of the body, the major information available is on the poly-morphonuclear leukocyte (PMN). At the light microscope level, both normal and abnormal granules have been shown to be present in the same cell. The abnormal granules may be present singly or multiply, and their staining characteristics have been shown to be the same as normal granules with the Romanowski stains. Histochemical studies have shown them to be peroxidase, alkaline and acid phosphatase, sudan black B, oil red 0, and PAS positive. They are negative to Feulgen, methyl green pyronine, and Prussian blue. The granules have been shown to vary in size from 1.5 to 4.4 μ. The initial reports described the abnormal PMN granules as having striations (formes myeliniques) which were generally membrane bound (BERNARD et al., 1960). Subsequent reports have, in general, confirmed this description (BESSIS et al., 1961; LUTZNER et al., 1967; DOAK, 1968; DAVIS et al., 1969; EFRATI and DANON, 1968; and DOUGLAS et al., 1969). WHITE (1966a) has shown that the abnormal granules are acid phosphatase positive at the electron-microscopic level (Fig. 3).

B. Granule Formation

BESSIS (1961) and MAURI and SILINGARDI (1964) have suggested that the abnormally enlarged granules of leukocytes may be formed by fusion of normal granules or by fusion of substances liberated by ruptured normal granules. LUTZNER et al. (1965) included fusion among their many hypotheses on the mode of formation of the abnormal granules. It is quite likely, however, that they referred to fusion of mature granules rather than to fusion of vesicles or spherules as discussed in the excellent reports of BAINTON and FARQUHAR (1966) and WETZEL et al. (1967) since their work was not published at that time. As an alternative to fusion, it has been suggested that an autophagic process might account for the formation of the abnormal granules. However, LUTZNER et al. (1965) stated that autophagy was unlikely to explain the ab-normal granule in all of the cell types in which they have been observed. While WHITE (1967) did not comment as to the mode of origin of the abnormal granules characteristic of the C-HS, he did propose that a secondary structure, a "sequestration vacuole", arose by fusion of normal sized mature granules in C-HS leukocytes. He suggested that the normal lysosomes fused as a result of leakage of enzymes through an excessively permeable membrane which encloses the abnormal C-HS granules. It is of interest, that WHITE (1967) failed to state specifically which type of leukocyte or if all types of leukocytes were involved in this process, since no other investigator (BESSIS *et al.*, 1961; BERNARD *et al.*, 1960; JANNINI *et al.*, 1963; DOUGLAS *et al.*, 1969; EFRATI and DANON, 1968) has reported them in human C-HS leukocytes. Furthermore, LUTZNER *et al.* (1965) did not report them in mink, or mouse leukocytes (LUTZNER *et al.*, 1967). DOAK (1968) observed a similar structure in a capillary endothelial cell and suggested that it arose from fusion of pinocytic vesicles, a process that has been shown to result in the formation of acid phosphatase containing lysosomes in macrophages (COHN and BENSON, 1965). However, he did not observe such structures in the leukocytes of C-HS cattle, and furthermore, suggested that the abnormal granules arose through the normal granule forming pathways in the cell.

If the affected granules are formed through the normal granule forming pathways of the cell, then there should be a logical explanation for the presence of these granules and normal granules within the same cell. It is now generally accepted that granule contents are synthesized in the endoplasmic reticulum and packaged in the Golgi area of the cell. Furthermore, it is generally accepted that there are 2, if not 3 types of granules present in polymorphonuclear (PMN) leukocytes, the cell type most extensively discussed in the C-HS. PEASE (1956) pioneered the studies on multiple granule types with his work on guinea pig marrow which was followed by the work of BESSIS and THIERY (1961) and by FLOREY's (1962) contributions on human and rabbit PMNs respectively. However, it was not until the report of BAINTON and FARQUHAR (1966) that a clear picture of granule development in the PMN was presented. They suggested that 2 types of granules were present, the first were azurophil granules which budded off the concave face of the Golgi complex as vesicles. Multiple vesicles then fused to form the complete azurophil granule which could be identified by morphological and staining characteristics. The second granule type was the specific granule which formed as small vesicles on the convex face of the Golgi and then fused to form a larger granule in a manner similar to that described for the azurophil granule. Thus, the granule complement of the mature PMN was comprised of relatively few azurophil granules which had been diluted out by subsequent cell divisions since the progranulocyte stage and the much more numerous specific granules which were produced by the cells throughout the various divisions which occurred during the myelocyte stage. This work was supported by the studies of WETZEL *et al.* (1967) who also suggested that a third granule type may be present in addition to the granules described by BAINTON and FARQUHAR (1966).

DAVIS *et al.* (1969), in a preliminary report, have shown that the azurophil or primary granules of normal mink (non C-HS) are laden with crystalloids which are not present in the specific or secondary granules. Furthermore, they have shown that the abnormally large granules in C-HS mink contain crystalloids and the normal sized granules do not. It now appears that the abnormally large granules in C-HS mink PMNs are those granules which are classified as azurophil granules in a normal PMN. This quite likely explains the fact that there are relatively few abnormal granules per cell compared to number

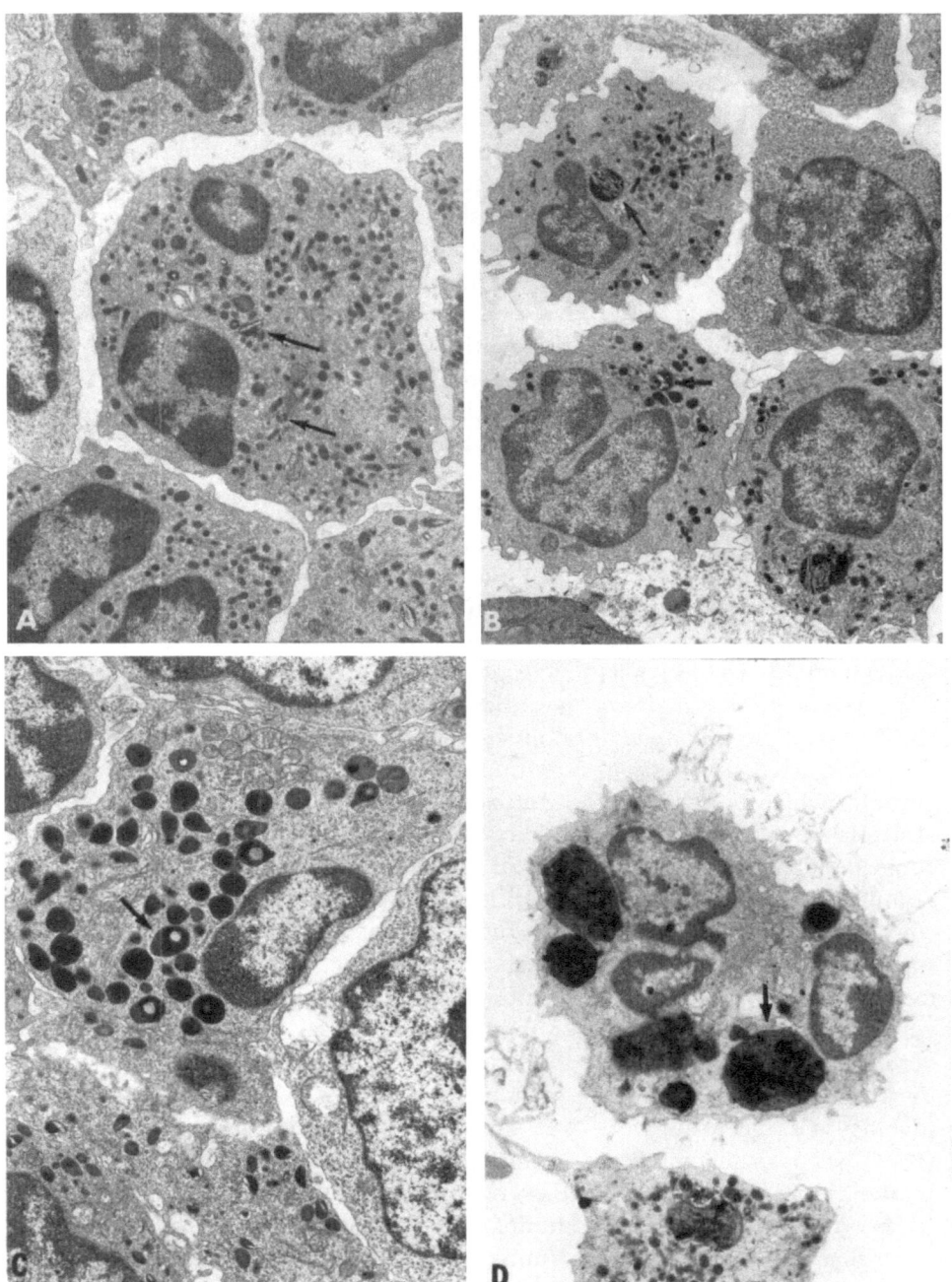

Fig. 3A—D. Comparison of aa (C-HS) and AA (normal) mink leukocytes from bone marrow. The cells were fixed with phosphate buffered 1.5% glutaraldehyde with 1% added sucrose, post fixed with phosphate buffered 1% osmium tetroxide, pre-stained with uranyl acetate and embedded in epon-araldite. Sections were post stained with uranyl and lead salts. A Mature neutrophils from normal mink. Primary (azurophil) granules are dense and contain one or two crystalloids (arrows). Secondary (specific)

of normal granules per cell, since the abnormal granules would be diluted out by cell divisions which occur after the progranulocyte stage. In addition, very preliminary findings indicate that the abnormal granules present in the PMNs of C-HS cattle and mice will also fall into the azurophil, or primary, granule classification.

While it is true that these are preliminary findings, they have provided the first plausible explanation of the data in numerous previous reports from this laboratory and others. The work of DAVIS *et al.* (1969) will be considered further under the section on cell function.

It should be clearly understood that multiple cell types are affected (LUTZNER *et al.*, 1965; KRITZLER *et al.*, 1964; PADGETT *et al.*, 1967; WINDHORST, 1966b) and explanations of abnormal granule formation should be consonant with this fact. Since the syndrome is inherited as an autosomal recessive trait in all species studied (LUTZNER *et al.*, 1967; PADGETT, 1968) and given the current one gene, one enzyme or polypeptide subunit theory, an explanation of abnormal granule formation should most likely be applicable between cell types. In various cell types as in the PMN, (pituitary, pancreas, adrenal, gastric chief cells, etc.), enlarged granules and normal granules have been demonstrated in the same cell in C-HS animals (DOAK *et al.*, 1968; LUTZNER *et al.*, 1965). These findings and those of DAVIS *et al.* (1969) suggest the possibility that the enlarged granules in all types of C-HS cells represent a specific population of granules.

The inference which can be drawn from these findings is that in all cell types in which normal and abnormal granules are present in the same cell, in C-HS individuals probably represent cell types which contain at least 2 granule types in normal individuals. Furthermore, the distribution of abnormal granules in the C-HS suggest that each granule type in a given cell is controlled by an individual gene. Such a hypothesis is supported by the studies on eosinophils where it has been suggested by WETZEL *et al.* (1967a) that the eosinophil contains a homogeneous rather than a heterogeneous population of granules. In all four species with C-HS, all eosinophil granules are abnormal in size suggesting that if the above hypothesis is correct there is only one granule type in eosinophils.

granules are less dense and contain no crystalloids ($\times$ 7,000). B Neutrophils from C-HS mink (intermediate to late stages of maturation). No normal primary granules are present, but instead, large C-HS granules (arrows) that contain dense material and crystalloids similar to those found in primary granules. The secondary granules are present in normal numbers and appear unaltered ($\times$ 5,000). C Eosinophil from normal mink (intermediate stage of maturation), containing moderately large specific granules which have a round core of variable density and a rim of different density (arrows) ($\times$ 7,000). D Eosinophil from C-HS mink. The specific granules are fewer in number and several times larger than normal (arrows). The cores exhibit pleomorphism and some forms suggest that fusion of individual granules has taken place ($\times$ 6,700)

C. Cell Function

1. Enzyme Distribution

As with granule formation, the PMN will be considered most extensively in this discussion since the majority of work has been done on that cell type.

Numerous investigators have proposed that enzyme heterogeneity exists among the granules in PMNs. However, localization of a given enzyme within a given granule type was more difficult to demonstrate. Wetzel et al. (1967b), Spicer et al. (1968), and Bainton and Farquhar (1968a), Bainton and Farquhar (1968b) have shown histochemically that the acid phosphatase activity of PMNs resides in the primary, or azurophil granules. In addition to acid phosphatase, Bainton and Farquhar (1968a) showed that 6 other enzymes were localized in the azurophil granules. Both groups of investigators relegated alkaline phosphatase to the specific or secondary granules.

More recently, Zeya and Spitznagel (1969) and Baggiolini et al. (1969) have separated populations of granules that correspond to the azurophil and specific granules. In addition, a third, somewhat more heterogeneous population of granules was isolated. The azurophil granules were shown to contain myeloperoxidase, lysozyme and 5 acid hydrolases. The specific granules were shown to contain alkaline phosphatase and lysozyme activity. The third granule population was shown to contain acid hydrolases but little or no myeloperoxidase (Baggiolini et al., 1969).

If the above studies, localizing acid phosphatase in azurophil granules, are correct then some previous studies on C-HS children require reinterpretation.

White (1966a), using electron microscopic histochemistry, reported that the abnormally large granules in peripheral blood PMN leukocytes of children with the C-HS stained heavily with acid phosphatase while the normal-sized granules stained irregularly, or not at all. He concluded from his findings that the membranes of the abnormally large granules were more permeable to the substrate than the membranes of the normal-sized granules. In the light of the work of Davis et al. (1969) demonstrating that the C-HS granules are large azurophil granules, and the foregoing work on the distribution of acid phosphatase it now appears that conclusions concerning membrane permeability based on acid phosphatase staining may be untenable.

2. Viral Diseases

White (1966a) reported finding "large, membrane-bound areas honeycombing the cells" which were apparently formed by the fusion of degenerating C-HS granules. Other investigators have not reported similar findings in electron microscopic studies of C-HS leukocytes. A possible explanation for the observation of White (1966a) may be the fact that virus-like particles were found in leukocytes from their 2 patients, White (1966b), Dent et al. (1966). If these particles were associated with or caused the degenerative changes it might account for the fact that they have not been observed by other investigators. However, it would certainly mitigate against their argument that the virus-like particles and degeneration are general phenomena associated consistently with the C-HS in children. In fact, DOUGLAS et al. (1969) and others failed to find evidence of virus-like particles, cytoplasmic sequestration or degenerating C-HS granules inducing areas of degeneration or autophagy in the surrounding cytoplasm in leukocytes of C-HS children. DOUGLAS et al. (1969) studied 4 C-HS children, 2 of which had a well documented mononuclear cell infiltrate in the tissues which was similar to the infiltrate in the tissues of the children studied by WHITE (1966a) and DENT et al. (1966).

The importance of WHITE's (1966a) work, if his interpretation is correct, is obvious for he has presented evidence suggesting that defective leukocyte lysosomes may allow the propagation or maintenance of an agent which is not usually found in normal leukocytes. Conceding the point that we are concerned with a specific agent in this case so that data on other agents may well not apply, it is still necessary to consider the available evidence.

As mentioned previously, C-HS children have apparently dealt with vaccinia, varicella, measles, and mumps infections as well as normal children. C-HS mink cleared a bacteriophage ΦX-174 as rapidly and as well from the peripheral blood as did non-C-HS mink (PADGETT et al., 1968c). IKEDA et al. (1967) found that the cytopathic effect and growth curve of bovine enterovirus (BV-1 strain) in peripheral blood leukocyte cultures obtained from C-HS and normal cattle were similar. Pseudorabies virus did not replicate in normal leukocyte cultures, nor did it replicate in cultures obtained from C-HS cattle. In addition, the extinction curves of pseudorabies virus were similar when leukocyte cultures obtained from C-HS and non-C-HS cattle were compared. The latter finding suggests that a virus that will not replicate in normal cells will not replicate in C-HS cells. Similar findings were observed with Aleutian disease where a clear cut difference in susceptibility has been reported by a number of investigators, but no difference in the peripheral blood titer of the agent (PADGETT, 1969). In the case of AD there is no *in vitro* method presently available to investigate the cellular response to the agent. However, *in vivo* studies indicate that the peripheral blood titers of the AD agent are not materially different (peak titer $10^{5.5}$ at 11 days postinoculation, declining to 10^4 infectious doses 28 days postinoculation) when C-HS and non-C-HS mink with persistent hypergammaglobulinemia were examined. It was observed that all C-HS mink were dead within 5 months postinoculation and the non-C-HS mink lived until they were sacrificed at 11 months postinoculation (PADGETT, 1969).

These findings are important in the C-HS, since, with the same level of circulating agent the mean time of death of the C-HS mink was less than one-half that of the non-C-HS group. It appears that the greater susceptibility of the C-HS mink is not due to faster replication of the AD agent or even to larger amounts of circulating agent. At present, it seems likely that the shorter death time is due to the inability of the mesangial cells to catabolize the macromolecular material deposited in the glomerulus (HENSON et al., 1968; HENSON et *al.*, 1969). If this is true, the susceptibility to this virus may ultimately prove to be due to a lysosomal defect, but not one that is associated with leukocytes.

3. Bacterial Diseases

Windhorst (1966a) and Padgett (1967a) were unable to demonstrate a defect in the ability of polymorphonuclear leukocytes obtained from C-HS individuals to kill bacteria. This finding was puzzling since Padgett (1967a) showed that the abnormally large granules in PMNs fail to lyse after ingestion of bacteria, whereas the normal granules lyse in the manner described by Hirsch (1962), Hirsch and Cohn (1960). Failure of the large granules to lyse has been confirmed in the studies of Root *et al.* (1968). However, considering these results in relationship to Bainton and Farquhar's (1968a) hypothesis that bactericidal components in PMNs are contained within the specific granules and the work of Davis *et al.* (1969) showing that the abnormal granules are azurophil in origin, one can now point out that perhaps no difference in killing should have been expected. It now appears that Padgett's (1967a) failure to find a difference in the amount of acid phosphatase, cathepsen, β-glucuronidase, lysozyme, phagocytin, and histone in C-HS and non-C-HS cells is not unreasonable. Furthermore, it may well be that the entire enzyme complement of the cell is present in normal amounts.

Despite this intriguing explanation, it probably is too early to disregard the possibility that the neutrophil is associated with the increased susceptibility to infection which is observed in individuals with C-HS. Windhorst's (1966a) work is available only as a preliminary report and Padgett's (1967a) work needs to be extended and confirmed. Furthermore, modifications of techniques to quantitate the bactericidal ability of cells *in vitro* have been developed during studies on granulomatous disease of children. Perhaps, it will be possible to show a difference which was not detectable previously.

IV. Immunology

Various investigators have studied the serum electrophoretic patterns of individuals with the C-HS. As would be expected in individuals with a large number of infections, they have generally revealed altered gamma globulin-albumin ratios, (Saraiva *et al.*, 1959; Jannini *et al.*, 1963; Hansson *et al.*, 1959; Iwai and Oyake, 1964). Henson (1969) found no difference in the serum electrophoretic patterns of homozygous recessive, heterozygous or homozygous dominant mink or cattle if they were not affected with secondary diseases.

Page *et al.* (1962) immunized one of his C-HS patients with mumps, diptheria, and typhoid vaccines and found that they produced a normal level of antibody. Both C-HS and non-C-HS mink have been shown to produce protective antibodies to botulism toxoid and distemper virus (Leader *et al.*, 1963). Saraiva *et al.* (1959) found that after vaccination with "anti-typhoid-paratyphoid" vaccine neutrophils from his C-HS patient phagocytized larger numbers of bacilli than they had previously. Experimental allergic encephalo-myelitis has been used to evaluate the delayed hypersensitivity response of C-HS and non-C-HS heterozygous and homozygous dominant mink (LEVINE et al., 1966). No difference in the time of onset of symptoms, the severity of the response or in the associated cellular infiltrate was found when the 3 types of mink were compared. DONOHUE and BAIN (1957) observed an encephalo-myelitis in their C-HS patient and suggested that it was probably due to a secondary chronic degenerative process. The work of LEVINE et al. (1966) on mink suggests that C-HS children, like normal children, have the capacity to develop an allergic postinfectious encephalomyelitis.

Although these studies suggest that there is no immunologic defect in individuals with the C-HS, further work is necessary before one can accept that conclusion without reservations.

V. Other Studies

A. Lipids

Abnormal serum lipid levels have been reported in several children with the C-HS. Low levels of cholesterol, phospholipids and the total lipoprotein fraction of the serum were reported by SARAIVA et al. (1959). KRITZLER et al. (1964) observed hypertriglyceridemia and low levels of sphingomyelin, lyso-lecithin, α-lipoproteins and esterified cholesterol. CAT et al. (1965) suggested that the C-HS and idiopathic hyperlipemia were associated. He found high levels of neutral fat but normal serum cholesterol values. The most extensive lipid studies were reported by KANFER et al. (1967), KANFER et al. (1968). They found approximately a 50% decrease in both sphingophospholipid and sphingoglycolipid in leukocytes from C-HS children when compared with those of controls. In addition, they reported a marked increase in the incorpo-ration of radioactive precursors (glucose U-^{14}C, inorganic ^{32}P) into sphingo-lipids and an increase in the ability of leukocytes from C-HS patients to cleave glucosyl ceramide and sphingomyelin. KANFER et al. (1968) suggested that their studies indicated an accelerated turnover of cellular constituents which parallels WHITE's (1966a) demonstration of cytoplasmic sequestration and degredation. The implication of this work is that there may be an ab-normality in the incorporation of lysosomal membrane lipids or an abnormality which results in excessive breakdown of lysosomal membrane lipids, either of which could result in a release of the lysosomal enzymes resulting in cellular degeneration and death.

There is reasonable evidence which argues against lipids being primarily involved in the C-HS. The children studied by BERNARD et al. (1960) and JANNINI et al. (1963) had no serum lipid abnormalities. Furthermore, studies on the leukocytes and serum of C-HS mink and cattle have failed to reveal a decrease in lipids as described above (PADGETT et al., 1969) and differences were not detected in mice.

B. Biomembranes

The possible mechanism or mechanisms responsible for the clinical manifestations and phenotypic expression of this complex and interesting disease
have been debated. An integral part of many of these explanatory hypotheses
has been the unit membrane, particularly as it relates to compartmentalization
of metabolic activities.

Recently, the argument has become one of increased stability versus increased permeability or decreased stability of the lysosomal membrane.
Morphologic evidence is presented in support of both arguments. White
(1966a) has suggested that increased permeability, resulting in leakage of
hydrolases and damage of intracellular constituents which ultimately results
in the formation of autophagic vacuoles, sequestration vacuoles and residual
bodies is a major feature of the disease. This concept is supported in a recent
report by Windhorst et al. (1969) of an apparent increased structural lability
of C-HS liver lysosomes subjected to conventional isolation procedures. In-
direct support for the concept of increased membrane lability is suggested by
the work of Kanfer et al. (1968), demonstrating increased turnover of phospholipid in isolated leukocytes and the work of Blume et al. (1968) in which
markedly increased levels of serum muramidase (lysozyme) were detected in
children with the C-HS. However, neither increased phospholipid turnover
nor increase in serum muramidase levels have been detected in C-HS cattle
or mink.

Decreased permeability or increased stability and a primary defect in
granulogenesis is the alternative hypothesis. The studies of Padgett(1967a)
and Root et al. (1968) support this concept in that they demonstrated that the
large granules failed to lyse after polymorphs ingested large numbers of bacteria. Moreover, Davis et al. (1969) have demonstrated that the large granules
are azurophil granules arising in normal pathways of granulogenesis rather
than by autophagy.

The compelling reason for assuming that a membrane defect is present in
the C-HS, however, is that no matter which of the above arguments is correct
(increased or decreased stability) both suggest a membrane anomaly of some
type. In addition, an abnormality of the structural protein of the membrane
could easily account for the formation of abnormal granules in the normal
granule forming pathway. One might readily assume that a membrane defect
would allow continued fusion of vesicles or granules after the time that they
usually mature or reach a stable state in normal cells.

However, preliminary studies in this laboratory, which were studies
designed to demonstrate a membrane defect, have been inconclusive. Red cell
structural protein prepared from C-HS cattle has an identical pattern in poly-
acrylamide gel when compared to normal controls (Holland and Padgett,
1969). Membrane lipids also do not appear to vary either qualitatively or
quantitatively when C-HS and normal cattle are compared. Moreover, studies
on polymorphonuclear leukocytes have not revealed major differences in
membrane components.

C. Hemorrhage

Approximately 25 percent of the children with the C-HS have had a hemorrhagic tendency (PADGETT, 1968). In five of the children this was severe enough to contribute to, if it was not the actual cause of death. A similar tendency has been observed in mink and cattle with the syndrome (PHILLIPS *et al.*, 1967) but not mice. However, there has been no consistent defect reported in the clotting mechanisms of man or animals with this syndrome. Moreover, preliminary studies show no granular defect in the platelet (DAVIS *et al.*, 1969).

D. Tissue Culture

Various investigators have reported the *in vitro* cultivation of cells from man and other animals with the C-HS (DENT *et al.*, 1966; PADGETT *et al.*, 1968; IKEDA *et al.*, 1967; DANES and BEARN, 1967; BLUME *et al.*, 1969; YOSHII and PADGETT, 1969). All have reported the presence of abnormal granules characteristic of the C-HS, regardless of the cell type cultivated. To date, spleen cells, skin fibroblasts, peripheral blood lymphocytes and peritoneal exudate cells have been cultivated. No investigator has reported the induction of abnormal granules in normal cells by C-HS serum nor the prevention of development of abnormal granules in C-HS cells by normal serum. The abnormality is apparently due to some defect in the genetic makeup of the cells. DANES and BEARN (1967) have reported that heterozygotes could be detected by use of skin fibroblast cultures. However, HURVITZ and RIPPS (1969) were unable to confirm their findings in C-HS mink and mice. WHITE (1966b) and DENT *et al.* (1966) have reported the presence of virus-like particles in a child with the C-HS. DENT *et al.* (1966) were unable to demonstrate similar particles in splenic cell tissue cultures taken from that child. BLUME *et al.* (1969) failed to demonstrate virus-like particles in peripheral blood lymphocyte cultures from a child with the accelerated phase of the syndrome and DOUGLAS *et al.* (1969) failed to demonstrate virus-like particles in electron microscopic studies of the peripheral blood leukocytes from the same child. IKEDA *et al.* (1967) have reported no difference in the response of C-HS and non-C-HS cultured leukocytes to the action of two viral agents. YOSHII and PADGETT (1969) found that cultured peritoneal exudate cells from mink with the C-HS were carried without difficulty for 20 to 30 generations. Control mink cultures were not materially different from those obtained from animals with the C-HS.

All of the tissue culture studies to date indicate there is no difference in the media required, cultural characteristics (except for presence of large granules), response to viral infection or longevity when cultures from C-HS and non-C-HS individuals are compared.

VI. Of Man and Animals

Throughout this assessment of the Chediak-Higashi syndrome the assumption has been taken that the inherited aspects of the condition in man, mink, and cattle are the same. However, all investigators who have worked on this disease have not taken a similar attitude.

Table. *Comparison of the Chediak-Higashi syndrome in man, mink and cattle*

Characteristic	Man	Mink	Cattle	Mice
Reticulohistiocytic infiltrate	yes	no	no	no
Aleutian disease	no	yes	no	no
Presence of virus-like particles	occasional	not observed	occasional	?
Cytoplasmic sequestration	occasional	no	no	?
Granular and cytoplasmic degeneration	occasional	no	no	?
Increased lysozyme levels	occasional	no	no	no
Serum lipid abnormalities	occasional	no	no	no
Autophagy	occasional	no	no	?
Increased membrane permeability	occasional	no	no	?
Autosomal recessive inheritance	yes	yes	yes	yes
Same distribution of abnormal granules	yes	yes	yes	yes
Similar abnormal granule morphology	yes	yes	yes	yes
Increased susceptibility to infection	yes	yes	yes	?
Hemorrhagic tendency	yes	yes	yes	?
Similar bactericidal capabilities of neutrophils	yes	yes	yes	?
Similar inflammatory response	yes	yes	yes	?
Similar results with tissue culture	yes	yes	yes	?
Immunologic deficiency	no	no	no	?
Partial albinism	yes	yes	yes	yes

If there is value in studying the disease in animals, it must certainly be derived from their utilization to develop and evaluate hypotheses concerned not only with this disease in man, but with basic mechanisms of cellular physiology and function. Furthermore, they should be of value in circumventing the inability to examine all parameters of the C-HS in humans and they will aid in the evaluation of the genetic and environmental factors associated with this disease.

The established differences and similarities are presented in the table. As can be seen from the table, the differences which have been noted between man and animals could, in general, be attributed to environmental factors or differences in species susceptibility to an agent or the drugs used to treat secondary diseases.

References

Baggiolini, M., Hirsch, J. G., DeDuve, C.: Resolution of granules from rabbit heterophil leukocytes into distinct populations by zonal sedimentation. J. Cell Biol. **40**, 529—541 (1969).

Bainton, D. F., Farquhar, M. G.: Origin of granules in polymorphonuclear leukocytes. Two types derived from opposite faces of the Golgi complex in developing granulocytes. J. Cell Biol. **28**, 277—301 (1966).

BAINTON, D. F., FARQUHAR, M. G.: Differences in enzyme content of azurophil and specific granules of polymorphonuclear leukocytes. I. Histochemical staining of bone marrow smears. J. Cell Biol. **39**, 286—298 (1968a).

— — Differences in enzyme content of azurophil and specific granules of polymorphonuclear leukocytes. II. Cytochemistry and electron microscopy of bone marrow cells. J. Cell Biol. **39**, 299—317 (1968b).

BARKVE, H.: Chediak-Higashi-Steinbrinck syndrome. A survey with report of a case. Acta paediat. scand. **56**, 105—109 (1967).

BEGUEZ-CESAR, A.: Neutropenia cronica maligna familiar con granulaciones atipicas de los leucocitos. Bol. Soc. Pediat. **15**, 900—922 (1943).

BENNETT, J. M., BLUME, R. S., WOLFF, S. M.: Characterization and significance of abnormal leukocyte granules in the beige mouse: A possible homologue for Chediak-Higashi Aleutian trait. J. Lab. clin. Med. **73**, 235—243 (1969).

BERNARD, J., BESSIS, M., SELIGMANN, M., CHASSIGNEUX, J., CHOME, J.: Un case de maladie de Chediak-Steinbrinck-Higashi. Etude clinique et cytologique. Presse méd. **68**, 563—566 (1960).

BESSIS, M., BERNARD, J., SELIGMANN, M.: Etude cytologique d'un cas de maladie de Chediak. Nouv. Rev. franç. Hémat. **1**, 422—440 (1961a).

— THIERY, J. P.: Electron microscopy of human white blood cells and their stem cells. Int. Rev. Cytol. **12**, 199 (1961).

BLUME, R. S., BENNETT, J. M., YANKEE, R. A., WOLFF, S. M.: Defective granulocyte regulation in the Chediak-Higashi syndrome. New Engl. J. Med. **279**, 1009—1015 (1968).

— GLADE, P. R., CHESSIN, L. N., WOLFF, S. M.: The Chediak-Higashi syndrome: Continuous suspension culture of peripheral blood leukocytes. Blood In press (1969).

CAT, I., MARIONI, L. P., GIRALDI, D. J., ALMEIDA, M. B., NETO, A. S., BRAGA, A. Q.: Chediak-Higashi syndrome with familial idiopathic hyperlipaemia. Lancet **1965 I**, 1398.

CHASE, H. B.: Personal communication (1969).

COHN, Z. A., BENSON, B.: The in vitro differentiation of mononuclear phagocytes. II. The influence of serum on granule formations, hydrolase production, and pinocytosis. J. exp. Med. **121**, 835—848 (1965).

— FEDORKO, M. E., HIRSCH, J. G.: The in vitro differentiation of mononuclear phagocytes. V. The formation of macrophage lysosomes. J. exp. Med. **123**, 757—766 (1966).

DANES, B. S., BEARN, A. G.: Cell culture and the Chediak-Higashi syndrome. Lancet **1967 II**, 65—67.

DAVIS, W. C., GREENE, W. B., SPICER, S. S.: Ultrastructure of bone marrow granulocytes in normal and Aleutian mink. Fed. Proc. **28**, 36 (1969).

DENT, P. B., FISH, L. A., WHITE, J. G., GOOD, R. A.: Chediak-Higashi syndrome: Observations on the nature of the associated malignancy. Lab. Invest. **15**, 1634—1642 (1966).

DOAK, R. L.: Ultrastructural study of the Chediak-Higashi syndrome in cattle. Masters thesis. Washington State University (1968).

DONOHUE, W. L., BAIN, H. W.: Chediak-Higashi syndrome. A lethal familial disease with anomalous inclusions in the leukocytes and constitutional stigmata: Report of a case with necrospy. Pediatrics **20**, 416—429 (1957).

DOUGLAS, S. D., BLUME, R. S., GLADE, P. R., CHESSIN, L. N., WOLFF, S. M.: Fine structure of continuous long term lyphoid cell cultures from Chediak-Higashi patient and heterozygote. Lab. Invest. **21**, 225—229 (1969).

— — WOLFF, S. M.: Fine structural studies of leukocytes from patients and heterozygotes with the Chediak-Higashi syndrome. Blood **33**, 527—531 (1969).

192   G. A. Padgett, J. M. Holland, W. C. Davis, and J. B. Henson:

Efrati, P., Danon, D.: Electron microscopical study of bone marrow cells in a case of Chediak-Higashi-Steinbrinck syndrome. Brit. J. Haemat. 15, 173—176 (1968).
— Jonas, W.: Chediak's anomaly of leukocytes in malignant lymphoma associated with leukemic manifestations: Case report with necropsy. Blood 13, 1063—1073 (1958).
Eklund, C. M., Hadlow, W. J., Kennedy, R. C., Boyle, C. C., Jackson, T. A.: Aleutian disease of mink: Properties of the etiologic agent and the host responses. J. infect. Dis. 118, 510—526 (1968).
Florey, H. W.: Inflammation. In: General pathology, ed. 3, ed. by H. W. Florey. Philadelphia: W. B. Saunders & Co. 1962.
Gorham, J. R., Leader, R. W., Padgett, G. A., Burger, D., Henson, J. B.: Some observations on the natural occurrence of Aleutian disease. „NINDB Monograph No. 2". In: Slow, latent and temperate virus infections, p. 279—285. Washington D. C.: U.S. Government Printing Office 1965.
Hansson, H., Linell, F., Nilsson, L. R., Söderhjelm, L., Undritz, E.: Die Chediak-Steinbrinck-Anomalie respektive erblich-konstitutionelle Riesengranulation (Granulogiganten) der Leukozyten in Nordschweden. Folia haemat. (Frankfurt) 3, 152—196 (1959).
Hartsough, G. R.: Personal communication (1969).
Helgebostad, A.: The Aleutian disease. Fur Trade J. of Canada 40, 10 (1963).
Henson, J. B.: Unpublished data. (1969).
— Gorham, J. R., Padgett, G. A., Davis, W. C.: Pathogenesis of the glomerular lesions in Aleutian disease of mink. Arch. Path. 87, 21—28 (1969).
— — Tanaka, Y., Padgett, G. A.: The sequential development of ultrastructural lesions in the glomeruli of mink with experimental Aleutian disease. Lab. Invest. 19, 153—162 (1968).
— Leader, R. W., Gorham, J. R., Padgett, G. A.: The sequential development of lesions in spontaneous Aleutian disease in mink. Path. Vet. 3, 289—314 (1966).
Hirsch, J. G.: Cinemicrophotographic observations on granule lysis in polymorphonuclear leukocytes during phagocytosis. J. exp. Med. 116, 827—834 (1962).
— Cohn, Z. A.: Degranulation of polymorphonuclear leukocytes following phagocytosis of microorganisms. J. exp. Med. 112, 1005—1014 (1960).
Holland, J. M., Padgett, G. A.: Unpublished data (1969).
Hurvitz, A., Ripps, C.: Cytoplasmic inclusions in cultured fibroblasts from mink and mice. Fed. Proc. 28, 2386 (1969).
Ikeda, S., Padgett, G. A., Gorham, J. R., Henson, J. B.: Comparative studies of the Chediak-Higashi syndrome: Bovine leukocyte-viral interactions. Exp. Hemat. 14, 66—74 (1967).
Iwai, T., Oyake, K.: A study of medical examination and treatment—an autopsy case of Chediak's anomaly. Acta paediat. Jap. 68, 163—167 (1964). [In Japanese.]
Jannini, P., Pinto Lima, F. X., Hubner Franca, H., Tricta, D. F., Tannos, D.: Sobre tres casos de anomalia leucocitaria identica a la descrita por Beguez-Cesar, Steinbrinck, Chediak, Higashi y Sato. Sangre (Barc.) 8, 138—159 (1963).
Kanfer, J. N., Blume, R. S., Yankee, R. A., Wolff, S. M.: Alteration of sphingolipid metabolism in leukocytes from patients with the Chediak-Higashi syndrome. New Engl. J. Med. 279, 410—413 (1968).
— Richards, R., Kampine, J. P., Handmaker, S., Yankee, R. A.: Alternation of the sphingolipid content in leukocytes from patients with Chediak-Higashi syndrome. Life Sci. 6, 2661—2664 (1967).
Kritzler, R. A., Terner, J. Y., Lindenbaum, J., Magidson, J., Williams, R., Preisig, R., Phillips, G. B.: Chediak-Higashi syndrome. Cytologic and serum lipid observations in a case and family. Amer. J. Med. 36, 583—594 (1964).

LEADER, R. W., PADGETT, G. A., GORHAM, J. R.: Studies of abnormal leukocyte bodies in the mink. Blood 22, 477—484 (1963).

LEVINE, S., PADGETT, G. A., LEADER, R. W.: Allergic encephalomyelitis in Chediak-Higashi mink: Encephalomyelitis, ganglionitis, and neuritis. Arch. Path. 82, 234—241 (1966).

LUTZNER, M. A., LOWRIE, C. T., JORDAN, H. W.: Giant granules in leukocytes of the beige mouse. J. Hered. 58, 299—300 (1967).

— TIERNEY, J. H., BENDITT, E. P.: Giant granules and widespread cytoplasmic inclusions in a genetic syndrome of Aleutian mink: An electron microscopic study. Lab. Invest. 14, 2063—2079 (1965).

MAGGI, R., GUTTIERREZ, E., PENALBER, J., DI MENNA, A., ROCCATAGLIATA, M., MATERA, F., ETCHEGARAT, E., MILLAN, J.: Sindrome de Beguez Cesar-Chediak-Higashi. Presentacion de nos casos. Arch. argent. Pediat. 48, 323—334 (1957).

MARSH, R. F.: Several pathological conditions in mink. N.E. Mink Farmer 12—13 (Jan. 1968).

MAURI, C., SILINGARDI, V.: A cytological and cytochemical study of Chediak's leukocytic anomaly. Acta haemat. (Basel) 32, 114—126 (1964).

PADGETT, G. A.: Neutrophilic function in animals with the Chediak-Higashi syndrome. Blood 29, 906—915 (1967a).

— The Chediak-Higashi syndrome. Advanc. vet. Sci. 12, 239—284 (1968).

— Aleutian disease virus replication in mink of different genotypes. Fed. Proc. 28, 2384 (1969).

— Unpublished data (1969).

— BURGER, D., GORHAM, J. R.: Viruses and the Chediak-Higashi syndrome. Fed. Proc. 27, 1826 (1968c).

— KANFER, J. N., BLUME, R. S., WOLFF, S. M.: Unpublished data (1969).

— LEADER, R. W., GORHAM, J. R.: Hereditary abnormal leukocyte granules in mink. Fed. Proc. 22, 428 (1963).

— — — O'MARY, C. C.: The familial occurrence of the Chediak-Higashi syndrome in mink and cattle. Genetics 49, 505—512 (1964).

— REIQUAM, C. W., HENSON, J. B., GORHAM, J. R.: Comparative studies of susceptibility to infection in the Chediak-Higashi syndrome. J. Path. Bact. 95, 509—522 (1968b).

PAGE, A. R., BERENDES, H., WARNER, J., GOOD, R. A.: The Chediak-Higashi syndrome. Blood 20, 330—343 (1962).

PEASE, D. C.: An electron microscopic study of red bone marrow. Blood 11, 501 (1956).

PHILLIPS, L. L., KAPLAN, H. S., PADGETT, G. A., GORHAM, J. R.: Comparative studies on the Chediak-Higashi syndrome. Coagulation and fibrinolytic mechanisms of mink and cattle. Amer. J. vet. clin. Path. 1, 1—6 (1967).

ROOT, R. K., BLUME, R. S., WOLFF, S. M.: Abnormal leukocyte function in the Chediak-Higashi syndrom. Clin. Res. 16, 335 (1968).

SARAIVA, L. G., AZEVEDO, M., CORREA, J. M., CARVALHO, G., PROSPERO, J. D.: Anomalous panleukocytic granulation. Blood 14, 1112—1127 (1959).

SPICER, S. S., HORN, R. G., WETZEL, B. K.: Ultrastructural and cytochemical characteristics of leukocytes in various stages of development. Biochem. Pharmacol., Suppl. 17, 143—157 (1968).

STEINBRINCK, W.: Über eine neue Granulations-Anomalie der Leukocyten. Dtsch. Arch. Klin. Med. 193, 577—581 (1948).

SUNG, J. H., MEYERS, J. P., STADLAN, E. M., COWEN, D., WOLFF, A.: Neuropathological changes in Chediak-Higashi disease. J. Neuropath. exp. Neurol. 28, 86—118 (1969).

WETZEL, B. K., HORN, R. G., SPICER, S. S.: Fine structural studies on the development of heterophil, eosinophil, and basophil granuloctyes in rabbits. Lab. Invest. 16, 349—382 (1967a).

Wetzel, B. K., Spicer, S. S., Horn, R. G.: Fine structural localization of acid and alkaline phosphatases in cells of rabbit and bone marrow. J. Histochem. Cytochem. **15**, 311—334 (1967b).

White, J. G.: The Chediak-Higashi syndrome: A possible lysosomal disease. Blood **28**, 143—156 (1966a).

— Virus-like particles in the peripheral blood cells of two patients with Chediak-Higashi syndrome. Cancer (Philad.) **19**, 877—884 (1966b).

— The Chediak-Higashi syndrome: Cytoplasmic sequestration in circulating leukocytes. Blood **29**, 435—451 (1967).

Windhorst, D. B.: Studies on a hereditary defect involving lysosomal structure. Fed. Proc. **25**, 358 (1966a).

— White, J. G., Zelickson, A. S., Clawson, C. C., Dent, P. B., Pollara, B., Good, R. A.: The Chediak-Higashi anomaly and the Aleutian trait in mink: Homologous defects of lysosomal structure. Ann. N. Y. Acad. Sci. In press (1969).

Yoshii, Z., Padgett, G. A.: Unpublished data (1969).

Zeya, H. I., Spitznagel, J. K.: Cationic protein-bearing granules of polymorphonuclear leukocytes: Separation from enzyme-rich granules. Science **163**, 1069—1071 (1969).

Author Index

Page numbers in *italics* refer to bibliography

Thompson, R. I., see
Kadowaki, J. 35, *56*
Thuline, H. C. 27, *60*
— Norby, D. E. 27, *60*
— see Chu, E. H. Y. 3,
52
Tierney, J. H., see Lutz-
ner, M. A. 180, 181,
183, *193*
Tjorstad, K. O. 113, *143*
Tonnelat, J., see Guinand,
S. 101, *139*
Touat, E., see Harte-
mann, J. 38, *54*
Treadwell, M., Cartwright,
T. C. 8, *60*
Tricta, D. F., see Jannini,
P. 176, 181, 186, 187,
192
Trujillo, J. M., see Ohno, S.
9, 11, *58*
Tucker, E. M., see Dain,
A. R. 22, *53*
Tucker, H. St. G., see
Koontz, W. W. 42, *56*
Tuffy, P., Brown, A. K.,
Zuelzer, W. W. 124,
143
Turner, C. D. 34, *60*
— Asakawa, H. 34, *60*
Turner, J. H., Li, C. C.,
Wald, N., Borges, W.
35, *60*
— see Hutchinson, D. L.
35, *55*
Turpin, R. 48, *60*
— Bocquet, L., Grasset,
J. 40, 49, *60*
— Lejeune, J., Lafour-
cade, J., Chigot, P. L.,
Salmon, Ch. 46, *60*
— Salmon, C., Cruveiller,
J. 40, *60*
— see Lejeune, J. 48, *56*
Tuuteri, L., see Furuhjelm,
U. 113, 114, 124,
129, *139*

Uchida, I. A., Wang, H. C.,
Ray, M. 37, 39, *60*
Ueno, S., Zuzuki, K.,
Yamazawa, K. 38, *60*
Undritz, E., see Hansson,
H. 177, 186, *192*

Vahlquist, B. 113, *143*
Van der Zwan, A., see
Stroer, W. F. H. *174*
Velez-Orozco, A. C., 38, *60*
Verdon, T. A., Jr., For-
rester, R. H., Crosby,
W. H. 113, 114, 124,
143
Verley, W. G., Hunebelle,
G. 63, *96*
Verloop, M. C. 104, *143*
— Bierenga, M., Dieze-
raad-Njoo, A. 104, *143*
Verri, B., see Massimo, L.
40, *57*
Verschuer, O. v. 51, *60*
Vervoorn, J. D., see
Beukering, J. A. 46, *52*
Veyrat, R., Maurice, P. A.
105, *143*
Vialatte, J., see Lejeune,
J. 42, *56*
Vianello, M. G., see
Massimo, L. 40, *57*
Viner, E. D., Frost, J. W.
113, 118, 124, 125, 129,
130, 131, 132, *144*
Vinijchaikul, K., see Fitz-
gerald, P. J. 63, 64,
67, 68, 94, *95*
Virolainen, M. 29, *60*
Vischer, D., see Schmid,
W. 41, 42, *59*
Vogt, D. W. 24, *60*
Vorder Bruegge, C. F.
see Mostofi, F. K. 99,
141
Vries, E. de *174*
Vries, M. J. de, see Bek-
kum, D. W. van 29, *51*

Wald, A. 94, *96*
Wald, N., see Turner, J. H.
35, *60*
Walker, B. E., see Leblond,
E. P. 63, *96*
Walthard, B. 102, *144*
Wang, H. C., see Uchida,
I. A. 37, 39, *60*
Warner, J., see Page, A. R.
177, 186, *193*
Wassermann, L. R., see
Stats, D. 135, 136,
137, *143*

Watters, Chr., see Black-
shear, P. L. Jr. *137*
Waxman, S. H., see
Gartler, S. M. 45, *54*
Weber, W. T., see Hare,
W. C. D. 25, 28, *54*
Weibel, E. R. 64, 67, 68,
96
Weir, W. C., see Stormont,
C. 21, *59*
Weiss, E., Hoffmann, R.
12, *60*
Wellings, S. R., see
Fujikura, T. 49, *54*
Westring, D. W. 110,
122, 124, 125, *144*
Wetzel, B. K., Horn, R. G.,
Spicer, S. S. 180, 181,
183, 184, *193*
— Spicer, S. S., Horn,
R. G. 180, 181, 184,
194
— see Spicer, S. S. 184,
193
Whipple, G. H., see
Lichty, J. A., Jr. 100,
140
— see Newman, W. V.
99, 100, *141*
White, J. C., see Dacie,
J. V. 104, *138*
White, J. G. 177, 180,
184, 185, 187, 188,
189, *194*
— see Dent, P. B. 177,
184, 185, 189, *191*
— see Windhorst, D. B.
188, *194*
Wiener, A. S., Moor-
Jankowski, J., Gor-
don, E. B. 31, *60*
Williams, D., see Alexan-
der, G. 22, *51*
— s. Ilbery, P. L. T. 23,
55
Williams, G., Gordon, I.,
Edwards, J. 12, *60*
Williams, G. R., see Keith,
H. B. 112, *140*
Williams, R., see Kritzler,
R. A. 183, 187, *192*
Wilson, J. G., Jordan,
H. C., Brent, R. L.
147, *173*

Subject Index

The numbers set in *italics* refer to those pages on which the respective catch-word is discussed in detail.

Index to Volumes 37—50

(Ergebnisse der allgemeinen Pathologie und pathologischen Anatomie)